Laminin

I dedicate this book to all the people who are ill, to everyone who has ever suffered mentally or physically, as well as to those who do not believe in God, or who believe that He never did and never will do anything in their lives.

M. KARNICKI

Laminin

Lodz, Poland, 2022

Translated by Joanna Zahorska

Typesetting by Maciej Torz

Cover design by Kuba Ferenc

©2022 M. Karnicki. All rights reserved.

"Only a man who knows what it is like to be defeated can reach down to the bottom of his soul and come up with the extra ounce of power it takes to win when the match is even."

Muhammad Ali

CHAPTER I

A day? A month? A year? Many years? How much time does it take to understand that every one of us got here for a reason? Can your dreams, various thoughts, or, perhaps, the requests and pleas hidden in them be heard by anyone aside from yourself? Are you the master of your own fate, or is your life a collage of random events that are absolutely meaningless?

* * *

Oh, if only I could begin this sentence in the style of one of the most prominent sportsmen of all time, and, according to many, the greatest master of boxing, Cassius Clay, better known as Muhammed Ali! It would go as follows, "I'm king of the world! I'm pretty! I'm a bad man! I shook up the world! I shook up the world! You must listen to me! I can't be beaten!"

Sadly, as fate would have it, I had to start in a different way. But was it really because of fate?

It was eight o'clock, an evening as any other – a quick action movie, a horror, or a good comedy. When you're twenty-three, that's how you spend your evenings, usually. Chilling with a good movie gives me much pleasure. I still love movies to this day. Back then, I didn't realize that watching movies would soon become the only activity that wouldn't cause me any issues, and the only positive time of my daily existence, usually lasting one hundred and twenty minutes.

Instead of studying for college exams, as usual, I'd go online searching for the right Hollywood production that would satisfy my needs and keep me distracted with some fictional characters' story. The upcoming exams aside, my greatest concern back then was how many pounds I'd bench-press on the next day during a training session at the gym. I had a regular student's worries that pertained to my weight, the size of my bicep, and what I was about to do with my girlfriend or my buddies come the weekend.

Hence, sitting in front of a laptop and rummaging through all possible websites that allowed you to download or see copies of the most recent American movies on the spot, I was scanning their casts.

"Who's it gonna be tonight? Di Caprio? De Niro? Or maybe Brad Pitt?" I asked myself.

Eventually, as usual, I'd quickly pick a specific title. Unfortunately, I can't recall what movie I was watching when my whole life turned upside down; I certainly know, however, that I had no clue what was about to happen that evening and didn't even imagine the avalanche of serious issues that was about to sweep me off my feet – issues that wouldn't only transform my life, but also that of other people.

As always, I'd make myself comfortable in my black faux-leather swivel chair, my legs crossed on the desk, American-style. Mom would always tell me not to do that, as it was not hygienic. Sadly, ever since I can remember, I've always had this habit and, most likely, nothing will ever change that. I guess you acquire some manners in the land where you were born. I reached into a bag of chips with one hand, and turned the movie on with the other.

After fifteen or maybe twenty minutes (or maybe it was already half an hour later), alarmed, I jumped to my feet abruptly. Back in that moment, I had no reason to be afraid of anything, I didn't get scared by anyone, and it wasn't because I recalled at the last moment that I was about to sit an exam on the next day while my notes were in shambles. For no reason, my heart started pounding like crazy. In a single moment, my entire world came to a halt, all my attention focused on what was happening inside my chest. Terrified at the condition my heart was in and the lack of any control over what was going on with me, I was trying to calm myself down somehow. Unfortunately, the more I was trying to make my heart slow down with my thoughts, the faster it went. I had no clue what was happening to me. It was like a herd of wild miniature horses galloping, the sound of their hoofs echoing across my chest; furious, they sped up with my every attempt at appeasing them. At one point, I felt the horses slowed down, giving my heart a moment of rest.

Still terrified and slightly overwhelmed with all the stress, I wanted to shout, "Dad! Something's happening to me!"

At that time, only my dad was home. I gave myself a second to calm down, as I thought the worst part was over. I rested for a couple of minutes, pulled myself together. The beating of my heart somewhat relaxed, yet I could still feel it speeding up a bit for some reason when I was focusing on it. My heart rate was very high on many occasions. Practicing sports on a daily basis, my pulse was often going high. This, however, was totally different. I thought I was just tired and that I must have overtrained. Back then, I was practicing pretty hard at the gym. Although I got very scared at first, I wasn't scared enough to stop watching the movie. For twenty-two years, I had had no health issues and the only ailments that I had been experiencing up to that moment, quite frequently, were the common cold and some mild spring-time grass allergy. That's probably why I continued watching the movie, already at ease. Sadly, a few minutes later, I felt the same situation was about to happen again. Another episode occurred. Again, with no warning, my heart started beating so hard and so fast, as if the horses left their boxes and threw themselves into a race after a false start. This time, it was severe and terrifying enough for me to start feeling panicky and afraid. Back then, I had no idea how to define what was happening to me in professional terms. I jumped to my feet. I was so laser-focused on my heart, racing like crazy for no reason, that the more I wanted to slow it down, the more it sped up. Fear was closing in on me, not the one I'd usually feel when being concerned about losing my loved ones, becoming crippled, or when hearing the sound of a hornet flying over me; it was a completely new fear that I had never experienced before.

I rushed out of the room to let my dad know that there was something very wrong and inexplicable going on with me. At the very same moment, my mom got home. My parents were petrified, as they had never seen me in that state before. The more they pondered on what to do and the more questions they asked me, the more severe my issue was getting. At one point, I could feel myself becoming short of breath and I started struggling for air. Everything was getting darker before my eyes and my vision went blurry. I sat down on a couch and after a moment, with hundreds of thoughts dashing through my head, I realized that I was probably going to pass out. Never before had I experienced that feeling, though I did witness other people under such circumstances. This time, I felt that I was the one about to faint. I could feel my body becoming powerless as I slowly slid off the couch. I remember as if it happened today.

Petrified, I cried out, "Mom! I'm blacking out!"

I was half-conscious, but I didn't black out. I could still see blurry silhouettes of my parents moving before my eyes, terrified but focused at the same time; they knew what to do. Without hesitation, they immediately called an ambulance. It didn't take long until it arrived at our doorstep; it seemed to me as if it teleported in no time.

Obviously, the state I found myself in rendered my brain completely confused, distorting my sense of time and space. Completely absorbed by what was happening to my body and trying, albeit unsuccessfully, to calm my racing heart down, I had to talk to the EMTs who had arrived, nonetheless. Sadly, the state I was in hindered my communication, forcing the men to direct a series of routine questions to my parents.

"Does your son have any chronic diseases? What did he eat and drink today? Did he take any narcotic drugs? Does he take any on a regular basis?"

My parents knew me pretty well and they had always trusted me. They knew I had never been interested in drugs or other mood enhancers. Since I always considered them not only parents but also my best friends, I could tell them anything, and they were well aware of that. They also knew that I would never fail or deceive them. When answering the EMTs' questions, they recalled a mild migraine I had been experiencing for some time, which was probably due to overload of the body and the spine after training at the gym. When taking my history, one of the EMTs checked my pulse. My heart was beating two hundred beats per minute. The measurement was indicative of severe tachycardia.[1]

Having conducted a brief examination, the EMTs had to decide what to do with me next. During the EMTs' visit, my symptoms subsided. Accepting my parents' answers as reliable and swiftly assessing the situation, the EMTs concluded that most likely, I had had a panic attack. Since neither I nor my parents had ever experienced panic, we struggled to comprehend the diagnosis issued that swiftly.

"A panic attack?" I asked.

One of them replied, "Yes. Don't get stressed up that much."

I thought, *What are you talking about, man? Stressed up about what?* I replied, "Just half an hour ago, I was chilling, watching some movies, not stressed up about anything."

The EMTs recommended me to relax more often and that was it. For my parents and I it was quite a shock. After this whole situation, which was tragic to us and to me in particular, the diagnosis provided by the EMTs seemed to us irrational or even ridiculous. We all knew that I was a happy young man in good health, fit, studying, with friends, a good job and in a happy relationship. Back then, I had no reason to get stressed up.

Since I was still tired, trembling all over, fearful of another seizure, and my parents didn't want to entertain the thought of

---

[1] Tachycardia, also called tachyarrhythmia, is a type of heart rate. disturbances. In tachycardia, the rate at which the cardiac muscle works is increased and reaches up to over a hundred beats per minute

anxiety seizure for even a moment, considering reasons for this situation that the EMTs didn't even mention, they decided they had to get me to the hospital.

The wry faces of the EMTs showed slight disbelief at my parents' readiness to nitpick. Aside from the alleged panic attack and the stress that they claimed was bothering me, the men insisted that I was fine; they didn't consider hospital treatment necessary, and so they refused to take me to the nearest medical center.

They informed us that had they done that, we would have had to bear additional costs not covered by my medical insurance.

Still sitting on the couch, I thought, *How come? I'm a student who started working for my parents' business on top of that, I do pay my monthly health insurance.*

Thankfully, I started feeling a little better as the conversation progressed; seeing that it all raised my parents' eyebrows and that they were about to kick up a fuss, I jumped the gun and decided that we'd drive to the ER by ourselves. The EMTs left our house while we were left much disgruntled. It was a prelude to what was about to happen to me later.

Immediately after the ambulance drove away, we ran outside. With slippers still on his feet, my dad started the car's engine. My mom locked the door to our house and we set off to the nearest hospital, the very same that the EMTs were about to return to. My dad was driving so fast that we managed to catch up with the ambulance. Since we had a green light on our lane, we were first to arrive, saving all the money an ambulance ride would have cost us, as we had been informed back at home by the EMTs – that's a joke. We got to the ER at the exact same time the ambulance did.

My dad and I took comfortable seats next to other people waiting in line to be called by name by a doctor. I remember that I wasn't the youngest bloke there. The other people who were sitting there, waiting for their turn, included a teenager with a messed up face, a small girl with an arm that was likely broken, and several homeless people squatting here and there on the floor, most likely faking various ailments just to stay in a warm place, buy a cup of cheap hot coffee from a vending machine, or to simply capitalize on the opportunity to have a chat with anyone. After all, it was difficult for them to find a sympathetic ear out on the street among crowds of commuters rushing to work, rarely paying any attention to the homeless.

At that moment, my mom approached the reception desk to describe what had happened and specify why we came there. As it turned out, the ladies at the desk were not in a good mood, most clearly discontent at the fact that they had to work the evening shift on that day. They gave my mom the look, as if making it known to her that our presence there was just another annoying nuisance. My parents and I soon realized that they took me for a faker who most likely arrived in with either an intricate plan to extort a leave letter for school from a doctor, or an intention to undergo a swift medical check-up without having to wait for a scheduled appointment. Sadly, such situations were and are still rampant; thus, having scanned me with their eyes like with some x-ray vision that showed them a picture of a young, fit boy that presented himself quite well compared to other patients, the ladies presupposed that I had come there with a malicious intent. My mother got overwhelmed with emotions and nearly snapped because of this entire situation, which was nothing short of bizarre. Fortunately, at that very moment, one of the EMTs who had come to our house earlier approached the reception desk and noticed my mom, who was about to explode in a fit of rage. He came near one of the medical receptionists and spoke with her. After a while, we were informed that a doctor would come to us soon. My mom thanked them cordially, and we all sat down waiting for our turn.

To our surprise, we didn't wait long for the doctor on duty. Perhaps it was just an hour, which is not a long time given the circumstances doctors on duty work in and the usual wait time at a hospital. The doctor took me aside and pulled a turquoise curtain behind me, separating us both from the rest, and started asking me a series of questions. I described minutely everything that had happened on that day.

He looked at me ironically and said, raising his voice, "You do realize that people are dying here, don't you, young man? Do you know that in the very moment when you called an ambulance, someone could've needed that aid much more than you did, and that they could've died?!"

Perplexed, hearing these questions, I was completely lost as to what I should say. Being quite witty, I was always good at making a clever comeback. Back then, however, it felt as if I got slapped, perhaps for perpetrating some truly horrendous act. I think that one of the effects this emotional paralysis had on me was that I still felt swept off my feet by the violent emotions that had been overwhelming me for a few hours. Never before had anyone evoked in me such a profound feeling of guilt. I took those words personally, although, in all actuality, I knew that the doctor was wrong big time. I knew that but for the situation I found myself in and my crippling exhaustion, I would've snapped back fewfold. After all, my parents had no choice but to call help. How could a person without any medical training know when to call help and when not to? If I were in their shoes, I would've done the same. Everyone would do the same when facing a threat. I decided that as long as we stay at the hospital, I wouldn't tell my parents what the doctor told me. I knew that had I done that, the evening would've been epically ruined; the only thing I wanted was for someone to finally give me some diagnosis so that I could go home and make that awful day come to an end.

Once my medical history had been taken, which was done much more swiftly at the hospital than back at our home, the doctor on duty checked my pulse and ordered an ECG. Then, he told a nurse to get hydroxyzine[2]. After I took the pill and some time passed, he checked my pulse again. My heart began calming down. Suddenly, my parents emerged from behind the curtain, having lost their patience. They asked the doctor what had happened and what was the possible cause of my health issue.

---

2 Hydroxyzine – an organic chemical compound; a sedative and an anti-allergic medication.

The physician replied, "It seems that your son had a panic attack."

Again, both my parents and I struggled to comprehend this diagnosis, and we didn't want to believe that the doctor simply confirmed what the EMT had said.

"How come? Why? I don't get it, doctor." I insisted. The only thing he replied was, "The cause lies somewhere else and, unfortunately, I cannot help you, young man."

How come? Aren't you a doctor? I thought.

My mom, who unlike me could think clearly, recalled that I had frequent headaches, as well as that recently, I had been experiencing them often and very regularly right after my training sessions at the gym. She added that I had occasional fits of pain that lately lasted for two or perhaps even three weeks straight. Having learned that, the doctor on duty asked me again in that loud, pretentious voice of his why I hadn't mentioned that before. This time, he was right; however, the state I was in wouldn't let me think clearly about all the things that justified my behavior in some way. I realized that I wasn't the only person who was handled by the medical staff in such an arrogant manner. In a distance, you could hear a conversation between an ill elderly man and some employee of the facility, coming from behind a curtain. I could hear clearly either a male nurse or an EMT asking that person, "If you have no family, no friends, and you have no car to drive home in, why on earth did you come here?"

That old man was probably just as embarrassed as I was, finding it difficult to come up with an answer. At that moment, I had a clear realization that it is only in some movies and TV series that hospitals are idyllic. In fact, it was not at all how I imagined such a place. I was accustomed to watching doctors who always had a bright smile on their faces, a kind demeanor, and a solution to every problem. These were the medical experts I knew from TV. The mundane reality proved completely different.

Maybe it's different here on a regular day, and in every other hospital it smells nice, there's shiny floors, charming person-

nel, and patients suffer less, and rarely die. All the people here just had a bad day, I contemplated.

Some time passed and I was taken for a head CT scan to check if nothing bad was happening inside. Waiting, again. Eventually, the doctor on duty came back to us with my ECG and CT scan results. According to these test results, neither my heart not my head gave the doctor any reason to order further testing or to continue to investigate what had happened to me that evening. There was only one diagnosis, and it was unquestionable – anxiety disorder.

After several hours spent at the hospital, tired with all the waiting for any results, we went home. Each of us had only one thought, *Anxiety disorder? What is that? What's that all about?* When we got home, it was already too late for doing any research and each of us went to bed. Although I wanted to fall asleep badly, I couldn't; the bewildering welter of thoughts wouldn't let me. Among all the things I brought with me back home from the hospital, lying on the bed next to me, there was my discharge summary that I had received before leaving the ER. Driven by curiosity, I was trying to decipher the preliminary diagnosis issued by the doctor when I encountered an obstacle – a medical history report written in Latin. *Have some sleep, man, it was a rough evening*, I thought.

Rubbing my eyes, I realized that there really was a Latin phrase under the diagnosis, reading "*Spondylosis regionis lumbo-sacralis suspecta.*"

Damn, why did you chose Spanish in high school? We're living in the 21st century! Who on earth still speaks Latin?! I asked myself.

Having swiftly translated the phrase online, I realized that the doctor who examined me diagnosed me with degenerative changes of the lumbar spine and recommended further care at the outpatient clinic with an annotation reading, "x-ray image of this part of the back."

How on earth has my incident anything to do with the lumbar spine and why hasn't the doctor on duty written anything about anxiety disorder in the diagnosis? He probably forgot how it goes in Latin, I thought.

I decided to leave it out of my memory together with everything that happened that evening.

Eventually, I managed to fall asleep and I woke up quite refreshed, feeling a zest for life. Unfortunately, during the day, I realized that something had changed in me with the anxiety and the panic. I could feel that I was different, that my perception of everything around me was somehow unnatural. The feeling I felt on that day was quite like that experienced by protagonists of sci-fi books or movies when the way they perceive the world becomes altered. Such characters, be it vampires or Spider-Man, would acquire heightened senses immediately after turning into beings with supernatural powers. They'd get razor sharp vision and enhanced hearing, rendering their surroundings easier for them to navigate and explore.

In my case, it was completely the opposite. Everything that was around me remained the same, but my attention was more centered on myself and my body. A part of me wouldn't leave me in peace, nagging me constantly that something was wrong. I raised both my hands to look at the palms and I got terrified. The sensation I felt at that moment could be compared to being born again. It was as if for twenty-three years I had been oblivious to the fact that I had arms and hands, and hadn't realized it until that very point in time. Suddenly, everything that was around me started irritating me. Looking around, I could see the difference; I could feel that from that moment on, I was someone else. The more I explored that state of mind and my thoughts, the more it seemed to me that my hands were not mine. I got really scared.

I decided to call Anna, my sweetheart, and tell her what she missed out on. Obviously, in a situation like the one that took place on the previous day, there was no time for that, and it wasn't a good time to stress her up and make her come to the hospital. That was clear. My parents knew all too well that I wouldn't want to bother her, and so they didn't inform her either. As soon as Anna learned about the EMTs' visit at my home, she got slightly disappointed and angry that I hadn't notified her earlier. Her anger didn't last long, though, as she quickly came to understand our decision. She realized that had she been in my shoes, she would've done the same.

A few days passed without me getting any more panic attacks. From the moment the doctor made me realize that that was the right diagnosis given the symptoms I was bothered by on that evening, I'd been using the terms 'anxiety' and 'panic'. However, I was still experiencing altered perception, feeling like my hands weren't mine, on a daily basis, which was causing me great discomfort. Nonetheless, I tried to live on and forget about everything that happened in order to return to my normal life as soon as possible. And I did. Just as usual, I continued to engage in my regular activities.

My parents and Anna were not as optimistic as I was, though, and regardless of it all, they were still trying to persuade me to get tested elsewhere; they deemed it not normal for a young, healthy, strong boy to experience sudden panic attacks or heart palpitation. Obviously, their hunch was right. I had that hunch, too, but it simply wasn't the right time for doctor-shopping and comping up with new diagnoses. That was how I looked at it. I was young, fit, and I wanted to live my life to the fullest. I considered the incident that had occurred merely a one-time thing, and attributed it to my training at the gym.

To me, strength training was something special; it became an inherent part of my life. This passion didn't appear out of nowhere. As a young kid, I was never fond of sports. I recall that back in elementary school, most of my peers were all hyped up at the thought of Friday swimming classes. However, I was just glad that the weekend was coming. To me, having to dive deep into ice-cold water was a torture. The very thought of cold water and the deep swimming pool would numb me out, rendering me unable to put a rubber swim cap on my head without aid. As swimming classes were the last class on Fridays, I was often rescued by my mom; she'd come watch how I was doing in the water through a glass wall, and lend me a helping hand with the cap. To this day,

I remember how much fun my buddies had at my expense. Not only did I struggle to keep up with their swimming skills, but on top of that, I couldn't even put my cap on.

I was standing out among my peers in a negative sense, always far behind them in team sports. This difference was clearly noticeable during PE classes. I'd always do poorly in disciplines like soccer or basketball, where it is not only the team effort that counts, but also the ability to force your way through. There was one reason behind my poor results: I was one of the smallest boys in the class. From an early age, my colleagues had been superior to me in terms of strength, weight, and height, so I didn't have much say in team sports. It wasn't until junior high that I started seeing the colossal gap between my physique and theirs.

When I was twelve, my family moved to another district in the city. This meant that I had to reckon not only with the fact of changing my place of residence, but also that of losing my childhood buddies and having to make new ones. Back in the late 1990s, the Internet was still fledgling in Poland, unfortunately, while cell phones with antennas longer than the phones themselves could only be seen carried by businessmen in American movies. For a young teenager who was afraid of his own shadow, that meant only one thing – losing his childhood friends.

I easily found myself in the new place and my new school, and it came easy to me to established new friendships.

However, in junior high, I experienced the immense disproportion and the gap between me and my peers. In the class I was in, I was the smallest. My classmates would often discuss my height and weight. One of the nicknames my colleagues gave me was very accurate – they simply called me Shorty. Luckily, I was never bullied by kids bigger than me, though the feelings I experienced during PE classes would often take a toll on my self-esteem. My chances in team sports were nonexistent. I think that my every contact with the ball during a game was a coincidence or simply the good will of my buddies, who would sometimes pass the ball to me so that I could feel like part of the team. Since our PE teacher was a woman, we were doomed to practice the sports discipline that was dear to her heart; sadly, it was volleyball, which we played during nearly every PE class. This soon became very dull. I could tell before each and every PE class what we were about to practice on that day. The prospect of waiting for my taller pals to pass me the ball while I was standing there like a bump on a log was very disheartening; I was willing to do anything to avoid attending PE classes. I soon ran out of the limited number of times where I was allowed to be "unprepared for class" without any negative impact on my grade. There were two, maybe three instances of unpreparedness allowed, and every new one resulted in a minus that our home room teacher would jot down in her notebook, which then affected your final grade. For this reason, I'd often pretend to be ill, or lie to the PE teacher claiming I forgot to pack the proper attire. I also happened to skip PE classes. I knew that there was no benefit I could reap from spending my time on physical education. There were also some positive moments during these classes, nonetheless. Fortunately, I wasn't always at a disadvantage. The roles would reverse in disciplines that require a player to depend on himself, in which case his height and, therefore, the reach of his arms, is not that decisive. In activities such as pull ups or table tennis I was undefeated. Whenever it was the time for physical fitness tests, I'd always stand out in some way. Pulling my bodyweight on a bar and timed running allowed me to improve my final grade, and thus catch up with my colleagues who were bigger and stronger than I was. Had we played table tennis during PE classes, most likely my final grades would have been even better.

My passion for table tennis started when they installed a ping-pong table in a small park in our neighborhood. Since the park was the main venue where I'd hang out with my new friends, wasting most of our days sitting on a bench for hours, we were all very happy that a bricked ping-pong table was set up there. As it soon turned out, of all the boys I was the one with the greatest flair for this game, though their skills were improving from one game to the next, too. I came to love playing ping-pong so much that I got my own table to practice with my dad, who was the only person

I couldn't easily win with. He turned out to be very good at it. He'd always triumph over me, even when using a piece of a plank instead of an original table tennis racket. Finding it hard to believe me, the guys would often visit me to play with my dad and see for themselves if my stories about his extraordinary skills were true.

This passion didn't last long, though, proving nothing more but a transitory enchantment. Time flied, and each of us had to go his own way to attend his chosen high school. From then on, we all had much less free time, but I'd still hang out with the boys at the park after school and on weekends, occasionally playing table tennis. Starting high school, I was well aware of my body size, but I also knew my strengths. It didn't come to me as a surprise then that I was one of the shortest, most minuscule students in my new school.

I found myself in the class of my dreams. I'm sure many guys my age fantasized about the situation I was in. I had only two male classmates, Grzes and Daniel, and as many as thirty female colleagues. High school is a time when every boy starts paying more attention to his looks and focuses more on the opposite sex. So neither the guys not I could have been in a better place.

That's ten chicks for each of us, we thought.

The first time I came to the class, I was overjoyed; not because the crowd of girls that made me unable to stop my eyes from jumping back and forth from one to another, but rather due to the fact that finally, for once, I wasn't the shortest guy in the class anymore. Daniel was a little shorter than I was, though more chubby. I could venture to claim that he was also stronger than I was. In turn, Grzes had that look of a regular high school student, much taller and heavier than the two of us. I assumed that after the miserable experiences I had in pervious schools, given the positive surprise our small 'harem' was, PE would be just as promising. I also hoped that perhaps in high school I'd have the chance to show off my good table tennis skills. Sadly, time has shown that I was in the wrong.

We'd practice PE together with boys our age from other classes. They were all quite decent, so we got along. Unfortunately, to my discontent, my posture was far from standard, as usual. Worse still, our PE teacher was not a creative type; showing little interest in coming up with diverse activities, he would give us a free hand to choose a discipline of team sports that we wanted to play during each class. Much to my misfortune, it turned out that most of the guys were volleyball freaks who'd often choose to pass the two-hour-long PE class doing exactly that.

I was 'overjoyed' every single time.

Excellent! Just awesome! I'd remark ironically in my head.

My colleagues soon realized I was a poor player, and so I was rarely picked for the team. From my perspective, the player selection process for team sports was nothing less of a circus. The PE teacher, whom the boys used to call 'coach', would usually appoint two team captains, adorning the chosen two with bands that went across the chest. In the moments when he was about to pick team captains, some would even look him deep in the eyes, begging him, "Pick me, coach!"

I found it hilarious. Some classmates were acting as if it was an extraordinary moment of their lives. The lucky one that was made a captain was tasked with choosing players for the team. As you can imagine, I've never been picked right at the beginning. Since the team captains were taking turns when choosing players, each captain was trying to cherry-pick the most valuable assets in the most reasonable way, so that his team was stronger than the other. Hence, they'd first go for the tallest and the strongest boys who had no difficulties spiking and saving. Every time, among the last few left who had to be assigned to one team or the other, there was I and my other classmate, significantly taller than me, named Michas. Due to his distinct womanly tone of voice and the clumsy way he moved, we considered him somewhat disabled. His motor coordination was massively impaired and, as if that wasn't enough, he suffered from uncontrolled bloating when doing sit-ups. When there came a day when Michas was picked for the team before me, making me the last one to be selected, a liability, I realized yet again that PE was not for me. Nonetheless, like in junior high, I was able to use my physical fitness to improve my final grade by jumping over obstacles, throwing a medicine ball, or, again, doing pull ups. I could do pull ups all day, probably because I was the lightest, while some of my colleagues who looked like full-grown men couldn't even do two reps.

In high school, physical appearance was highly important to boys, as an athletic physique not only meant a better shot at winning the hearts of female colleagues, but also boosted overall self-confidence. My high-school years were a time when fights would often break out between male students, while mugging out in the city streets were all too common. There was a degenerate lurking in a park next to the school, waiting for students who were walking home alone. He was like a wild animal, crouching and hiding in the bushes on the lookout for his potential prey. Much older than we were, he was a boy on probation with a bad record of numerous cases of theft and assault. He would attack defenseless high school students who had to take the route across the park to get to our school. The infamous thug was stealing teenagers' cash and cell phones. Back in those days, virtually every other student had a cell phone, making it easy for the thief to make quick money by selling his loot to fences. Aware of what was happening at the nearby park, the school principal took relevant measures to solve this problem. The police were put on the case, while the entire situation got covered in the local newspaper. Shortly after, the perpetrator was arrested.

I was attending a high school located in a district called Baluty, whose bad reputation had been known for generations. Theft and mugging were an inherent part of that area. Therefore, sooner or later, I was bound to get mugged out in the street, too.

My parents would always tell me to never play wag and to study hard. They didn't consider skipping school acceptable. Although I rarely engaged in such antics, one day, Grzes, Daniel, and I decided to skip classes. Daniel lived outside the city and always headed in a different direction than we did; for this reason, we would split in front of the school and each of us would go his own way. Since Grzes and I were heading in a similar direction, we continued our escape together, quite content. One time, since we had a lot of free time, we chose not to take a bus, but to go the distance of a few bus stops on foot instead. And so we did. Soon after, we realized that was a mistake. As it turned out, from the very beginning we were watched and followed by two local youngsters. We reached a large, busy intersection with a traffic jam of cars and buses, swarmed with people. Despite all the bustle, the assailants didn't abandon their plan. We realized that they weren't going to give up and that most likely, we'd have to defend ourselves. We decided to split. The two strangers did the same. One followed Grzes, the other went after me. Grzes and I figured that it would be best to get close to each other again. As soon as we did, the two aggressive guys were already in front of us.

"Now what, you dickheads?" one of them struck up a 'polite' and 'peaceful' conversation.

"Who do you support?" the other cut in, asking about our soccer club preferences. "Hand up your cash and phones!" he added.

These guys must be in the same business the park mugger is, I thought.

In these circumstances, you have a thousand thoughts all at once. Most of all, I wanted to remain calm and think positively, but the palpable tension was getting into us bit by bit. Both Grzes and I had a similar thought, *Attack? Punch? Maybe one of us gets one of them and the other hits the other one?*

As far as Grzes could stand a fair chance of fighting one of the aggressors, I knew I had none. My jacket made me look slightly bigger, but I was aware that they were both much taller than me and one of them was considerably bigger than my buddy, too. Some part of our male pride didn't let us try run away or ask anyone for help. Looking at each other and peeking at our attackers, we were waiting for their move, ready for the worst to happen. Then, one of them told me to give him my cell phone.

"It's yours if you find it!" I replied.

I had a backpack with coursebooks and a jacket. I didn't have any cell phone, hence my reply. He did notice, though, that one pocket of my pants had a wallet in it.

He 'asked' me if he could have it, saying, "Give me that or I'll fuck you up!"

I found him quite convincing and, sensing that there was no other option, I handed my wallet to him. The mugger took my last twelve *zlotys* out of it and decided to keep the money along with the whole thing. Grzes, however, incurred a much greater loss. He had a brand new cell phone. He hadn't even enjoyed it for long. He had to give it away to these guys. After the successful robbery, they turned on their heels and started away, leaving us alone. We were so disappointed with the fact that we hadn't even tried fighting back. Our pride was hurting for some time after that. Although I didn't lose as much as my classmate did, I was very sorry, as my wallet contained a unique sticker depicting Uruguayan actress Natalia Oreiro, and I was nothing short of in love with her.

Grzes and I knew that this incident could've ended quite differently for both of us. Had we gone through the park on that day, it could've been a completely different story. Regardless of it all, we took that event to heart, as it bruised our male egos painfully. At the same time, it marked the beginning of a change in our high school lives.

From then on, we both had the same thought resounding in our minds, *I have to change something about my life*. Grzes decided to put some work into his physique and started exercising passionately with weighs at home to become a bit bigger. In turn, I wanted to feel safer, so I started thinking about learning self-defense to be able to defend myself if I were to be assaulted ever again. Sometime later, I joined taekwondo classes. Our third classmate followed in my footsteps and signed up for a course in Thai boxing. For me, the beginnings were extremely hard and painful, even. Up until that point, I had had nothing to do with physical exercises as tedious as these were. Initially, I wasn't doing that great. You couldn't even compare PE classes at school to the warm-up before the main training session of the Korean self-defense course. The warm-up alone, which lasted for over ten minutes, would put me through the wringer, leaving me completely deprived of any strength and willingness to continue the training. It took my body several weeks to start adapting to such a high physical workload. Over time, I grew accustomed to that course and I came to be quite fond of it, and thus also of having my butt kicked during the class. Each time, I'd go home all bruised. Taekwondo is a martial art that consists mainly in striking with your legs. As you can imagine, the strength of the leg is more destructive than that of the arm, with each well-aimed kick leaves significant damage. Although I was doing my best to not get hit, I didn't always succeed. My forearms, which I'd often use quite clumsily to keep my guard in order not to be hit somewhere else, were constantly covered in green-and-purple bruises. Despite the never-ending contusions and bruises, I drew much satisfaction from doing martial arts. Since my motor coordination and body awareness were always quite good, in a very short time I got flexible enough to do splits. Stretching was a highly significant and essential element of the Korean training. In short time, it allowed me to perform kicks just like my favorite action movie actor Jean-Claude Van Damme did. Back as a kid, I loved watching him, particularly fight scenes with him, as well as his famous kicks that he dispatched his biggest adversaries with. My training sessions consumed me to the point that on my way home, I'd additionally do an hour of leg stretching to become even better.

I trained that specific martial art for two years, with classes held two or three times a week; they made the time left before my exit exams pass much faster. Unfortunately, in the third year of high school I had to discontinue training due to the upcoming exit exams. This is how my Korean martial art story ended. After the exams, like most high school students, I went to college. I got admitted to the College of Tourism and Travel. In the Polish education system, PE classes usually end with the graduation from high school. To my surprise, the curriculum for the major I decided to pursue had obligatory PE classes. Fortunately, I could choose from several options available. The offer was neither overly extensive nor enticing. I had to make up my mind at the very beginning, so that the college authorities could put my name on a list for a specific class. There were three options to choose from: team sports, swimming classes, and aerobics for female students or gym for male students. The choice was simple. My gut feeling told me that the name "team sports" was nothing but a cover-up for one thing – volleyball.

Although many years had passed since elementary school and I finally taught myself how to swim and put a swim cap on without assistance, I concluded that water was probably still ice-cold. Sadly, I had no other option and I had to go with the gym. The final year of high school and then a nearly four-month-long summer break before choosing college made me very lazy. Though from time to time, I was still playing table tennis with my friends from junior high in the park, it was not often enough to allow me to call myself a physically active person. In college, there was no room for any excuses that would help me avoid exercising due to improper attire, for instance. It was obligatory to get a credit for PE. With no such credit in my student's book, I wouldn't be allowed to complete my freshman year. I had to come to terms with the fact that there was no way I could avoid the gym. It was definitely not my cup of tea.

It's just a gang of sweating dudes staring at themselves in the mirror! I'd tell myself. *Where are the girls?* I kept asking in my head, regretting that putting my name on the list for aerobics was not an option.

I found it completely impossible to start being comfortable at the gym. My college buddies were doing their best to persuade me to try any workout gear with the hope that perhaps I'd find some of it likeable. Sadly, there was nothing that could make me catch the bug. Eventually, to make time pass faster, I had to mount one of the machines at the gym. I decided to go with a stationary bike, spin the pedals a bit, and somehow make my way through to the end of the class. It turned out to be a great idea. Time really flied faster. As you can expect, I wasn't content with the fact that I had to get up in the morning and get on a bus once a week specifically to watch the clock at the gym for an hour, pedaling at the lowest resistance settings.

Spinning hundreds of miles on the gym equipment, waiting for the compulsory training to end as soon as only possible, several months flew by before I even knew it. One day, everything turned upside down because of one moment that I found to be very peculiar. I remember like it happened today: during my gym class, I was sitting on a bench, leaning my back against the wall, watching my colleagues working out. Then, a student who was attending this class with us sat right next to me. I had seen him around the campus before, but we had never talked. We were sitting like that, next to each other, for a couple of minutes. At one point, we both cast a glance at each other, looking into the reflection of each other's eyes in a gigantic mirror wall that was in front of us.

Suddenly, the boy said, "Man, you're skinny!"

Utterly stunned, I only nodded. I looked at my reflection and his body, which was not fit at all; comparing our silhouettes I realized deeply that in fact, he was right. I was very lean for a freshman. At the height of five feet, eight inches, I was slightly below one hundred and six pounds. That was way below the standard BMI. On that day, I was wearing a t-shirt, sweatpants and shoes I formerly used to have on when practicing taekwondo. I took another look at my reflection in the mirror. I pondered for a while. Suddenly, my outfit brought to my mind the old days and I recalled how much effort and sweat it cost me to practice hard, wearing these very clothes.

One thought came to my mind, *That boy's right. I need to do something about this.*

After my freshman year ended, my life gained momentum. It was the beginning of great changes that transformed my previously lazy life. My friends back from junior high Franek and Rudy asked me to come with them to the gym. I didn't refuse. I decided that this time, I wouldn't be going long distances on the spin bike. I had a different goal – to buff up.

We would all start a training session with a brief warmup. With some recollection of the key components of how to warm the body up that I had learned during my training back in high school, I implemented some of them to get prepared for lifting weights. Since my buddies had been going to the gym on a regular basis, they were well-versed in the art of working out. Had I not spent an entire year staring at the clock at the college gym, I would've had it much easier at that moment. Watching my friends, I copied the way they were exercising. I didn't consider it fascinating or feel special about it until the light-weight training was over and it was time for the legendary bench pressing. Since forever, I had always associated a weight bench, ubiquitous at all gyms everywhere, with the specific type of a venue a gym is. I recall beefy peers from my high school bragging to one another how many pounds each of them could bench-press. Very often, during recess, they'd show off their skills on a regular bench in one of the school corridors. Although I had many occasions to test myself on that bench, I never had.

Franek and Rudy were much bigger than I was. Rudy was about six feet, three inches tall, and nearly twice as heavy as I was. The two of them were repeatedly pressing a barbell one hundred and ten pounds heavy. Each of them could also easily bench-press one hundred and thirty pounds, which was far less than the body mass of either of them. They were having serious troubles handling a bigger load. It was my turn. For the first time, I lay down on the bench. I boldly put my hands on the bar, which was hanging right over my face.

It'll kill me, I thought.

The guys were standing right next to me to spot in case I didn't have the strength to lift the load on my own. Initially, I put only sixty-six pounds on. I believed that I had to do it. I yanked the barbell off the rack and started lowering it slowly towards my chest. Very soon I realized that the weigh was not that heavy for me, and I started swinging it up and down with ease.

"Put on twenty-two more!" I asked.

My friends knew that a barbell eighty-eight pounds heavy was equal to eighty percent of my entire body mass. We all assumed that I was probably incapable of handling that. However, it turned out that this load was not much of a challenge for me, either. I could easily do a few series of reps. Since I liked that a lot, and the masculine element hidden somewhere deep inside me was screaming for more, I asked the guys to put on twenty-two pounds more. When lowering a load equal to my entire body mass, I felt that was quite heavy. At one point, I realized that I could have some difficulties lifting it back up. I gritted my teeth and, mustering all the strength I still had inside, I managed to press the weight upwards and re-racked the bar. Although I paled in comparison to my friends, I realized that given my body weight, it was still quite amazing that I successfully lifted a weight equal to my entire body mass. My buddies were stunned, too, wondering how I managed to do that. From then on, I had a new goal. I wanted more.

Throughout the summer break, I continued to delve deep into the weightlifting world. From one workout session to the next, I was getting stronger and putting heavier plates on. My weight didn't change much, though. There came a time when the guys gave up on training and I was left by myself on the battlefield. Since I've always been somewhat introverted, I concluded that I'd continue training alone – at home. I bought a weight bench, a barbell, and some weight plates. I found myself increasingly absorbed and fascinated by working out. Having purchased some gear for home use, I got completely obsessed about training. There was nothing else that I considered as important as honing my physique. Lacking the experience and knowledge in the field of weight training, I was busting my guts every single day.

At the beginning of the second year, I came back to college somewhat transformed. My posture was slightly different, but my weight remained roughly the same. This time, when choosing a PE class option, I didn't even hesitate to pick the gym. Some of my colleagues were quite impressed by my transformation and my new attitude to fitness. The tables had turned – some of those who had been working out hard during the previous year now took my former spots at the gym where I had been watching the clock from. From that moment on, I didn't have to force myself to pass the PE class; I considered it a warmup before the training that awaited me at home. After a few weeks, I was already friends with two guys from the gym. They were attending the same college and I used to pass them by in lecture halls. You could tell by their physique that they had done some hard work in the training room. Seeing how hard I was pushing myself, they noticed that aside from increased strength and minor changes in my appearance, my weight remained low and I still looked very lean. For this reason, they encouraged me to change my diet, and buy some protein and carb supplements that would make me gain mass in no time.

It didn't take me long to decide. Much impressed by the physiques of my new buddies from the gym, I wanted to look like them. So I bought the supplements that would supposedly help me attain my dream body shape.

For an entire year, I was training at the college gym and also by myself in the comfort of my home. Having learned more from my friends, I managed to take on over twenty-six pounds in just eight months. The increased daily food intake and my proper weekly workout plan allowed me to acquire a body shape that I found nothing short of impressive. From then on, strength training was an obsession of mine. I'd lock myself in my self-arranged training room and for that moment, I'd become oblivious to the whole world. Ceasing to work out was not an option. I went so far as to feeling the compulsion to train even when I fell ill or had a mild fever. One of my greatest desires was to reach the point where I'd bench-press the magic number of two hundred and twenty pounds. Few of my colleagues from the campus could take such a great weight on. The only ones who succeeded had an extensive experience in training at the gym (many years in some cases) or were bestowed by mother nature with great innate strength. Attaining that goal was all the world to me. I was working out passionately to reach it as soon as possible. I was so obsessed by it that I didn't even take into consideration the possibility that I could sustain an injury.

One day, I hurt my wrist at work, which made it impossible for me to continue lifting weights. It took me little time to come up with a solution. I strengthened my wrist with some cardboard and bandages, and, giving it little thought, I started bench-pressing. Although the pain was immense, back then, I considered training to be of key importance, regardless of its effects on my health.

Within three next years of my weightlifting endeavor, not only did I manage to bench-press the magic number of two hundred and twenty pounds that I desired so much; I also became so strong that I could do several series of reps with the barbell. Both my friends back from junior high and my college buddies couldn't believe how it was possible for me to bench-press that load while weighting slightly over one hundred and thirty-two pounds. This made me very self-confident to the point that I was finally able to hold my head up wherever I went. Although I remained lean, I knew what I was capable of. Though always a humble guy who never competed with his friends in any way, deep inside I was proud that the ever-shortest 'Shorty' managed to cut his buddies down to size; despite still being almost twice as big as I was, they just couldn't bench-press that load.

In my life, there never was any room for rivalry. I learned that at school, being a good boy who'd somehow always find himself at a disadvantage. My peers participated in the rat race that was supposed to reveal which one was the best. Be it playing soccer or working out, it was rivalry all the way. My friends would often go to the gym in pairs of two or larger groups, for it was the only way they could motivate one another to train. They would spot for their buddies, and strive to outperform them later on. As for me, however, since I acquired the knowledge necessary for training, I never wanted to join people at the gym again. I simply didn't feel the need to do so. What motivated me was my desire to change my looks; I didn't need any rivalry to do that.

It was never my goal to surpass my colleagues in any way; on the contrary, in times when I proved better than others at something, I gave way so that others could feel joy and satisfaction, too. This was often the case with my buddies while we were playing table tennis, for instance. And yet, my life's story soon made me take up the gauntlet and fight the greatest adversary that ever crossed my path. Several weeks went by from the time of the panic attack that made me end up in the ER. Though my loved ones encouraged me to have some additional testing done, I wouldn't budge, wanting to forget about the recent events as soon as possible.

During the first year of my master's degree, I wanted to focus on studying and working in the family business. For many years, my parents had been running a small company that allowed us to make a decent living of it. They always strived to provide my sister and me with the best living conditions. After many struggles, having retired from their previous jobs, they managed to build a small successful family business that allowed them to live a better life, but also help many people in need. It could be said that children of successful individuals tend to be bratty and spoiled, spending their parents' hard-earned money like water; however, I was far from that stereotypical picture. I knew how hard my parents were working to make sure we lacked nothing. I never asked my parents about too much. Though I knew they'd do anything for me, I was often too embarrassed to ask them for anything. My parents' business didn't involve only their intellectual effort, but also daily physical toil. As a twelve-year-old boy, I started helping my parents at work. Seeing them both having to tackle heavy packages of goods, I wanted to help them at any cost; primarily, to make it easier for my mom, who was performing a 'man's job'. Although I strongly refused, my parents would always pay for my assistance. My mom would put my modest compensation for the work done into an envelope. I resisted, but she would do that anyway. My parents have always been altruistic – if there was an opportunity to help someone, they did. Very often, they'd help my sister's buddies by offering them several-hour-long shifts for a very good pay. Later, as years went by, my friends would get an easy option to make money. The guys would eagerly come help us out, as they knew they'd be well rewarded for those several hours, often getting as much as they would've earned for a few days in a full-time job in any other business. One time, I asked my parents why did the guys get so much money for helping just for a couple of hours. The reply was simple.

"Remember that what matters the most in life is not the money, but the man," my mom said.

"It won't make us poor, and the boys did a good job," my dad added.

These words taught me a lot and became a kind of a guiding principle for me.

One day, I'll be just like them! I decided. Although I could say that the opportunity to earn money from the youngest years for gigs at the family company weren't the best approach to raise me, since I didn't have to look for other ways to earn money, I did learn to value it and respect both work and people, nonetheless. I remember some of my peers who, unlike me, had to toil hard in a strawberry field in their youth to make a couple of *zlotys* for their whims. Having worked for several hours in the field, they'd ride back home on their bicycles, stealing a few flower bouquets on their way from an elderly man who was trying to sell them by a busy road. Dashing downhill on their bikes, they'd lean down and reach out to grab the flowers standing in a bucket of water. Pedaling as fast as possible, they'd ride off leaving the old man behind, most likely tarnishing the only way he could make a living. They'd give the flowers they had stolen to their mothers on Mother's Day, for instance, giving not a single thought to what they had done. Today, some of them surely recognize the errors of their youth while their moms remain oblivious to this day as to how did their sons get them the flowers.

Unlike many of my peers, right after graduating from high school, I had no idea what I wanted to do in the nearest future. I had no specific plan for my life. Since one of the most popular undergraduate courses back then was in Tourism, I decided to follow this path. As it turned out after I had studied it for three years and completed the bachelor's degree, I didn't feel like continuing this major to my master's. I still had no idea how to self-actualize or what my future plans would be. However, I did know that I should help my parents run their business. Therefore, I decided to take a part-time course that would prepare me for running my own business endeavor. I chose a major in Management at the University of Lodz. On weekdays, I was working at the family company and on weekends, I was attending classes at the university. In Poland, you have to pay a tuition fee to take a part-time course. I was one of the few students who didn't have to grind away in a nine-to-five job every week to be able to afford studying at a university. As a co-owner of the business set up by my parents, I had quite a lot of free time. Perhaps too much. The assumption was simple. My parents would help me cover my tuition fees, and I would gradually familiarize myself with how the company operated while acquiring knowledge intended to make it easier for me to run the family business down the line. Unfortunately, the major I picked and the knowledge my lecturers delivered had little in common with what my parents were dealing with. I was very disappointed, as I soon realized that I wouldn't learn much during this course. Nonetheless, I did know that I had to study hard and that once I started the course, I had to finish it. At the faculty, I saw many students who made the wrong choice, studied for a semester or two, and then changed the major for a different one, thus losing all the money they had invested so far. Often these were young people with parents who were sponsoring their opportunity to acquire knowledge and get the degree. In my case, it was fairly similar; however, I knew that the hard-earned money of my parents who were covering my tuition fees shouldn't go to waste. Although I felt that it wasn't the right place for me, I knew that I had to keep studying. This was my decision because, after all, studying allows you to expand your horizons.

    The beginning of my master's course was a time when I was expected to start showing a strong commitment to work. However, my hobby continued to be my entire world. Instead of dedicating more time to growing my parents' business to spare them the burden of my responsibilities, I was focused on my looks and the training I had to do. I adored going to the gym, but frequent meetings with my buddies or my daily trips to my girlfriend Anna's house were even more important to me.

    Anna was my second-greatest 'obsession' – right after the gym. I would always tease her, saying, "The greatest loves of my life are pizza, a barbell, my dog, and then you come in."

She would get highly irritated with this line, but I do believe she knew I was joking. She knew how deeply I fell in love with her on first sight. It is very difficult to find the right words for what I felt for her. A "true love" is probably the best way to put it.

As a young boy, I wasn't as lucky as my peers were. I was infatuated with different female friends (but especially with Natalia Oreiro); however, never before had I truly fell in love in any of them. Since for most of my life I wasn't particularly attractive to my female colleagues, who would usually fall for boys bulkier than me, I stood little chance of getting into a relationship. Very often, I was questioned by my family, "And you, young man, do you have your eyes set on any particular lady? When will you bring a lady friend home?" I'd get highly irritated with that. I think that I wasn't the only boy to be asked such questions nonstop. I remember that back in high school, I prayed while gazing at the stars, "God, please make it so that I get a girlfriend and then everyone leaves me alone."

Sadly, my wish didn't come true; most likely because I hadn't been going to church that much. I noticed that the fair sex was interested in me when I was in college. This was certainly to a considerable extent owing to my training, which significantly transformed my body and made me more self-confident. Back in college, I'd often hang out with female colleagues, and there were many of them. I started dating girls, buying them flowers. I felt that I became more attractive to women than ever before, and although they did make some immoral offers, for some reason I knew deep in my heart that I shouldn't exploit that.

"There are more ways we can spend some nice time together other than just holding hands. Come to my place, you know where that is," one of them said.

I passed on the offer.

"You're an idiot," my buddies told me.

There were many girls like that, but none of them made my heart skip a bit. That didn't happen until I saw the most wonderful creature on earth.

When I was in my third year of the undergraduate course, I got a call from my friend Tomek, who lived permanently in the United Kingdom. Since his driver's license was taken away, he had to come to Poland to re-sit the exam. He asked me to give him a lift to the examination center.

It was a time when I was getting ready to get my driver's license. Most young people do so right after they turn eighteen. However, I had a habit of always getting down to things with some delay, and the driver training course was no different. For some reason, I didn't feel any drive or pressure to get behind the wheel as soon as possible. When I decided to do so, I struggled. I tried to pass the driving test four times, and failed each time (while getting a full score from the knowledge exam).

"I don't want to, I don't feel like doing it," I replied to Tomek.

Tomek had a limited time, as he had to get back to England soon. He wanted to forget what happened as soon as possible and immediately get his lost driver's license back so that he could return to the UK. For this reason, he signed for a fast-track knowledge test that could be taken on a preferred day without having to wait for some date in distant future. Only fifteen lucky people who were in a hurry and managed to get in line were allowed to take this test. To this end, you had to start keeping your place in the line as early as possible. This is why Tomek decided to take his spot as early as four a.m. As you can imagine, I wasn't in a hurry at all, and the idea of waking up at night to take the test on the next day seemed unrealistic to me.

"What do you mean you don't feel like doing it? Come with me."

"Four a.m.? Have you lost your mind?!"

Eventually, I gave in and decided to go with him.

"I'm doing this only because of you," I told him.

As it turned out later, it was one of the best decisions of my life.

Not only was I lucky enough to nail the questions and get a full score from the knowledge test, but I was also hit in the heart so hard I didn't know what was happening to me.

In the center, Tomek and I took our seats waiting for the noon, when the test was supposed to begin. It turned out that we weren't the only people there who were keeping their place in the line from early morning hours. By eleven o'clock, we had already had a full group of fifteen that the regulations required.

One hour before the test, one of the people waiting in line had to leave for some reason. Then, out of nowhere, the vacant place of the fifteenth test-taker was taken by the most beautiful girl I've ever seen. I got infatuated with and hypnotized by her face. Her height, dark hair, blue eyes, and white smile... In our all-male company, the impression she made while standing in line couldn't have gone unnoticed. I imagined every guy in that moment saying to her in his mind, *Look at me! Look how cool I am!* From the moment she joined the line, time started flowing even faster and even more pleasantly. The girl retrieved some chocolate and started sharing it with all the fifteen of us with a smile.

Perfect, I thought.

Obviously, I didn't mean the taste of the chocolate, but that modest girl whose looks were nothing short of incredible, smiling to every person standing in line, winning them over instantaneously.

This was a new experience to me, since though I've always been smiling and kind to people, I'd keep my distance. On that day, she was radiating joy, optimism, and love for the entire world, which she spread among the entire line of tired people waiting for the exam. Before the test, every person awaiting it had a brief word with her and exchanged looks. However, I couldn't overcome my shyness except for uttering the words "thank you" when offered a piece of chocolate. During the exam each of us took a seat in front of a computer, fixing eyes on the screen. I knew that questions were the same as previously, and that my presence there was a mere formality, as I'd get the full score. For this reason, instead of stress that would otherwise surely start gnawing at me, I felt discomfort because I couldn't catch a glimpse of the girl, not even from the corner of my eye.

The test questions were displayed on the screen. Instead of replies pertaining to traffic regulations, all I could see was, "A. Chocolate, B. Blue eyes, C. What's her name? D. She didn't even look at you, so don't bother."

Since I was perfectly prepared for the knowledge test, despite my head buzzing with thoughts about the beautiful stranger, I managed to pass it.

Tomek passed the test, too. It was time to go home. When we were leaving, we learned that unfortunately, the girl didn't make it, as she was one good answer short of passing the test. Seeing the sadness on her face and tears in her eyes due to the defeat, I mustered the courage.

"Don't worry, next time you'll make it!"

She looked at me and smiled. I went red in the face and, holding my head low, I left. Tomek and I said goodbye to everyone and got back home.

Weeks went by and I couldn't stop thinking about the girl with chocolate.

One day, after I finished classes at the university, I went to a bus stop. It turned out that I was late – the bus was gone. The next wasn't coming in fifteen minutes. To my misfortune, of all the buses stopping at the campus, there was only one that was going my way. I decided to not wait idly at the bus stop and to go a couple of blocks on foot to have the possibility to catch some other bus lines going in the direction where my home was. Having walked a couple of miles, I was getting close to a bus stop on a street leading to the Driver License Testing Centre, where one month earlier I passed the knowledge test. Suddenly, less than a hundred feet away, standing at the bust stop was THAT GIRL. The closer I got, the more I felt overwhelmed by stress, though it was quite a nice feeling. I wondered if she'd remember me at all. I'll never forget the big, genuine smile that lit her face in the very moment I got close. Content, I realized at that point that she didn't forget. I approached her.

"Hi."

"Hi," she replied.

I was happy that I happened to meet her again, especially since I had already written that off as a dead loss.

"It's remarkable that we meet again," I added.

"Yes, you're right, it's remarkable, especially given that on this very day, I've passed my driving test."

I congratulated her and, asking about the details of the driving test that she had just passed successfully, I asked what her name was.

"I'm Michal," I introduced myself, extending my hand towards her.

"Anna."

Our conversation on that day wasn't long. I knew that I couldn't make her stay at the bus stop for ages. We were both waiting for buses that were going in completely opposite directions. Although we talked only for a couple of minutes, I had a feeling we knew each other since forever. In that moment, all I wanted was to make it last as long as possible. Sadly, the bus Anna was waiting for appeared too soon. I could only watch the bus driver close the door behind her. Raising our hands up, we both waved to each other goodbye through the window. I was highly dissatisfied, but I still smiled to not let it show.

On my way home, I was wondering why once again, I didn't do anything more to have a greater chance of having a longer conversation with Anna.

You could've asked for her phone number! I thought.

Fortunately for me, when we met at the bus stop, someone called her. During that call, I eavesdropped on her mentioning the name of the high school she was attending. It was the only chance and the only clue I had, and I could use it to find Anna. I got home and started rummaging through a social media website that allowed me to identify students from that specific school. It didn't take long for me to find her. I was completely overwhelmed with joy.

In the evening on the same day, I decided to contact Anna. Since I didn't want to scare her off, I came up with a story. I DM-ed her that I was looking for a colleague of mine named Piotr. As I didn't want to create any fictional characters, I used a full name of my classmate back from junior high who was allegedly attending the same high school she was, which obviously wasn't true.

"Oh, hi, what a coincidence! You won't believe it! I'm looking for someone, his name's Piotr T. and he's from that high school. Do you know how can I find him?" I DM-ed her.

Anna was very pleased. She was a bit surprised to discover shortly afterwards that there was no such person at that high school, and that actually, I hadn't DM-ed her by accident. Once again, I congratulated her on the passed exam and after that, there was not a single day when we didn't exchange a few words.

Days went by and we were constantly chatting online about every subject imaginable. Eventually, we decided to meet and go on our first date. I'll never forget that wonderful day.

I was very excited and stressed up at the same time. Though we knew a lot about each other from our online conversations, I was concerned that this time, Anna would see me from a completely different angle, and that probably, our entire relationship built so far would cloy in her eyes and become meaningless to her. I was wrong. On that day, we both realized we couldn't jeopardize it. After talking with Anna for an entire day, I walked her to a bus stop. Our hair and faces got all wet in drizzling sleet. Waiting for the bus, we were looking deep into each other's eyes. Anna was a bit clod, trembling a little – the walk was long and the air was freezing. Watching tiny ice crystals resting on her long lashes creating a play of light and shadows in her teary azure eyes, I was well aware that she was very cold. I dreamed of hugging her and keeping her warm. Unfortunately, we both knew that some rules that we had been taught entire life should not be broken. I could feel Anna wanting the same thing as I did, but on our first date, we had to keep up the appearances of being people of high principles. It was time to say goodbye to Anna. I didn't know exactly how to do it. She gave me a small kiss on the cheek. Overjoyed, I went home.

From that moment onwards, our lives changed. We stated going out on dates more often and spending more and more time together. Months went by and eventually, there came a time for the first passionate kiss. To me, it was a one-of-a-kind moment, but not because Anna and I had been putting that important step forward off, but because for the first time in my life I was truly in love and I had never felt like that about anyone else. Kissing Anna was something magical to me; at the same time, it all probably opened the door to what both of us had to face shortly afterwards. The consequences we suffered turned our previously carefree lives upside down, brutally changing our plans together. Like every young couple in love, we could imagine our ideal future. Anna always dreamed of getting married young, having a bunch of kids running around the house and a stable life, as most young women do. In contrast, my dreams were never that specific; I knew, however, that I wanted to be happy and to spend the rest of my life with my girlfriend.

I dedicated each and every free moment to meeting with Anna. My feelings for her were growing day by day until they turned into nothing short of an emotional obsession. I wasn't obsessed about my sweetheart in an unhealthy way, though; on the contrary, I'd simply consider it overprotectiveness.

Although there were many instances where my jealousy of Anna took over and I was unable to hide it, I knew I could trust her. She had quite a lot of male acquaintances and male friends she always held dear to her heart, and I considered them all my competition. I was jealous to the point that I found suspects even among my own close buddies I had been friends with since junior high. I think, though, that this symptom of jealousy was caused by the fact that never before had I been so involved with anyone like I was with Anna.

I feared that someone could hurt her and so, on many occasions, instead of fulfilling my duties at the university or at work, I'd cut out early to make sure she got home safe. Anna lived outside the city. To get to her apartment, she had to go a couple of miles across fields and woodlands. My mind would come up with various unpleasant images. Aware of cases of young women being kidnapped or assaulted, often in daylight, I was pretty worried about her. For this reason, I'd often talk to her on the phone when she was on her way home or simply shuttle her around once I finally managed to get a driver's license for which I had been waiting for ages.

I got that document after putting the driving test off for quite some time. I was forced to do so due to an incident that I'll remember until the end of my days. One Saturday, I decided to surprise Anna and visit her before noon; better yet, had everything gone as planned, I'd have been the first person to see her right after she woke up that day. I went to a bus stop near my house. In front of the bus stop there was a flower shop where I'd buy one rose whenever I was going to meet Anna, asking the floral clerk to shorten the stem so that I could hide the flower in my pocket and surprise my girlfriend when she least expected it.

"You want it cut as usual?" the kind female clerk asked me.

"Of course!" I replied, smiling.

In my experience, the city bus services were never keeping it up with their own timetables. However, I didn't expect things to be better on that day. When the effective temperature is five degrees, everyone hopes that a bus would come on time. Sadly, it didn't.

With frost and sharp snow blown right in my face, scratching it painfully, I couldn't waste time hesitating. I didn't even think for one moment to get back home. I had one thing in mind: to wake up my girlfriend in person with the scent of the rose. I decided to take a brisk walk passing two bus stops on my way to catch other bus lines that would allow me to continue my trip. I walked a little less than a mile to reach a bus stop. Waiting for a transit that could take me closer to the road leading to Anna's, I was gazing at my watch begging the fate to make any bus arrive as soon as possible. I knew I didn't have much time to catch the only bus serving outlying suburban areas, shuttling residents from Anna's village to downtown and back. In contrast to the municipal bus services, that bus was dead on time. I was well aware that if I didn't make it, I'd lose the only (and the fastest) conveyance. I looked at my watch every ten minutes but none of the buses listed on the timetable appeared on time. Having waited for half an hour, I finally saw a large red-and-yellow vehicle emerging in the distance.

I got on the bus, which then took me to another location where I could catch another bus line that would take me to my destination. Fortunately, this time, the other bus appeared quite quickly. When I was on my way to a bus shelter where I was supposed to take the final, outbound bus, which was the only and the fastest means of getting to Anna's village, I spotted it leaving. When I got off, not only was I frozen to the core, but also devastated. I knew there was nothing else I could do but march on for a lengthy distance towards a hub where tram tracks would lead me out of the city. However, while still standing at the bus shelter, I realized that I couldn't take it any longer; I wouldn't make it on foot all the way. I knew I had to make myself warm. There were some taxis parked nearby. I checked my wallet and concluded that I could probably afford getting to Anna's faster, and in much warmer circumstances.

Shivering, I ran to one of the cars. I got in, and in a shaky voice, I asked to be taken right to Anna's door. We set off.

Although my body was painfully cold, I was glad that I still had some time to wake my woman up. Passing by several bus stops on our way, I noticed through the window the tram that I'd have had chased after had I not decided to take the cab. I realized that I made the right choice. However, a moment later, I was somewhat regretful about getting out of bed at all.

At one point, a man in a car in front of us fully applied his brakes on a red light. The taxi driver was forced to follow suit. Unfortunately, the cab skidded, and the driver had to do a specific maneuver to avoid ramming straight into the back of the car in front of us. With the wheel all the way right, he caused the cab to go towards a street lamp on the side of the road at full speed. Seeing what was about to happen, I knew we'd crash into it with the side I was on. We hit it.

Somewhat scared, I started acting as if I was surprised by this situation. Under the driver's rearview mirror there was an exceptionally pretty rosary, swinging left and right. The taxi driver was more disturbed and spooked than I was.

"Fuck!" he yelled.

He apologized to me for what had happened. Although the hit was loud, it had virtually no effect on us. As it turned out, the car or, rather, the right wheels of the car got cushioned by a small mound that was closer to the road than the street lamp. We got out to check the condition of the cab. Fortunately for the driver, the only damage it sustained was inflicted on the hubcap and a fender of the vehicle. We got back in.

"Well, let's go, shall we?" the cab driver suggested.

I nodded approvingly. He informed me that on our way, we'd have to stop for five minutes at a self-service car wash to clean the hubcaps. When we got there, the cab driver realized that the only means of payment accepted by the car wash machine was coins, and he didn't have any in his wallet. I gave him all my coins so that he could wash the wheels and assess their condition more accurately. Beneath a layer of mud that got washed off, the cab driver spotted a new issue that could have resulted from the accident; however, for some reason, he decided not to tell me anything more about it. He apologized and informed me that he wouldn't be able to take me to my girlfriend's, and he dropped me off at a place from where I still had a couple of miles to go. Since we had a minor incident, he also decided to give me a small discount for the ride. We parted ways. Due to these circumstances, the sum I paid for the cab was roughly the same amount I would have had spent on a suburban bus. Nonetheless, before getting into any cab in the future, I'd take a good thought. Luckily, in this spot, I didn't have to wait long for the final bus bound for Anna's village. It took me to a bus loop where from I had over a one-mile-long walk across the woodland and fields, which was my girlfriend's regular route that she had to take on a daily basis. Sadly, my journey lasted much longer than I planned and this time, I didn't arrive on time to wake my sweetheart up. Luckily enough, though, I delivered the flower intact.

I knew already what I had to do in the nearest future.

I had no more excuses.

That's enough! I thought.

I was very happy when I got my driver's license. I knew that from then on, I could visit Anna whenever I pleased. As a young bachelor in love, I considered it the best thing I could have done; all the more given that my girlfriend lived over twelve miles away. Having obtained the document, I could finally purchase my first car. My parents decided to help me and bought me a small, vintage, second-hand vehicle. Overjoyed, my dad and I went to the city outskirts to collect my first car. As soon as we bought it and got back home, I immediately set off to Anna's. Driving my own car made me happy and I couldn't wait to see my girlfriend's reaction. Since it was my second lengthy trip on that day, I was very careful behind the wheel. Despite maintaining all the focus and keeping my senses razor-sharp despite all the stress, my first ride to Anna's proved disastrous for me. Halfway, I found myself on a poorly developed street I had been often taking with my dad who'd occasionally give me a lift to my girlfriend's. You couldn't drive at a high speed on that street, as there were speedbumps installed every forty-four yards. Having driven over a couple of those, I noticed a small black kitten standing on the side of the road close to the next speedbump I was about to go over. Having little experience behind the wheel, it didn't occur to me to use the horn. What is more, I didn't think of simply steering the car more towards the middle of the street, or to the other lane.

"Go, please! Go! Beat it!" I shouted.

The small animal couldn't hear me. It was still standing in that spot as if it was glued to the road. Although I was going over the speedbump as slow as a turtle, I had a feeling that the cat was waiting for me there to commit suicide for some reason. When I was going down the speedbump, I felt that I went over another bump. I realized that was the cat. Finding no courage to look in the rearview mirror or to just stop the car, I drove away. Since I always loved all animals, and I grew up with a dog and cats, I was very hurt by what happened. I drove over to my girlfriend with my eyes all watery, overwhelmed with anger and resentment towards her and everyone who had been pressuring me for years to get a driver's license. These bad emotions didn't last long, though.

From then on, having the opportunity to spend more time with Anna, I was somewhat neglecting other important responsibilities, such as my work in the family business, studying, or house chores in general. The more often I was meeting with my girlfriend, the less often I'd meet my friends from junior high. I wasn't the only one having that problem, though. It affected all the guys. The more of us started relationships with girls, the less time we all had for one another, as each of us wanted to spend it with his sweetheart. Obviously, as soon as there was an opportunity, we'd meet up, as before, but accompanied by our women. I preferred meetings with Anna to everything else; however, there was only one thing about me that others might have considered a greater priority of mine than Anna was. This was training, obviously. Many saw it to be a great passion of mine with some hidden objective, while others considered it pain and suffering. Regardless of what any third party thought about it, I loved my hobby and couldn't image my life without working out. And yet, soon after, everything had to change.

Several weeks after the event where I was diagnosed by the hospital staff with a panic attack, I was suspecting my body of developing a case of tonsillitis or flu-like bronchitis. There was nothing weird about that, since I would often get various infections, particularly those of the upper respiratory tract. Up until that point, I had always gone through them quite smoothly, experiencing just slightly raised temperature and other symptoms typical of infection or cold. That time, however, it was a completely different thing. For some reason, my temperature was a hundred and four degrees Fahrenheit, and I felt just awful. I was switching back and forth between convulsions and cold sweat, flushing with hot fever, weak to the point I thought I would die.

The fever continued for an entire day. In the evening, as usual, the thermometer showed over one hundred and four degrees. Anna and I didn't need much time to reflect on what to do, and we rushed to the ER. Because on that evening I had my friend Tomek over, who would often vacation in our country, he offered to give us a lift to the hospital. We didn't say no to that. Although I was in a very bad condition, no exceptions were made for me at the hospital - I had to show my ID and describe to the ladies behind the front desk what brought me there during their night shift.

Struggling with the extremely high fever that made me lean on the desk for support, I replied, "I feel very bad, I'm probably dying, ma'am!"

The woman scanned me with her eyes from head to toe, and then cast a mocking glance at Anna and Tomek.

"You sure are! Sit down, young man. A doctor will come see you in just a minute," she smiled ironically at us.

Despite my poor health, I was conscious enough to recognize that yet again, I had been handled with distrust at a place where people should be offered help.

"Did you sense mockery in that lady's voice, too?" I asked my companions.

"Man, look... How was she supposed to react?" Tomek replied.

"I don't get it."

"Look at yourself! 'I'm dying, ma'am'? I would've died laughing, too," he commented.

I realized what he meant. To him, the way I worded how I felt at that moment was completely inconsistent with my physique. Both Tomek and the medical receptionist could take it as a great joke. I didn't find it amusing, though, as just a few weeks prior, I was in a similar situation. It opened my eyes to the fact that hospital staff rarely see a young, fit person in need, and so they cannot fathom that an athlete could suffer from any ailment or a disease. Therefore, the course of my previous visit was not accidental. In that moment, I realized that cases of young people dying because they didn't get any help at a hospital, which I had heard of repeatedly on TV, are not necessarily a mere fiction intended to captivate the audience; these stories were true.

Shortly afterwards, I was approached by the doctor on duty.

"What brings you here?" he asked.

Barely mustering some strength to speak, I told him I felt very bad, that I had a sore throat, over a hundred and four degrees that I was trying to bring down throughout the day to no avail using home remedies, and that I suspected that I had tonsillitis. I mentioned that I was aware that when you have a fever that high without any temperature drop for a longer period of time, you should call an ambulance or go to a hospital.

The doctor took my temperature and said, "You don't have tonsillitis, but I can see signs of acute bronchitis. You do have a fever, but I don't see it necessary to bring your temperature down to normal."

I was handed acetaminophen, which I took with water. Highly enfeebled, I assumed the man knew what he was doing.

Getting up off the couch to head towards the exit, I heard the doctor saying, "One more thing, young man. Next time, before you decide to come to this hospital, be aware that people are dying here, and in the time when I'm attending to you, I could save someone's life."

Once again, I was stunned. I had a *déjà vu* moment. On the next day, my temperature started dropping, thank God, and I couldn't believe that I had heard these words again in the only place where everyone, regardless of their age, should feel free to seek help.

After an over week-long stay in bed with high temperature, my state improved significantly and I returned to the world of the living. I still had that bothering, odd, unnatural sensation that appeared with the panic attack. All the time, I was having weird thoughts and sensations that wouldn't leave me alone. When I was looking at my hands, not focusing on anything specific, I was suddenly getting overwhelmed by a sensation of being trapped inside a suit that wasn't mine. It was as if I put on a diving suit or a spacesuit, the only things I could see through the glass visor of the helmet being the surrounding reality and my hands. Although I found it highly inconvenient, I had to hope that everything would go back to normal soon.

One day, I was doing some house chores with my parents and we were introducing some changes at home. Since my elder sister had left the nest, I could take her room, which was much bigger than the one I had been occupying up until that point. The change of the space called for a change of furnishings, too; for this reason, I had to put together a brand new furniture set. When I was installing a drawer slide, I cut the skin on the tip of my thumb. Feeling the pain, I put my thumb into my mouth. Then I took a look at the slightly cut finger. When I saw the minor cut on the skin and the blood that was flowing out, I suddenly realized something bad was happening to me again. In one moment, I got an awful stomach ache and nausea. Then, I felt something much worse was about to ensue. As in the case of the panic attack, I could feel myself blacking out. And there we go again; the overwhelming feeling I had at that very moment was certainly the state that precedes fainting. I realized that I was blacking out, though in truth, I was conscious all the time. I couldn't catch a breath and everything went black for me. However, I could hear everyone around me, and I knew exactly what was going on. For a couple of minutes I couldn't see anything. My parents took my inert body on a sofa where after a few minutes I already started regaining consciousness. I was convinced that the issue was gone and that certainly, it wouldn't happen again. Highly shocked at my strong reaction to the small wound and the sight of blood, I started wondering what was that all about and why did I react like that. After all, seeing blood was nothing new to me. Fights at school, taekwondo training sessions, and action movies that I had been watching passionately, they all had me accustomed to seeing things much worse. Some part of me was telling me that there was something bad going on with me, but I didn't want to get even more immersed in grim thoughts. I calmed my parents down a little; yet again, scared by my state, they wanted to call an ambulance. The funny thing was that despite the triviality of that entire incident, we actually started debating whether making such a call was a reasonable thing to do. My two previous visits at the hospital, the response of the medical staff, and their two attempts at guilt-tripping me because there could've been some other patient dying, made us all change our approach. The hospital personnel playing on people's emotions like that, which was my experience up until that point, was the reason why we opted out of another appointment.

1:0 for healthcare services, I thought.

Days went by and I still didn't see any reason why I'd have to start looking for an answer for what had happened over the last couple of weeks. I hoped that soon everything would come back to normal. I was convinced that my weird sensation of being trapped inside my own body was simply caused by overtiredness, the training, changes related to entering a new stage of my life, starting a master's degree or beginning to work at my parent's company.

And yet, my loved ones were still upset due to the several previous incidents. My parents and Anna strongly insisted that I went anywhere to have some additional testing done. However, they did know that I was as stubborn as a mule, and that seeing a doctor was the last thing on my mind.

Ever since being a child, I hated medical appointments. From an early age, I considered seeing an internist a waste of time and I had to be taken there by force. Up until I turned twelve, I had to be led to an outpatient clinic by my mom by hand while my peers, particularly girls, were doing great at such venues by themselves.

I was never afraid of that place; I simply didn't see any sense in me visiting an elderly medical doctor. Throughout my life until that point, I had been associating a doctor with a retired old lady with reddish hair who wears cylindrical glasses. Sitting behind a desk and soaking a giant stamp in ink, she was smashing a stamp on patients' prescriptions, saying, "Next!" I always had a feeling that the internist I was seeing was working two jobs, and that the clinic aside, you could also meet her sitting at a station at a post office, performing the very same tasks.

I soon realized that it wasn't only her; every other doctor usually prescribed the same medication or supplements for a cold or inflammation. With or without a drug prescription, my every seasonal disease lasted exactly just as long: from seven to ten days. The older I got, the harder it was for my mom to talk me into going to see a doctor. Obviously, my attitude was completely different when I needed a doctor to give me a leave letter for school so that I could be granted exemption from PE class or other classes.

Although I'd always steer clear of outpatient clinics, soon there came a time when I had to change my habits.

One weekend, I took a ride with my dad to the nearby mall to do some shopping. From an early age, I'd occasionally go with my dad to wander hypermarket halls and aisles together aimlessly. We'd gaze at the shelves with articles, and if we came across something interesting, it could end up in our shopping cart later on. Most often, we'd go to stores with home appliances or consumer electronics. I was very fond of these trips with my dad, taking pleasure in those moments when we'd both lay our eyes on some piece of equipment, pondering whether it would look cool on a shelf back at our place. On that day, as always, I was very happy to go on a spontaneous trip with my dad. I didn't know, however, that in just a moment, my nightmare would return to pay a call. While we were getting closer to our destination, we were listening to some good old music from the 80s (as we always did). Whenever I was going somewhere by car with my dad, we would always have the kings of that era killing it on the back seats - Bryan Adams and Jon Bon Jovi, entertaining us on every mile. Fair weather with a clear sky, rays of sunlight penetrating the car interior through glass windows, falling on both of us – it all set us in a good mood, as it seemed that we'd spend some great time together. Unfortunately, in just one moment, when I was listening to one of my favorite tracks, I felt that I was being swept off my feet by a wave of odd thoughts and sensations similar to those that had overwhelmed me back when I had the anxiety seizure.

I was somewhat scared, but I didn't alarm my dad that there was something wrong going on. When we were arriving at the shopping mall, I had a feeling that my mild anxiety and the recollections of the previous experience dissipated, and thought that everything would be just fine. We set off to roam the stores. Our first target was a very popular German electronics store that we'd often visit. Entering the store was a little unpleasant for me as I felt as if I was stuck in a spacesuit. We split so that each of us could freely scan countless shelves stacked with electronics. Strolling the alleys, I noticed a product that caught my undivided interest. Suddenly, a whirlwind of racing thoughts appeared in my head and once again, I started feeling anxious. I couldn't control them. Holding the product that I was interested in, I was staring at it completely disassociating from reality. It was as if for a few seconds I was elsewhere and the world around me didn't exist anymore. If someone tried to catch my attention in that moment by waving his hand before my eyes, I'd probably fail to even notice it. All my thoughts were fixated on one thing – my body.

The more I pondered on what was happening to me, the more anxious I got. I realized that my heart rate was growing to catch up with the racing pace of my intrusive thoughts. Paralyzed, I was standing in one spot, listening closely to my body, waiting for what was about to unfold. Within a millisecond of that nightmare, I realized that every deeper thought like, *How could this be happening? What's going on?* was escalating the entire issue. This state became even more aggravated when I saw my hands, causing me exasperation and mental discomfort. I was doing my best to calm down.

You're fine, everything's fine. Breathe. Think about something else.

The more I tried to stop thinking about what was happening to me, the more my mind would become consumed with the galloping thoughts. It was like falling into a spider's web with no chance of getting out – the more you toss around trying to fight it and free yourself, the weaker and less likely to escape you become. A perfect trap. I could feel my heart beat becoming faster and faster, and I knew it could end up pretty bad; this time, however, I wasn't in my room but at a shopping mall swamped with hundreds of people. I could imagine myself lying between racks, my dad and the store clerks kneeling above me, waiting for an ambulance. With this picture in my head, I started feeling faint. I realized the situation I had experienced back when I was putting furniture together was about to reoccur.

What the hell is going on with you? Save me, God! What's wrong with me? I thought.

These were nothing but empty words though, and not a calling to God; just like the phrase "Jesus Christ!", commonly used nowadays, for instance, when we get scared or when we're ecstatic about winning a lottery. When it dawned on me that my situation was dreadful, I decided I had to go get my dad immediately. I ran to him and told him we had to leave straight away.

"What happened?" he asked.

"I think I'm having another anxiety seizure."

We quickly got to the exit. As soon as we left the shopping mall, I took a deep breath. At the very same moment, the intrusive thoughts disappeared from my head. I sighted, relieved. It was as if I had been drowning in a sea of bad thoughts when suddenly, a lifebuoy ring was tossed and I got pulled back into the vessel of reality, where I was safe. To me, it was all hard to fathom.

After getting back home, my loved ones and I were wondering what was it all about. Why would a young man experience such reactions and unsettling states? After all, I had been living a life of a strong young man with no reason to be concerned. On many occasions, both my mom and my girlfriend saw me struggling with weightlifting during training, my face getting all purple with strenuous effort. Because of this, they assumed that my recent health problems were caused by training.

Both of them, my mom in particular, were telling me repeatedly, "What's it all for? You're ruining your life! It's all because of the training!"

Although my parents and Anna wanted to force me to go to the doctor, despite the shopping mall incident, I still considered it unnecessary.

Everything changed though in the moment when I experienced the same seizure once again, this time while attending a lecture. Its course was very similar to that at the store. All unsuspecting, I was sitting in my row among other students when suddenly, for no specific reason, I started feeling anxious; I could feel my heart beating faster and faster. This time, somewhat more composed, I knew that I couldn't let myself get stranded in thoughts and that I had to try stop that state from escalating; I was well aware of the consequences - had I failed, I would be lost. Terrified at the prospect of yet another seizure and the situation I found myself in, I feared what my colleagues' reaction would be like. Then I snapped out of it, simply stood up, packed my stuff, and left the lecture hall. I ran out of the university building and got into my car. I could feel my body and mind gradually calming down; everything was going back to normal. I realized that things were going south and that there was something bad happening to me; something that was beyond my control. From then on, I knew I had to seek help.

My family, Anna and I gave it much thought as to where I should go. We still had many reservations over how the previous visits at the hospital went, which left us all disappointed and shocked, and we felt discouraged from revisiting that place. We ascertained that the staff working there was not that eager to investigate the causes behind my odd symptoms and that I'd certainly end up suspected of simulating some disease, again. We didn't have a clue as to what to do, where to seek help, since up until then, none of our relatives had ever had similar health issues. Sadly, there was no doctor in our family, either; no one to give us directions. We had to rely solely on a PCP, and that was the first person I decided to turn to.

Back then, I had been already registered together with my parents at an outpatient clinic situated a couple of miles away from our home. The reason for giving up the clinic in favor of a different one which was located farther from our house was quite simple – we wanted to keep up with the times and trade the elderly female doctor (whom I suspected of working another job at a post office) up for a relatively younger team of PCPs and medical experts; this was exactly what the newly opened and well-equipped outpatient clinic offered us. Unfortunately, it soon turned out that you can't judge a book by its cover, and I had several unpleasant situations at that place, too.

During our first visit to the outpatient clinic, it made quite a good impression on both my parents and myself. This clean, well-kept venue offered not only laboratory tests that were performed virtually instantly, but also appointments with a wide range of specialists covered by my medical insurance plan (aside from paid private ones, obviously).

From then on, I treated every instance of the common cold, flu-like inflammation, or grass allergy contracted during my bachelor's degree at that clinic.

Although I couldn't draw any comparison between their team of PCPs and the elderly lady with cylindrical glasses, I still had an impression that they all graduated from the same medical school. The model for solving my problems with cold was still on the same level. I concluded that since it's not rocket science and the same antibiotics, probiotics, and a few dietary supplements are prescribed on a loop, medical studies are not at all as difficult as commonly believed.

Where did you make a mistake? I thought. I was envious that PCPs had it so easy at work.

There came a time when I was about to see an internist at the clinic, hoping that doctors would prove me wrong and show me that their medical knowledge was much broader than I thought. Typically, I'd be scheduled a preliminary appointment with a young doctor whom I called Dr. Armani. In contrast to the family doctors I had been seeing so far, he was always smartly dressed, usually wearing a neatly tailored suit jacket when meeting with his patients. Since the reason for my previous appointments with the family physicians was related solely to common ailments that affect everyone, particularly in the fall and winter season, I could never say anything bad about the job they were doing. It all changed, however, with my first visit at the internist's office that was due to an issue which does not affect every young, fit man - and it was not the common cold.

I made an appointment with Dr. Armani at the clinic. With some trust for that doctor built over my previous visits paid because of the common cold, I hoped that he'd help me solve my problems. There, in his office, I gave him a detailed description of all that had happened until that point.

Having little life experience, I hoped that Dr. Armani would prescribe a miracle cure for my ailments, and that the anxiety diagnosed earlier by the EMTs and the doctor on duty would simply disappear. Unfortunately, I was deluding myself. Not only did my internist have no magic pill that would make all my problems go away just like that, but he also had no idea that could help me solve the mystery of my extraordinary condition. While recapping the circumstances that affected all the recent events, I hoped that Dr. Armani would suddenly stop being a regular PCP stuck behind the desk and turn into a real medical detective. In my imagination, I saw him taking his stethoscope off of his neck with one swift move, and replacing it with a fedora hat whose fabric and pattern matched those of his stylish jacket; putting the stamp for validating prescriptions aside, he gracefully retrieves a giant magnifying glass from his pocket. I imagined the doctor, whom I knew very well, leaning forward thoughtfully, considering my case while breathing in smoke from a wooden pipe he was sucking on like some eccentric 19th-century detective. Sadly, reality turned out to be brutal; the doctor had absolutely no interest in playing the role of a Hercules Poirot of the medical realm. Avoiding my gaze and fiddling with a ballpoint pen with both his hands at once, he fixed his eyes on it with his head held low, copying the diagnosis that had been issued earlier. At that moment, I realized that my problem was bigger than I thought, and that solving it would not be easy for me. There was nothing more I could do than to ask what I should do given my circumstances.

"You need to seek the help of a psychiatrist," he said.

"A psychiatrist?!" I couldn't believe it.

Up until that point, my only association as regards a psychiatrist was that of a mental asylum where individuals suffering from severe mental disorders are put in. I had heard of cases of patients with schizophrenia or various deviations treated by psychiatrist.

But ME? I thought.

I concluded that my family doctor overstepped the mark a bit. *YOU go see a psychiatrist! There's nothing for me there,* I contemplated.

Suddenly, I recalled the identical diagnosis the doctor on duty from the ER wrote in Latin in my patient record. I told Armani about it; without commenting on it, and without formulating any opinion on this matter, he simply started filling out a referral for lumbar spine radiography, as previously recommended by the doctor on duty. I thanked him for these exhaustive directions and left the clinic.

Having returned home, I didn't have much to tell my loved ones about; they saw I was concerned. We hoped that I'd have found the answers to my questions the clinic; as it turned out, it wasn't as easy as I imagined. I had no other choice but to follow the clues I got from the healthcare staff. Therefore, a couple of days later, I went to get lumbar spine radiography. After a few days, I received an x-ray image including an impression and I went to see Armani again to verify the results. This time, I didn't fool myself he'd transform into a detective. The only thing I dreamt of was for him to find anything that could be the cause of my problems. As it turned out, everything was just exactly as it should be; he claimed that both the image and the radiologist's impression showed my spine to be in an excellent condition. Concerned, I desperately wanted to find what was the reason behind my ailments. For me, the previous suggestion to seek a psychiatrist's help was not enough. I simply couldn't comprehend why Armani claimed that it was the only solution, and the right solution, on top of that. There was a part of me that could understand him, since upon hearing myself – a young, fit man providing a detailed description of sensations, particularly that of being trapped inside my own body – I came to understand that anyone could misinterpret that. However, my intuition was telling me that the problem lies somewhere else, and not in my mental state. For this reason, when I saw that Armani wouldn't turn into a detective or investigate anything, I thought that if not him, I'd have to be the one to take matters into his own hands. Sitting in front of the doctor, I swiftly put all the recent events and symptoms together like pieces of a puzzle. Back then, the only things I could come up with were elevated heart rate, which manifested during every seizure, and persistent headache lasting several weeks, which had been tormenting me back before I called the ambulance. I thought that perhaps it was the right path to follow to find the solution. Hence, I asked Armani for a referral for further heart testing. Having trained at the gym for several years, I was well aware that my heart was often forced to work faster to handle a lot of physical effort. With no objection, Armani stated that it was a good direction and that I should have my heart checked by an expert. He didn't seem to have anything against it, but I could tell by the grimace on his face that he issued another document reluctantly. I had an impression that I exhausted my limit by getting a referral for an x-ray. As for the headache, the doctor read the interpretation of my previous check-up at the hospital and told me that I could get a more specific test done using an MRI scanner. I was content at the thought that I somehow managed to squeeze out of Armani at least one idea that seemed quite good to me. Sadly, as it soon turned out, the PCP couldn't issue a referral for a more specific test for me. Only a neurologist could do that. I asked him why that was.

"These are the rules and we must follow them," he replied.

Hence, I also got a referral for an appointment with a neurologist. By the end of our meeting I felt weird, as if I had asked too much of the family doctor. Never before had I been forced to do that; it was something completely new to me. I thanked him for the appointment and got back home.

This time, I returned somewhat optimistic, though if not for my eagerness to continue the search, most likely, I'd have returned emptyhanded. That thought made me a little concerned.

With these two new options of seeing neurology and cardiology experts, I deeply believed that the nightmare I was experiencing would soon come to an end.

Unfortunately, it turned out that I had to wait for quite some time to see these specialists.

With little life experience, neither my loved ones nor I were aware that in order to get an appointment with a medical expert, you had to wait; not two days or two weeks, but even up to two months and longer. Naturally, as many other people, I could make the waiting time shorter by going for the optional paid private appointment, though it always costs lots of money. The price for a visit at an office of a doctor or a professor specializing in a specific medical field ranged roughly from one hundred to two hundred *zlotys*. Those 'exceptional' individuals whose name was well-known in the world of medicine charged even up to five thousand *zlotys* for an appointment. That was more than a semester tuition fee of my part-time studies; it was nearly forty percent of the minimum salary in Poland at that time. Not to mention that an appointment with many medical specialist cost just as much as monthly earnings of people in Ukraine, for instance.

Although I found myself among those lucky people who could afford a private medical appointment, I didn't want us to spend our hard-earned money on my trips to a doctor's office. My parents were trying to force me, a stubborn, full-grown man, to see as soon as possible someone who'd make my problems go away - to no avail. Despite the great discomfort and concern about my health, upon hearing how much getting an appointment straight off would cost me, I dug my heels in and decided to schedule a free-of-charge appointment with a doctor, as most people do, and patiently wait for my turn. Since throughout that time I was experiencing anxiety and elevated heart rate, I decided to see a cardiologist first.

While waiting for the day of my appointment, I continued living my regular lifestyle, which included attending classes. Unfortunately, that wasn't easy. Wherever I'd go, be it university halls or the movies with my girlfriend, I had to account for a possible anxiety seizure. Though I was doing my best not to think about it, I knew that there was a bomb ticking inside of me, which would explode when I least expected anyway.

Although I was surrounded by my loved ones, friends, and my girlfriend, I felt very lonely with my inner struggle. Every time I'd put my sensations and what was happening to me in words, none of those close to me could understand.

I felt that I was becoming a completely different man with every day, more and more focused on what was going on inside of him, concentrated on his heart beat, concerned what his own extremities looked like. I would dissociate from the world around me. Many times, when sharing moments with Anna, I'd lose my sense of time; not because time flies when two young sweethearts come together, but because of some unidentified internal reason that would come snatch me away from the present moment and pull me deep into the ocean of reflection.

What's happening to me? Why? I'd ask myself.

Often, gazing for the hundredth time at my hands raised before my face, wondering why that view was making me so uncomfortable, I'd scare my girlfriend, who would shift her teary eyes away from the TV, sensing that something bad was eating me alive on the inside. Over time, all these negative sensations that were tormenting me exacerbated, making me less and less present in the lives of others. My parents and Anna were struggling with my somewhat different state of being on a daily basis, whereas my childhood friends had never experienced that version of me before.

Tomek, owing to whom I became Anna's boyfriend, Franek, who helped me begin my journey with weightlifting, and three other companions were a team that we had formed back when we were twelve. Each of us was different, his individual traits a benefit that added to our crew. I met the guys back in junior high and from then on, we stuck together not only in the class, but also after school on a bench in the park, where we would hang out, strengthening our ties.

Day by day, year after year, we were growing up as best friends. We'd spend every free moment together discussing various topics, wondering who we'd become in the future. We would talk life and the challenges that it was testing us with every single day. Together we tried stimulants and alcohol for the first time. By watching one another and observing our habits, we were summoning our own reality into being. Though we parted ways in high school, when each of us chose another school and made new acquaintances, we all knew deep in our hearts that we felt best as part of our old crew. While growing up together, we were having our first big problems, first love interests.

As Bryan Adams sings in his song *Summer of 69*, *"We were killin' time, we were young and restless, we needed to unwind. I guess nothing can last forever."* When we entered adulthood, the first of us to leave and go abroad seeking the taste of an independent life and a job was Tomek. The rest of us went to college. Our friendship was still not in danger. Despite Tomek's absence and, sadly, the growing number of responsibilities that each of us had, we continued to hang out together in our free time. Tomek would fly back to the country to see us whenever he could. While undergraduate studies brought us even closer together, each of us was also making new friends in college. Many situations and events that happened in that period had a considerable impact on our relationship, such as me meeting Anna thanks to Tomek or the 'accidental' finding of a girlfriend for our friend Damian, to which I contributed a little. Shortly afterwards, she became his wife. The guys and I celebrated together passing our exit exams in junior high, then in high school, and then getting our degrees in college. It seemed nothing could stop us, nothing could break us apart. Time showed that it was otherwise. On many occasions during our summer trips together, we would raise bottles of beer for a toast, saying, "May we all meet again in ten years' time! Bottoms up!" These words grew on me, taking on a different meaning as time passed. When I told them that something bad was going on with me, they struggled to comprehend. Most likely they thought that I was overreacting to some trivial issues. They knew I was dating Anna, that I was working, studying, exercising at the gym; therefore, they assumed that things weren't as bad for me as I claimed. Hence, they couldn't understand why I started gradually ghosting on our regular hangouts.

Indeed, despite the symptoms that kept on tormenting me, which appeared out of the blue, I continued to pursue my passion for training at the gym. Although the sensations that wouldn't resolve spontaneously were preventing me from enjoying daily life to the fullest, I didn't give up, and I didn't want to give up on my hobby, either. Without any certainty as to whether that problem was of a cardiological nature, I kept on doing the entire strength training routine. Later on, I didn't have another anxiety seizure or panic attack at home, but for some inexplicable reasons, most often, I'd get palpitations and anxiety while away from home. For a young man, it is a very difficult experience to become overwhelmed with anxiety in the least expected moments and, on top of that, in front of his buddies who know him from their childhood years. On several occasions, while visiting various places or even when getting some groceries at the store with my friends, I had to pretend I had to go to the bathroom while in truth, I'd go out to get some fresh air in an open space, which would placate me and soothe the emotions that were emerging suddenly and for no reason.

The more often I experienced this type of situation, the more often I didn't want to go out with my buddies. I started then to minimize a bit the time spent with them. This solution wouldn't work when it came to Anna, though. I imagined that had I began withdrawing from our relationship, it would disintegrate, and I didn't want that to happen for anything in the world. As for my friendships, I was certain that nothing could tear us apart; I considered every one of my good old pals a brother, and I knew that if up until that point nothing made us part ways, a brief vacation from social life wouldn't change anything in this regard, either.

The end grade you get at your master's degree and the final examination in defense of your master's thesis largely depend on your note-taking skills, but most of all, on your attendance and focus during classes. In my case, during the first year of my graduate course, I couldn't fully concentrate on studying or participate in college life in its broad sense. It was caused by the symptoms that I was experiencing.

Due to all the permanent, negative feelings that took hold of me with my first anxiety seizure, as well as those that caused me panic and palpitations when I least expected it, I started seeking doctors' help and waited patiently in line to see a cardiologist. Sadly, quite soon and, yet again, when I wasn't expecting it, a new problem emerged, forcing me to see an expert faster. One day, when I was taking notes while attending a lecture at the university, suddenly, I felt it got quite cold under my left armpit, and I realized it was wet. It wouldn't seem anything odd at first, given that every third student was probably struggling with hyperhidrosis, particularly those who were overweight. In my case, however, the cold sweat appeared only under my left armpit, leaving a huge wet stain on my shirt, whereas the right one was completely dry.

What the hell? I asked myself.

Luckily for me, I didn't get an anxiety seizure at that time, but I did ponder throughout the rest of the lecture on what was happening to me and why did I sweat so much for no reason, and only under one armpit, on top of that.

After I got home, I tried to find the answer to my question online. Having entered the phrase, "sudden cold sweat", a long list of diseases unfolded before my eyes, each of them likely to include causeless sweating. By that time, the only sweating my body had ever produced was the natural one caused by physical effort. Despite the immense physical exertion that had been part of my life from the time I was twelve, be it when carrying heavy boxes at my parents' company, or practicing sports later down the line, I had never struggled with excessive sweating. On the contrary; unlike my peers, who'd often turn men's locker rooms into a gas chamber, my sweat was unnoticeable. Delving deeper into the search results, I found out, among others, about anxiety and nausea indicative of heart diseases. Since all these negative symptoms had been affecting me lately, I got scared and decided that I couldn't wait any longer to see a specialist. My loved ones and I started looking for a doctor who'd examine me sometime soon at a paid appointment.

To our surprise, finding a professional offering paid visits proved more difficult than we thought. As in the case of a regular free appointment, you had to wait for a long time for a private one, too. Meanwhile, my entire family learned about my issues. It turned out that a good friend of my uncle Andrzej's was a cardiologist who worked mostly abroad, but back then, he was staying in Poland for some time. My uncle suggested he could contact him and tell him a word about me; maybe his friend would agree to see me and examine my heart?

My uncle got highly involved in this matter; from the very onset of my ailments, he began searching for some information about it on the Internet. Whenever we met, he'd tell me about his suspicions as regards the causes of my problems. Although these ideas were not always accurate, I was very grateful to him for taking an interest in my problems. To me, uncle Andrzej, who won with brain angioma, was a good example to follow. Back then, as a young man, he was unaware that there was an insidious monster growing inside of his head. That tumor was highly likely to cause sudden death; the only hope lied in a risky surgery abroad, which was a risky, not thoroughly effective procedure. And yet, my uncle decided to fight and put himself to the hardest trial of his life. Aware of the fact that if the surgery failed, he would lose his wife, children, and all his loved ones, he took a shot. His strength and, perhaps, faith in God allowed him to overcome the growing angioma. Unfortunately, the risky surgery took an irreversible toll on his health. To this day, he struggles with hemiparesis of the left side of the body. Although life dealt him a heavy blow, and he had to toil every day to perform all his daily tasks, he was committed to try solve my problem.

Following my uncle's intervention, the cardiologist he was acquainted with slotted me in. I was glad, as the waiting time for an appointment got significantly shorter. Accompanied by Anna and my mom, I went for the long-awaited visit.

Meeting him was a completely new experience; for the first time ever, I had a new, positive feeling about it, as the doctor proved to have impeccable manners. He got up behind his desk, approached me, and introduced himself while shaking hands with each of us. This was something new to us all, since usually, the doctors we had been seeing so far wouldn't even open the door for their patients with a smile; they'd just sit behind their desks, shouting, "Enter!" or "Next!", and that's all. I was also surprised by the form of the diagnosis and the way in which the cardiologist conducted the history-taking process with me. I described everything I had experienced up until that point, and the doctor didn't cut me off – not even once. Listening closely to my monologue, without taking his eye off the laptop screen, he was typing swiftly on the keyboard all the information that caught his attention. Content with how this was going, I was happy that finally someone was listening to me, and I felt that I was in the right place. When I finished talking, the doctor proceeded to examine my heart. I was glad that such a test could be done at his office right away, without waiting or changing the venue. I lay down on the couch, and the cardiologist did an ECG and a cardiac echo. My ECG reading was normal. It showed normal cardiac axis and moderately increased sinus rhythm. The results that the doctor presented to me having performed echocardiography showed that my heart was working properly, too. Left ventricular systolic function and diastolic function normal, pericardium is unremarkable, heart valves are competent.

My results showed no left-ventricular segmental contractility dysfunction. According to the expert, the dimensions of my muscle that was pumping blood into all blood vessels in my body were normal, just like the overall test results. Although comprehending most of these specialist terms providing an overview of the condition of my heart was beyond me, I felt as if I was attending a lecture at a medical school. I soon realized that the doctor was simply informing me that my heart was working properly and that it was fine. On the one hand, I was ecstatic to hear that this key organ of my body was doing well, as that clearly proved that I could keep on training. On the other hand, I still had no answer to my burning question, "Where do all my ailments come from?"

To my surprise, the cardiologist entered into a lengthy discussion about me with my mom and my girlfriend. Together, they arrived at a conclusion that I wasn't satisfied with. They inferred that I was exhausted and that my self-esteem was too low. It was clear from their discussion that I was overly concerned with my physical appearance, and that I was dedicating too much time and effort to strength training. I had an impression that the most important women of my life wanted to hear from the expert that it was the strength training that my issues actually ensued from. They both considered lifting weights risky and, on top of that, evil. They hoped the doctor would at least tell me to give up training for some time. Since my heart was in good health, the doctor swiftly connected the dots and proclaimed his opinion.

"I think you should talk to someone," he said.

Then, he wrote a phone number to one of his colleagues on a piece of paper.

"What's the purpose of seeing another cardiologist?" I asked him.

"She's not a cardiologist. She's a psychiatrist," he replied.

Shifting my gaze from his eyes to my mom's, and then to Anna's, I was sitting there, silent, without saying anything. I knew that the girls were worried about me, and that they were desperately trying to find the reason behind my ailments. The only thing they came up with was my daily training routine. Upon hearing yet another doctor claiming that I should start seeing a psychiatrist, my mind drifted away to some faraway place. Seeing me sad and slightly disappointed with the course of the appointment, the cardiologist tried to show me some emotional support.

"Keep lifting weights. I wish I could look like you. I really don't know what is it about your body that bothers you. I'm sure my colleague will help you. It's worth giving her a try."

Listening to the people who were there with me at the office, I didn't know what they were saying to me and I couldn't comprehend it.

They're mad! I thought.

Indeed, I've always been bothered by comments made by my acquaintances or family members I saw only occasionally, hearing, among others, "Michal, my boy, you're so skinny,", "Do you even eat?" Some of my dim-witted aunts would also ask, "Will he be taller?"

Though I'd always get irritated with such questions, I was deeply convinced that such comments from the past couldn't have left scars on my heart causing all the negative symptoms I had been experiencing recently. We thanked the doctor for the very pleasant appointment and left the office.

After seeing the cardiologist, naturally, I told my uncle (among others) about how it went. However, I didn't tell anyone about the opinion I was dissatisfied with and the advice that I should go talk to a psychiatrist, which had become a standard recommendation by that time. My intuition was telling me that my issues had no mental basis; and yet, I'd give more and more thought to seeing a psychologist or a psychiatrist. Aware of the fact that no one of the healthcare staff I had encountered had identified me with any potential diseases, concluding that the issue was a matter of my mental health, I decided to put off the appointment with a neurologist I had a referral for. Nonetheless, a lot of time passed before I finally called the number my uncle's friend had given me. Reassured by the most recent expert opinion, I stopped being afraid of having some serious illness that I had been visualizing in my head.

Though it had no effect on the frequency of my anxiety seizures or my derealization caused by feeling trapped inside a spacesuit, the opinions issued by the medical professionals I encountered made me feel 'safe', regardless.

Hence, I began adopting a positive outlook and gave up on investigating my problems on the Internet, which I had been recently using solely for reading articles on websites dedicated to health conditions. Sadly, positive thinking was not strong enough to tame the inexplicable symptoms that were wreaking havoc in my life.

Although it was very difficult for me to keep on studying and helping my parents with the business, I kept on putting the appointment with the psychotherapist off. I hoped that my worries would go away on their own over time. Unfortunately, the more I was putting it off, the more often they tormented me. Going to the movies with Anna, which we both were very fond of, had to wait, since we often had to leave the auditorium halfway through the movie because of me or, on some occasions, as soon as the screening started. Anxiety seizures were ruthless. Over time, they became more frequent, coming at me when I least expected it. Though I was trying to stop it every time, it was tilting at windmills. Bit by bit, I was losing my will to live. I didn't feel like getting into the car and visiting my girlfriend. Our family and social life suffered because of that immensely, too. Although Anna didn't have to give up on family gatherings or hang outs with her friends, she did in order to spend as much time as she could with me. Sadly, I was incapable of giving her anything else than myself, locked behind closed doors. Seeking escape from my worries, I found a refuge at my home, where, after my first anxiety seizure, I didn't experience another one. I'd leave home only when necessary. It was my defense against the unexpected anxiety seizures. In a single day, my perfect plan to just wait until my problems go away went right out the window.

As usual, to get to the university, I had to leave my comfort zone and get into my demon of speed – a small, slim Renault Clio after a facelift. It was my first car and I loved driving it. Unfortunately, on that day, my joy of driving turned into a completely new experience. Halfway to the university, as usual, without any warning, I started feeling anxiety growing within me.

Please, no! Not in the car!

I pulled over on the side of the road. I switched on the hazard lights and turned the music up to focus on something else. I wanted to use the bass coming from the speakers to calm my heart down, which was beating stronger and stronger, as if about to burst out of my chest.

I rolled the windows down. In the moment when I felt cold drizzle drops on my face, blown inside the car with the wind, I cooled down. On that day, I realized that the joke was over and that regardless of anything, I had to talk to a psychotherapist.

For most students, the end of the academic year was the beginning of a three-month-long summer break – after successfully passed finals, that is. As for me, for obvious reasons, I wasn't fantasizing about my dream seaside vacation. Aside from the finals that had to be passed, I also had to face my weaknesses.

June is a time when the concentration of allergenic pollen that wouldn't leave me be was always the highest. In that period, a package of tissues was my best friend. On many occasions, the June grass pollen floating in the air would make me cry a whole glass of tears as if it was a big, well-sliced onion. Swollen nostrils, slightly reddened due to tampons inserted there, were giving my problem away to every person I encountered. The allergy itself could drive me into a state reminiscent of drunkenness, and when combined with the derealization that I started experiencing, it made me feel as if I was exploring the surface of the Moon like Neil Armstrong. To alleviate my suffering, I'd usually go see Dr. Armani to get a prescription for some anti-allergic medication. On that day, I had to pay him a visit, too.

As usual, my PCP prescribed me the medication I needed without any issues. Sometime earlier, I noticed that writing prescriptions was the simplest, the least demanding, and the least stressful task a patient can ask his PCP of. At one point, I was positively shocked when Dr. Armani asked me if I had made any progress toward finding the origin of my ailments.

"How are we feeling today?" he asked without referring to me specifically.

"Same old, same old. I'm still looking," I replied while fighting with an urge to cry out, *You are the one who's job is to identify my disease! What are they paying you for?*

Refraining from a pointless discussion, I informed Armani about my recent appointment with the cardiologist, my latest acquisition – irregular excessive sweating, and my anxiety that began surfacing while I was driving. I also shared with him my decision to see a psychotherapist he suggested I should meet with.

Armani advised me to get an appointment with a specialist who was meeting with his patients at that very clinic once a week. I already had the psychiatrist's phone number that my uncle's friend had given me, but it made me glad, regardless.

Great! I thought.

Since a visit at the clinic meant there was no need to go a long distance to see an expert, and thus there was no risk of getting any anxiety attack while driving, I gladly accepted the offer. I left the office and walked to the front desk, where I booked an appointment with the man who could help me, hypothetically.

Obviously, I also had to wait some time for that appointment, too. Luckily, that didn't take forever.

However, before my meeting with the psychiatrist took place, I took a hard look at my life. I was thinking for a very long time what would I talk with the psychotherapist specifically about. My life up until that point was too perfect for considering anything in it the cause of my ailments or at least the grounds for any mental issues. That was what I thought.

My childhood was nothing but perfect. A loving, supportive family. Lots of friends. I lacked nothing. I did lose my guinea pig when I was eleven. Her name was Cupcake and when she died after nine years, which is very long for these animals, I mourned her along with other family members. No, no, no! That's not the right track, I thought.

I'd consider growing up, my teenage years, and undergraduate studies excellent, too. I never had any painful failures, I never lost any of my loved ones, and I never experienced any trauma. Well, aside from a few days, due to the cat that got run over.

What the hell am I supposed to talk to him about? Oh yeah, I almost forgot – my complex. But does it even make any sense to raise a subject that isn't bothering me at all now, which seemed to be the cause of my problems according to my sweetheart and my mom? I kept asking myself.

Eventually, there came a day when for the first time, I was about to stand face to face with the man specializing in deep-seated issues invisible to the eye of every medical doctor.

Since time was ticking away and choosing a noncommercial appointment would mean I'd have to wait weeks on end, I availed myself of the option that was most convenient for me; I made a paid appointment with a psychotherapist at my clinic. On my way to see him, I continued to wonder how the visit would go. Eventually, I reached my destination.

Concerned, I was looking at my watch every five minutes, tapping my foot. Unfortunately, the analyst of the depths of the human mind didn't turn up on time. Accustomed to living in accordance with college rules, I thought for a second that under these circumstances, I could leave the clinic without any dire consequences; this would be putting the 'academic quarter' rule to use, which prohibits a lecturer who arrives fifteen minutes late (or more) to class from disciplining a student who decided to blow his lecture off. Sadly, I found myself in a different situation and concluded that I was the one who cared more about making this appointment happen than the man whose job was to help me. So I waited. Twenty minutes later, I heard steps. A silhouette of a middle-aged man dressed in a green coat emerged from around the corner.

"Are you here to see me?" he sked me.

"I am," I replied.

Opening the door and pulling up a sleeve, he looked at his watch and quickly realized that he was late.

"We both got here just in time," he said.

"How come?" I asked.

"It's exactly twenty-five past two," he explained.

I looked at his face in an attempt to decipher whether he was using irony to add some comedy in an attempt to mitigate the bitter aftertaste of his late arrival. There wasn't any trace, not even a slightly raised corner of his mouth; the expression on his face was that of deadly seriousness. I didn't comment on that. He didn't make a good first impression on me. And that was how the personality analysis began; but not that of MY personality. From the first moment when we met in front of the office, I knew that man wouldn't help me. He continued showing me how well aware of his lateness he in fact was by not taking his coat off and keeping his red leather messenger bag hanging off his shoulder; he took his place behind a desk, asking me to take a seat. I sat on a chair that looked like one from a class at school, whereas the desk we were sitting at vis-à-vis, surely served previously at a school. That was my impression. Accustomed to the look of a psychiatrist's office from American movies, I found it a bit disappointing. On my way there, I imagined myself lying on a couch in a very comfortable position, talking; the psychotherapist was sitting at some distance away from me in an armchair that was rocking gently back and forth; he was in the American figure four position[3], displaying a relaxed, self-confident attitude. With walls stacked with

---

[3] The American figure four sitting position – with one ankle over another knee.

colorful psychiatry books, the room was supposed to be dimly lit with an intent to soothe the patient and help him unwind.

Yet again, reality turned out to be brutal.

The situation I got myself into was more reminiscent of a high school student inquired about his home assignment by a tutor; the turquoise interior and the strong, cold light cast from above onto the desk fired my imagination.

At one point, I felt as if I was being interrogated by a police officer; not only because the ambiance of the room was feeding these pictures to my mind, but also because of the way in which the psychiatrist started conversing with me.

"What happened to you? How did that happen? Are you sure you didn't take anything?" he kept on bombarding me with questions, peeking hastily at his watch every minute, and jotting down some notes with a pencil.

Having been interrogated, after describing for nearly thirty minutes everything that had taken place up until then, I learned that it would be helpful to take some medications. Since our session was coming to an end, the expert concluded that we could agree on the further course of action during the next one. Realizing that we were both in the wrong place and at the wrong time, I thanked him for the appointment and told him I'd book the next session at the front desk. I was bluffing, obviously. I knew that that man had nothing he could give me, and I didn't want to give him a second chance. I'd always navigate life guided by my intuition. If I didn't like something at first impression, very often I just wouldn't continue. I felt that wasn't the place where I'd get help.

Hence, my first psychotherapeutic session ended in a bitter aftertaste lasting for a while. I had no other option; I knew I had to go to someone else. While doing some online research yet again, I stumbled upon a very crucial piece of information. A very wise man wrote that if there was no 'chemistry' between a patient and a psychotherapist, the psychotherapy or general treatment would probably fail. At that moment, I realized that I had done the right thing by discontinuing sessions with the expert at my clinic. I recalled that I had received a phone number to the cardiologist's colleague during my appointment. Recalling his accolades for that lady, I didn't seek other options. I decided to use her phone number, call her and book an appointment. As usual, I had to wait some time until the day when the psychiatrist could see me finally arrived.

She was seeing her patients in an apartment situated in an old tenement house in the downtown area. The place she lived in and the office where she admitted me was more like the pictures created by my fertile imagination. From the moment I walked in, I found the tidy and beautifully arranged apartment very pleasing. The office where I was then invited to had an air that was reminiscent more of a psychotherapist's workplace than an interrogation room at a police station.

What caught my attention instantaneously was numerous wooden statues of African deities that the office was filled with. Though some could feel overwhelmed by the way this interior was decorated, it was much to my liking. There was some scent of incense in the air coming from behind me, stimulating my sense of smell quite intensely. Another thing that was inconsistent with how I imagined the office would look like was an elegant wooden desk we sat at, facing each other. The ambiance aside, which was slightly different than my idealistic expectation, the therapist made a quite good first impression on me. At the very beginning of our meeting, we already found some shared interest. It turned out that she had been practicing aerobics and cycling for some time to stay fit. Despite being middle-aged, she found it very satisfying; she clearly knew how to strike a discussion with me. Perhaps it was just a psychological maneuver on her part, intended to build a good foundation for our future conversations. If that was really the case, it surely did work. I felt more at ease and ready to tackle anything she could surprise me with. Although the first appointment was solely a 'meet and greet' where we talked for an entire hour without even mentioning the issue that brought me to her office, I had to pay for her time she gave me, regardless. I wasn't very content about that, since I might have as well taken Anna for dinner to discuss the problems of the contemporary world or find another topic for consideration. Either way, I was doing my best to comprehend, telling myself this is most likely what a relationship with a good psychotherapist starts like. In spite of it all, I booked another appointment.

The week of my life that followed brought absolutely no progress. The day of the second appointment arrived. The African deities had an even more positive effect on my psyche. Sadly, the airborne scent in the chamber of secrets was starting to get on my nerves a little. This time, the psychiatrist decided to listen closely to my monologue about my problems. The sweat that I was describing, which had been manifesting for no reason in my interactions with others, was evident. Looking deep into the expert's eyes when talking about the anxiety seizures that had been tormenting me for the previous several months, I felt that I wasn't sharing my story in vain, and that she would help me. Having listened to almost everything I had to say, the psychiatrist told me something that didn't make me smile.

"I think you're suffering from anxiety disorder."

I wasn't surprised. This time, however, I prepared myself for the appointment. For some time, since everyone diagnosed me with mental disorders, I had been exploring the subject. I managed to find some information about symptoms typical of the so-called depersonalization-derealization disorder, which I mentioned about during our conversation. A man struggling with this condition feels as if he was living in an unreal world. The feeling of derealization that he experiences can be caused by the brain trying to protect itself from stress overload. This condition is often a symptom of schizophrenia, which very often develops in young people, but it can also affect individuals of good mental health in periods of overtiredness, such as tackling major life challenges, for instance. Everything I was experiencing and everything that was reflected in my life were fitting that illness perfectly. Considering my previous training and the objectives they involved, I was willing to accept this situation.

"There's one more thing, doctor. I feel trapped. It's as if I'm wearing a spacesuit and when I go under shower and close the glass door of the shower cabin behind me, I am breathless and feel even more trapped inside my body. When I look at my hands, I get that feeling that they're not mine. The longer I look the more anxious I get. I'm scared and I don't know what's happening to me," I said, locking eyes with the psychiatrist.

For a couple of seconds, the room went silent. I had an impression that the psychiatrist zoned out for a moment. Waiting for her to say something specific that would guide me out of my agony, I noticed her face changing like in slow motion to show utter astonishment. At that moment, her facial expression was telling me one thing: What are you talking about?

Then, I heard a question that every semi-intelligent person would take for a reason to worry even more, and, at the same time, to change the doctor again.

"A shower cabin? What makes you scared in a shower cabin?" she asked me.

Due to my lack of self-confidence, which had been taking control over my life day by day, I found myself unable to tell her what I was thinking. Yet again, I felt I wasn't in the right place where I could get help. I knew, however, that I had to keep that relationship going and that if I really had some mental issues, no one else would help me. The psychiatrist assured me that I didn't look schizophrenic and that my symptoms were not evidence of anxiety disorder, and it was definitely not overtiredness. She explained to me roughly where anxiety disorder comes from and defined all my ailments as somatic (physical) and psychosomatic. She also gave me a diagnosis – stress.

"A stressful lifestyle affects almost everyone these days. A constant rush or a difficult, demanding work cause much stress that then bit by bit destroys lives of many people around the globe. Often these people are very young, like you are. Stress can cause many symptoms similar to the those of various diseases known in contemporary medicine. From duodenal ulcers to the symptoms that you're experiencing. The amount of stress you've accumulated unconsciously, and that you're even unaware of, has given rise to anxiety that caused somatic symptoms that alone trigger more fear within you. We term this issue anxiety disorder," she summed up.

I wasn't pleased with the diagnosis I got, as put simply, deep inside, I felt that my symptoms were not caused by stress. Although I did have some bad moments in my life, I had always been an optimistic young man with much humor and an aloof attitude towards everything. I'd often turn things into a joke and, not concerned by anything, I'd put off many tasks for later. Though I was born in the 1980s, when permissive parenting wasn't as popular as it is today, I was lucky enough to get raised in that fashion, too. The psychiatrist had her vision about and assessment of my situation; still, I didn't believe in her diagnosis of anxiety disorder.

In an attempt to console me, she suggested antidepressants that would help me build the foundation for psychotherapy. She claimed that in order to launch an in-depth analysis of my personality, I'd first have to tame the symptoms that were tormenting me. I thought that it was the psychotherapist's job to do that instead of stuffing me with mood-improving pills. I did listen to her, though, and consented to this form of treatment. Although many people associate pills prescribed by a psychiatrist only with a mental asylum, my take on this matter was completely different. Having watched many documentaries on, for instance, Discovery Channel, I knew that many Americans were taking the 'happy pill'. I was aware of how many people were on Prozac[4], the drug used for overcoming depressive disorders highly popular in the media owing to its mood-lifting properties. Most of these people didn't even see a psychiatrist once. I was given a medicine called Seronil[5], which is the same chemical compound that the Americans take under the brand Prozac. As most antidepressants, this drug was supposed to boost serotonin levels when taken daily. Serotonin is a neurotransmitter produced by the body that regulates mood. Since the body's reaction to drugs of this sort can

---

[4] Prozac (fluoxetine) – an organic chemical compound used as an antidepressant.

[5] Seronil (fluoxetine) - a drug with antidepressant properties from the group of selective serotonin reuptake inhibitors.

vary, I was administered a very small dose for starters. At the same time, I was also prescribed a pill called Afobam[6], which I was supposed to take only in the event of a severe anxiety seizure that would spiral out of my control.

For the next few weeks, I was meeting my psychiatrist for a follow-up visit to see how the selected drugs were affecting me. She informed me that antidepressants start working after two weeks, whereas their full capacity shows after two months. And it did, indeed.

Over time, I started noticing my condition improved dramatically. Anxiety seizures wouldn't afflict me as frequently as they did before. I continued to attend lectures; still, there were times when I had to quickly leave the lecture hall as my heartbeat was gradually rising. However, I didn't have to skip all classes on a given day; I'd just rush into a restroom with my pills instead. Having washed an anxiety pill down with tap water, and splashing some cold water on my face, I'd look into a mirror and tell myself, "Easy there, you can do it!"

Perhaps it was just a placebo, or maybe the drug really started working in a blink of an eye; for some reason, I felt that I'd make it this time and that it would be easier on me. I knew, though, that the medication I got had an addictive effect and that I shouldn't overdose. For this reason, I left it all in the hands of time and waited until Seronil started doing its job at full capacity. Having treated myself with that antidepressant for over a month, I noticed that my anxiety seizures largely subsided. Sadly, other things didn't. My feeling of derealization wouldn't leave me be; I still had the persistent feeling of my entire body being trapped inside a spacesuit, whereas looking at my hands continued to generate the same level of distress.

"Happy pills?" I asked myself.

Despite it all, the significant improvement and my belief that the medication worked made me want to live again. I was glad

---

[6] Afobam (alprazolam) - a tranquilizer from the group of benzodiazepines [sold under the brand name Xanax in the U.S. – Translator's note].

that at least one of those inexplicable symptoms started disappearing and that I could go back to being social again. I did my best to make up for all the time I had wasted on fearing yet another surge of anxiety. Although I could still feel some of it simmering beneath, I was able to go with Anna to the movies or with my family shopping again. I didn't forget about my buddies, either. We could hang out more regularly again, and Tomek, who quite often accompanied me whenever he was back in the country, couldn't hold back his laughter whenever I was checking my t-shirt under armpits for stains. He'd roll on the floor, especially when I did that in a public place. Surely it must have looked hilarious and many could think, *What a freak!*

Only I knew that there was still something wrong going on with me. Though the psychiatrist was trying to tell me that with time, everything would go back to normal, something would keep on bothering me. I also felt that our sessions were heading in the wrong direction. As time went by, we were seeing each other less and less often, while every subsequent visit at the expert's office consisted solely in checking my current state and writing a prescription for more meds.

"How are you feeling today?" she asked me.

Leaving out my symptoms, which I didn't manage to fix with the 'happy pills', I replied, "Fine."

Upon receiving a prescription for several weeks to come, my visit at the psychotherapist's office was usually over. For some reason she didn't begin a psychotherapy with me, though whenever I touched upon that subject, she'd claim, "You're not ready yet, but if you want to, we can kick it off!"

Yet again, my intuition was telling me something was off. I realized that there must be a reason why the psychotherapist didn't want to subject me to psychotherapy. "Maybe she's already concluded based on my stories that I don't need it at all," I thought.

After my last visit, which took less than twenty minutes and culminated in a prescription, I had to pay over one hundred *zlotys*, as for all the previous visits. I arrived at the conclusion that in all actuality, the psychotherapist was running a quite successive business. As she informed me earlier, pharmacotherapy could take from six months up to two years. Upon careful consideration I did the math and figured that I could continue this line of treatment by myself, as Americans do, supervised by my PCP, Dr. Armani, and if anything went south, I could always go back to see her. I shared with her my idea of taking Seronil on a regular basis without her oversight, which she wasn't that fond of. She told me that it wasn't the best plan, since a patient on antidepressants should be supervised by a psychiatrist, and not a PCP.

Maybe she was right but, despite it all, I decided to take the risk and become responsible for myself and my actions further down the line. We parted ways without any attempts by the psychiatrist to make me to change my mind.

The 2011 academic year was very important to me, as it was the end of the sixteen years of my education. The only thing left to do was to pass the final examination in defense of my master's thesis. Although I didn't feel happy because of the antidepressants, I knew that they'd allow me to graduate safely and without any sudden seizure. Nonetheless, before I managed to make it until the end of the year, I had to face adversities that some force kept on putting in my way. For most people, the spring snowmelt signifies the end of winter and the start of new life in the world of flora and fauna. Very often, motorists associate this period with the upcoming time of changing from winter to summer tires. That day, which I wanted to spend hanging out with Anna, as usual, turned into a valuable experience. I got into my car to visit her. The road I'd always take to get to Anna's was very picturesque. Though I could have taken a different one, which was a couple of miles shorter, running across the city, I always preferred a longer one that cut through fields and woodlands. In spite of my allergy, which wouldn't leave me be when most plants were coming back to life, I loved driving to my Anna's. I've always been very fond of nature and wildlife. Offering views of undeveloped lands, particularly woodlands, the route connecting our homes would always make it easier for me to unwind. I knew that road like the back of my own hand. From the time when I got my first car, not a single day passed by without me driving to Anna's. With due consideration of the speed limit that applied on most of the route, occasional roadside checks by the police, and wild animals frequently strolling from the fields to the woods and back, I'd always cover the distance most carefully.

This time was no different. While driving at the maximum speed allowed on the pothole-ridden asphalt road, not only did I try to take the utmost care not to fall into a deep hole that formed with the passing of winter and the snowmelt, but I also maintained focus on what was happening to the side of the road and around me. It might seem that antidepressants make a man stupefied and, hence, he shouldn't necessarily be driving. In my case, the pills worked wonders without compromising my perception in any way.

Very often, I'd 'enjoy' the 'pleasure' of braking firmly before a family of wild boars running out of the woods unexpectedly or a roe deer dashing in search of food, oblivious to traffic. On that day, as a result of my still poor experience as a driver, my car simply failed me. Shimmering in the golden rays of sunlight, the asphalt road was forewarning me, but I failed to react, regardless. The sun was trying to send me some signals, too, scattering millions of shiny diamonds across the paved surface; still, I didn't slow down. Driving forward with a smile on my face, thinking about what Anna and I would be doing on that day, I came very close to the side of the road; the asphalt, previously illuminated with the light shining through the trees, suddenly made way for complete darkness. It was like entering a pitch-black tunnel formed by vast amounts of branches, hanging heavy with their winter burden of unmelt snowcaps, not letting even the smallest ray of sunlight through. Although the previous part of the road had been warning me on every mile, I failed to recognize that. Out of the blue, the car started acting funny, rendering the steering wheel in my hands useless. I was turning the wheel right and the vehicle would go left. Sitting in the uncontrollable car that was speeding like a sled on ice, I realized I was about to end up in the woods in no time.

"Oh, fuck!" I yelled.

Within literally just a few seconds that I had for taking any action, I pulled the emergency brake and tapped the brakes trying to save myself. Neither was helping. In a blink of an eye, I found myself on the opposite lane, heading towards some trees. With my hands clenched on the wheel, I closed my eyes in the final moment. BAM! I hit them.

When it was all over, I opened my eyes slowly and I saw in front of me snow-clad pine branches that luckily didn't pierce my windshield through. Judging from the slightly tilted position of the car and the feeling of sitting inside of it somewhat higher than usual, I concluded that I ended up in a small ditch. I knew that this wasn't good. Aware of the fact that having no control over the vehicle, I could have hit someone on the way, I started scanning the scene around me, although I knew all too well that there were no pedestrians on that road at that time. The amount of snow still covering that shadowy spot somehow cushioned the impact so that I didn't sustain any injuries. Still overwhelmed with stress, my heart rate elevated, I looked around the 'cockpit'; my gaze was caught by a keychain depicting Saint Christopher, the patron saint of motorists. I kept it in the car only because my mom asked me to; she gave it to me. With little thought, feeling immense anger at the situation that unraveled, cussing left, right and center, emphasizing my state of mind at that moment, I cast another glance at Saint Christopher.

"Thanks, Chris," I said ironically, not particularly believing in such things.

I realized that probably, I won't get out of that shallow ditch unaided. Still, I managed to start the car; I put it in reverse and tried to get it out. In vain. The car wouldn't move. I got out to assess the situation from the outside. The hood and the bumper scraped off beyond repair.

"Damn it!" I cried out.

The first thing that came to my mind was to call dad. I called him to get some help. As I wasn't that far from home, my dad decided to come and assess the situation. I was waiting for him standing on the side of the road. Every now and then cars would go past at high speed. I put aside the fact that none of them stopped to even ask me if I was okay. What concerned me much more was how was it possible that no one else skidded. Obviously, I didn't wish that on anyone, but I had no clue how could that be.

Waiting for my father, I noticed an elderly man emerging from the nearest property by the road, heading my way.

He approach me asking if I was okay and if there was any way he could help.

"Thank you, sir, I'm fine. I'm afraid we wouldn't be able to get my car out in just the two of us," I replied.

After a while, some car pulled over next to us. The elderly man's neighbor was sitting inside. He rolled the window down and asked me:

"What happened? I'll get you out!" he added swiftly, giving me no time to reply.

Again, startled, I was glad that the locals proved to be so kind. *There are still some good people in this world,* I thought.

"Wait here! I'll be back with an excavator," he added and drove off to get the big equipment.

An excavator? Not bad, I thought.

I was standing with the elderly man by my car, waiting for the excavator to arrive. Cars were still passing us by, their drivers completely ignoring the two of us, stranded in the woods next to a ditch-stuck car.

"Thank you for showing some interest in my minor accident."

"My pleasure, young man. You know, two years ago, I was in a similar situation. Two young people slammed into that giant tree over there, close to my fence," he said pointing with his finger to an old, colossal aspen tree.

"What happened?" I asked.

"I came to their aid, just like I came to yours today."

"They must've been surprised just as I was, right?"

"No. It was ME who was surprised. When I came close to one of those young men, the other sneaked up on me from behind and in one quick move, he sucker-punched me with a metal pipe several times, breaking several of my ribs, and shouted, 'No stress, old man!' Then they got into the car, started the engine and drove off."

Shocked by the story, I asked why did he lend a helping hand to me on that day.

"Aren't you afraid the same thing will happen again?"

"No, I'm too old to be afraid and besides, every Catholic should do precisely what I did and help another person regardless of consequences, even if it means you step in the same river twice."

After a while, the man's neighbor appeared with a big yellow excavator. We tied a rope to my car.

"Get behind the wheel, young boy! We'll get you out!" he shouted.

It didn't take long. In just one moment, the immense power of the engine hoisted my vehicle back again onto the paved road.

"Thank you so much, sir. How much do I owe you for your help?" I asked, taught to act with courtesy. I believed though that the man was just as altruistic as his elderly neighbor was, and that he'd probably refuse any monetary compensation.

"I'll take only as much as you're carrying around in your wallet," he said while getting off the excavator.

I smiled to share his dark sense of humor, expecting him to smile back. Then I realized that he wasn't kidding. I glanced into my wallet.

"I'm afraid fifty *zlotys* is all I have," I replied.

"That will do. Give me what's in there!" a grimace appeared on his face.

Having taken the money, he got into the excavator and drove off. I cast a look at the elderly gentleman. Without commenting on the situation, locking eyes with him, I had a feeling we were thinking the same thought.

Shortly afterwards, my dad arrived. He assessed whether my car was in a good enough condition to continue the trip. Though the bumper and the hood were damaged and required replacement, the vehicle proved fully operational. That small incident and the damage sustained by my ride didn't discourage me from continuing my trip. Although my dad recommended that I go home, I decided to go to Anna's. Driving across the woodlands, as usual, I was passing by a Franciscan sanctuary. I had never visited that place and on that day, I concluded it was the right time to stop by the church and express gratitude for going out of the accident unscathed and without harming anyone on the road. Maybe it was my internal need or the elderly man's words that made me think in a bit different way. All in all, I stopped by the monastery and, without stepping out of the car, I took Saint Christopher again in my hand and said, "Thank you."

I started the engine and went straight ahead. That day taught me a lot, but even a crashed car was not good enough reason to make me change my plans. Just as fast as I crashed it, I forgot about it all; nothing could stop me from heading forward to meet with Anna. We had been together for only three years but to me, every moment we could spend together was still like the first time we went out.

"Man, you're so unreasonable, my boy!" I could see these words in my dad's eyes once he heard I was going to stick to my plan; he shrug his shoulders and shook his head disapprovingly.

He'd always tell me, "Do today what you're supposed to do tomorrow." I knew that I should've listened to him and turned back to have the car checked at a repair shop but I was convinced that I could put that off until later. Putting everything off was nothing new to me. Part-time studies meant lots of free time for me. Although I should've used it reasonably for the good and growth of our family business, I knew that I'd still have the time to contribute to my parent's endeavor further down the line by bringing in something new at a later date. I spent most of the time building a relationship with my girlfriend and honing my physique at the gym.

Nonetheless, there came a time that made us all put our tedious tasks aside for some time and focus our all attention elsewhere. My gran, who most of her life had lived in Germany, returned to her homeland in her old years and moved in with us. She was eighty-six, and living alone at that age is highly risky.

Although for many years, we all had been asking her to stay with us, she never wanted to. It was very important to me, since she was the only grandma I had. My other one died when I was a little boy, and I didn't even have the chance of meeting my two grandpas, as they passed away before I was born.

"Sweetie, when I'm old and infirm, then I'll move in," she'd always reply in the same fashion.

We weren't surprised. Despite her age, my gran was invincible. At eighty-something, she would hop on a stool like an eighteen-year-old girl to clean all windows vigorously. Accustomed to her lifestyle so far, she couldn't imagine moving out. Like the saying goes, "old habits die hard." Sadly, in life, even the most resilient person has her end. Since for some time, my grandma had been complaining about pain in the hip, she underwent an endoprosthesis surgery abroad. Then, there came a time when she started feeling old, and we could finally receive her at our home and offer her a room we had prepared specifically for her. Unfortunately, we couldn't enjoy her presence for long, as for some reason, instead of becoming less and less swollen after the surgery, her leg got even thicker, causing her awful pain. Despite wrestling with my numerous health issues, my parents began running from one doctor to another seeking help for my gran in our home country. Finally, they stumbled upon a doctor working at the hospital of the Ministry of Interior and Administration, who was highly empathetic towards them and my gran, and who decided to help her; he started from ordering MRI scans. Sadly for us, the testing results got misplaced, and the person responsible for producing the images was away for vacation. From one day to the next, gran's health deteriorated significantly. Seeing how deeply in pain she was and how big her leg had swollen, my parents couldn't wait any longer. Gran was transferred to the Military Medical Academy Memorial Teaching Hospital.

There, she was swiftly provided with intravenous analgesia, which was clearly not strong enough to soothe the pain. Seeing how immense was the suffering she had to endure, my parents pleaded with the hospital administration that she be operated on on a fast-track basis. We were waiting for her leg surgery scheduled for a couple of days later for some reason, which was incomprehensible to us amidst all that tragedy. We wouldn't leave gran alone for too long. Both her relatives and friends were visiting her while she was dying in agony.

One day, I came with my mom to see how she was doing. As usual, mom would go consult the situation with the attending physician, while I'd stay with grandma. I sat by her bed. She was conscious but in all her suffering, with the lots of analgesics she was on that were rendering her stupefied, she was not very aware of her surroundings. I took her by the hand, but she barely reacted to my touch.

"Why are you doing it to her? She's been standing by you all her life!" I asked God.

Ever since I can remember, my gran's utmost priority was praying the rosary. There wasn't a day that she wouldn't talk to God. In church, she'd always sit in the first row and cry huge tears, as if she was a little girl weeping after falling down and bruising her knee.

"Grandma, why do you always cry when praying to God?" I asked once, back when I was a small boy.

"That's just the thing I do, sweetie. He suffered so much for all of us," she replied.

Back then, when asking my gran that question, I didn't understand her reply. Seeing her suffer on the hospital bed I was highly resentful towards God.

"Where are you now when she needs you the most!?" I asked angrily, my eyes watering up.

At the same moment when I was lost in grief, crying with my head supported on her bed, a female doctor came in with a group of over ten medical students. The doctor stopped next to me, while the group of young learners dressed in white hospital garments filled my gran's room like a football team rowing up to sing the anthem.

"How are you feeling today?" the doctor asked my grandma, taking her bedside card off.

Hearing no reply and seeing that the suffering woman didn't react, the doctor asked her the same question again. It was so ridiculous to me; her repeated question was echoing in my ears. I answered it for the patient, tears in my eyes:

"My grandma's not well, as you can see with a bare eye!"

After a moment, the doctor put the card back where it belonged and with one swift move, she took away the duvet, revealing to me and everyone else gathered in the room the naked body of my relative. I was stunned. The feeling that flooded me in that moment was unspeakable. The immense pain due to seeing my only grandma probably for the last time, my internal argument with the Lord, the disrespect that my relative was shown on her deathbed, and, thus, the disrespect I myself was shown - it all generated lots of negative emotions inside of me. Having uncovered the patient, the woman leading the group of students told them to watch my gran's naked body closely and take notes. I snapped.

"You must be kidding me! Do you have to do this now, in my presence? That's just sick! It's my grandma!" I shouted, covering her undressed body up.

I had a feeling that after some thought, the doctor realized she had indeed done something inappropriate, and that it could have waited.

"Come. We're leaving," that was all she managed to say to the students before departing.

To me, it seemed perfectly logical that the entire situation was immoral and unethical. I could hear one of the students currying favor with his superior and female colleagues by saying under his breath, "What a loser!"

I cracked. I felt overwhelming rage and a desire to hurt him. I left the room and rushed to catch up with that student. I grabbed him by his arm and turned him towards me. At that very moment, the entire group including the female doctor turned towards me, too.

I looked the boy in the eye aggressively and told him I'd be waiting for him in front of the hospital.

I saw he stopped feeling like laughing anymore, all of a sudden. In that moment everyone, especially ladies, started calling me an audacious thug. They turned their backs to me and walked away, following their leader.

I was standing there in the middle of the hall with other patients strolling in their robes, watching the group of students disappearing in the distance. Having given more thought to that entire situation, I came to the conclusion that the way I acted was overly aggressive.

That's not me! What's happening to me? I wondered.

Finally, there came a day when grandma had her hip reoperated. The medical staff informed us that if the endoprosthesis was removed, gran would be wheelchair bound for the rest of her life. This was not a problem for my parents and they gave their consent.

"A wheelchair is no big deal! We just want her to live," they told the doctors.

Sadly, after the second hip surgery it turned out that the reason for the calcification of gran's pelvis and hip was a type of cancer that remains untreatable to this day – multiple myeloma. My parents were shocked at this news. They realized that the experts who performed the first surgery in Germany probably mistaken this cancer for some other disease, and that was why they undertook the procedure in the first place; or, perhaps, they knew it all along, but didn't even mention the true reason behind grandma's issues. To this day, they're tormented by the thought, "what if?" One thing is certain: had we all known about the cancer, we wouldn't have let our beloved grandma go through all that suffering. Shortly after the re-operation, she passed away.

Time went by and Dr. Armani had nothing against prescribing me more supply of Seronil. Although when appearing at his office to collect the prescription for the meds I'd often touch on the subject of my feeling of derealization and frequent sweating that occurred even during these appointments (which had not happened previously), he had no idea how to help me. Despite my description of the relations I had with most recent psychiatry experts, he believed I should continue this line of treatment. I felt quite resentful towards him, as despite the recurrent visits, he didn't even try to link my symptoms to any other cause. It could look as if I was looking for some other diseases in myself, which I didn't want, naturally. At one point, I started believing that was just how it was supposed to be.

Why do you keep nit-picking, you moron!? Armani is surely right. He's a doctor, after all! They all were right! If they weren't, they wouldn't have diagnosed me with anxiety disorder, would they? I kept asking myself, and my loved ones, too, in an attempt to deceive my intuition and reason.

I tried to develop a great respect for doctors and accept their opinion. I thought that they must be right and that my issues surely would simply disappear over time. Unfortunately, time showed it to be otherwise.

Thanks to antidepressants, I managed to reach the finish line and successfully pass the final exams in defense of my master's thesis. Although I didn't graduate from college with honors, I was proud of myself for bravely persisting to the very end, for obtaining the master's degree, and for completing my education despite the adversities I was wrestling with. After taking Seronil for a year, I arrived at the conclusion that I didn't need it any more. My anxiety seizures disappeared completely, and that drug didn't fix my other comorbid issues in any way. On the contrary; I had a feeling that it was somewhat restricting my ability to express my true emotions. At my grandma's funeral I was suffering but I could feel that my tears were somewhat forced, which was terrifying. I recalled the psychiatrist's words that when going off the antidepressants, I'd have to do that progressively, like when first taking the pill, to make my body accustomed to a small dose. I asked Armani for a package of Seronil for the last time and got off the med gradually by cutting the dosage from an entire pill down to a quarter and then to the final tablet that was intended to end my entire 'happy pill' experience.

Over time, I accepted the theory and the diagnosis that experts issued during all my appointments; I gave up on reading the online content for days on end, and decided to take up my normal lifestyle again. Enjoying every moment free from studying, hanging out with my girlfriend or my buddies, I wasn't aware that the worst was about to come.

I entered the new stage of my life with recurrent bronchitis. At least that was the diagnosis I'd receive every single time not only from Armani, but also from his colleagues who'd occasionally see me at the same outpatient clinic. After a month or two, I'd contract another viral infection of the upper respiratory tract for some unknown reason. Lying in bed every two months with a fever, a massive cough, and muscle pains, I could only wonder how much time it would take me to rebuild strength and get back into shape at the gym. I couldn't even be bothered by the huge amount of work in the family business that my parents had to take up on themselves in my absence.

"Sick, again? That's no news!" my buddies would mock me.

And rightly so. All too often I was coming down with something, whereas their seasonal ailments would always end on day four of a runny nose, not preventing them in any way from fulfilling most of their everyday duties.

My common cold would often turn into a horrible sore throat and an entire kaleidoscope of other illnesses that rendered me not fit for performing daily tasks, leaving me no other option but to lie in bed. It could seem that from my teenage years, I had been catching cold quite often, probably more often than my buddies, but it was never that often and not that strong. Where I come from, there's a very popular saying that goes, "A runny nose lasts seven days when medicated, and a week if not medicated." I could consider this to be true, since indeed, in my previous years, that was my experience. Now, however, "seven days" was always just a warmup before a nearly three-week-long inflammation that I'd get more and more often. My PCP and his colleagues must have been happy to have work to do and patients to attend to, but my presence in the office would never put a smile on their faces.

"Why do I get inflammation so often?" I asked.

"You need to take care of your immunity," they replied.

"Fine, but how do I do that?"

"You need to eat healthy and eliminate stress from your life," they concluded.

Having received such a reply from the PCPs, I didn't know what to make of it.

All that stress talk again? They're mad! How am I supposed to get rid of all the stress when I'm suffering from something all the time? I pondered.

On this pessimistic note, I entered the year two thousand twelve. For many people, particularly enthusiasts of conspiracy theories, it was supposed to be the time when our planet would finally stop spinning. According to some who explored the culture and customs of the ancient Mayan civilization, 2012 was supposed to be the year when with the end of that Indian tribe's calendar, The earth was said to experience a geomagnetic reversal that would mark the end of our life as we know it. Though many investigators of end-of-the-world theories made a mistake also on that occasion and the human race was not annihilated, the 'geomagnetic reversal' did affect me regardless, and my apocalypse was truly near.

Waiting for my body to regenerate and for my health concerns to leave completely, I was still dedicating most of my time to shaping my physique. All types of exercising have always been the greatest source of endorphins that simply made me happy. However, day by day, I could feel something changing inside of me. Quite rapidly, I cut the five training sessions I had been doing for a couple of years on a weekly basis down to three. Despite the lower intensity of my workouts, I felt it was still too much.

It was only then that I admitted the diagnosis previously formulated by the cardiologist and my friends, who all stubbornly stressed I was exhausted, was valid. I realized that this could be due to recurring bronchitis that wouldn't leave me be for some reason. This fatigue worsened over time. I felt myself gradually losing my motivation to act and to do my training.

Am I slowly burning out? I asked myself.

And yet, despite it all, I didn't stop working out. It wasn't only a way for me to generate positive emotions; recently, it allowed me to forget about my problems for a moment, and take my attention off of derealization and the sensation of being trapped in my own body. At least for the ninety minutes of my training session, I could feel as if I had my own body under control, and that I was still myself, as if nothing had ever happened. To avoid thinking about my issues, I was spending as much time as possible with my sweetheart. I was deeply in love and I knew that I wanted to spend the rest of my life with Anna. Since I had been in a relationship with her for four years already, I felt that it was the time for the next step, and that I should muster the courage to propose to her sometime soon. In my head, I already had a plan that I wanted to execute at the end of the year.

Anna reciprocated my feelings and was spending her every free moment with me. She was very caring and committed to solving my problems. Standing aside, she could see me evolve and watched all my ailments developing over time.

"What's with all the flexing of your neck that you've been doing recently?" she asked me one day.

"I don't know, I guess I must've overdone it at the gym," I replied.

Indeed, as if it wasn't enough, my neck had been feeling funny for some time. I tried to 'adjust' it by turning the head right. Wherever I went and whatever I was doing, everyone would ask me, "Why are you tensing your neck so much?"

In moments like these, I didn't know what to say back.

"Something snapped there," I'd reply, trying to steer away from this topic.

From then on, I felt like Neil Armstrong attempting to fix an oxygen cord that was pinching him in the neck by jerking his helmet. The more often I moved my neck, the more irritated I got that nothing was helping.

Time flew by fast, as usual, and my new ailment stuck with me. Anna and my mom had yet another grounds for accusing me of overtraining and forcing me to stop weightlifting, which they considered from the very beginning not the best pastime I could have chosen for myself.

"You'll see you'll hurt yourself with these weights!" they'd repeat notoriously.

As usual, my intuition was telling me that there was something else, something very bad behind the recent issue; this time, however, I decided to listen to the hunch of my women and I made an appointment with Armani. I was already accustomed to the look my PCP would give me, as if wanting to cough up, "What have you come up with this time?"

With little to no difficulty, I asked for a referral for a cervical spine x-ray and for another referral for a visit with a physiotherapist. Luckily for me, I didn't have to wait long and quite soon, I managed to make an insurance-covered appointment with a female specialist who was working at my clinic. Before going there, I had an x-ray of my neck done, the interpretation of which I read aloud in Armani's presence. As it turned out, the x-ray results didn't show any changes in the structures of the neck.

The day I went to the physiotherapist gave me a completely new outlook on my entire situation. Although the lady I had an appointment with confirmed the absence of any lesions in my spine, when she was looking at the recently produced image, she gave me a new hint, suggesting a possible cause of my ailments.

"You're very tense, and anxiety and various forms of derealization can also be caused by the spine and its degenerative diseases," the physiotherapist said, massaging by back.

"How come? So why did the doctor who has his office on the first floor didn't mention that one year ago, when I started taking antidepressants?" I asked. "He knew that I was training. They all knew!"

The woman massaging me went silent but continued doing her job. After being massaged for forty minutes, I didn't feel fixed, sadly, only disgusted with the lack of knowledge among the 'experts' who had diagnosed me earlier. As it turned out, it was not possible to get all the structures of my body potentially responsible for my ailments fixed and massaged in the course of a single visit. For me, that was quite logical and natural. Therefore, I made another appointment with the masseuse.

Unfortunately for me, this time I had to wait a bit longer. The more time I was wasting on waiting for yet another appointment, the greater impression I had that something was destroying me from the inside. More and more often, I'd skip a training session.

"It's Wednesday today? Oh well, I'll train tomorrow!" as that's what my decision making was like.

I felt increasingly more tired and, at the same time, too demotivated to do anything that required any commitment from me. I started watching even more movies than before. That didn't require too much physical effort from me, only a laptop and a comfy bed. I was trying to participate in social life with Anna and our friends in spite of it all, but I wasn't getting the best results, since from one day to the next, I was feeling more and more odd and run-down. This is why I felt most comfortable spending most of my time at home. This way, I became infected with another passion: boxing. Though back in childhood, I happened to watch a few fights with legends of this beautiful game, it didn't fascinate me back then. It wasn't until 2010 that I saw the first fights of heavyweight champions the Klitschko brothers. I found myself fascinated with this discipline and from then on, I never stopped following their careers. From then on, I kept track not only of the struggles endured by masters in this weight class, but also of those fought by most boxers climbing up the ladder, waiting for that most important fight of their life. I was fighting my battle, too; I wanted to get my former wellbeing back. Unfortunately, over time, it only got worse.

One day, after training, I lay down on the bed with my laptop. All of a sudden, I felt weird tingling in the back of my head, which couldn't mean anything good was about to happen. It was as if some gas bubbles in a bottle of mineral water trying to escape upwards as the cap is being turned open. Although the entire sensation lasted only for a couple of seconds, I froze, focusing all my attention on that which came in just a moment. Agitated, I felt the tingling anomaly creeping all the way up the top of my head. I expected the finale would be no fun.

"Oh, snap!" I cried.

Never before have I experienced such an abhorrent sensation. It was as if someone was injecting a huge, long needle into my brain.

"God! What's happening to me?" I asked the Lord, though I wasn't calling to him, really.

From then on, I started fearing for my health even more than ever before.

Prior to my second appointment with the physiotherapist, not only did I experience the sensation of wearing a heavy spacesuit, but I also several sporadic 'needle injection' sensations in my head, each highly unpleasant. Three weeks later, still manipulating my neck muscles that wouldn't give me a break, I got into a car and headed for the second appointment. On my way, I wondered how to put my symptoms in words so that the female doctor wouldn't think I made up something new.

Surely she must be in contact with Armani, I thought.

For some time, when paying him a visit, I could feel he considered me a hypochondriac who keeps bothering him incessantly, if not with the common cold, then with some other imaginary problems.

"What do you make of the prickly sensations in my head?" I asked.

"I've no idea. The spine certainly gives no such symptoms, though," the masseuse replied.

I felt deeply disappointed with this opinion. Helpless, I lowered my gaze at my feet. Some part of me wanted very badly all my ailments to be caused by strained spinal muscles, which could still be fixed given my young age. At least that's what I thought. As usual, the massage didn't make my problems go away. It didn't bring me relief - not even for a second. I booked another appointment with the young masseuse scheduled in the distant future, but I wasn't sure if there was any point doing that again.

Meanwhile, someone made a certain suggestion to me. Most of the people around me had known for some time that I didn't feel well.

"Hey, how about energy therapy?"

I concluded that wasn't a bad idea.

Why not? I thought.

Back then, I didn't know yet that in my country, there was a ranking system for the best-known and most-efficient 'healers'. With little thought, wanting to get rid of my ailments as soon as possible, I went online to seek an energy therapist whose office was closest to my location. After making a call, I learned that I could book an appointment for the next day.

"Awesome!" I said.

Conventional medicine, take notes! I smiled at that thought. When I arrived in the waiting room, a lady who had her appointment scheduled right after mine told me that it wasn't energy therapy I'd subject myself there to, but the so-called chakra therapy.

"Oh snap! What's that?" I asked, slightly concerned.

"You'll certainly learn about it in there. However, all I can tell you is that the energy source for each one of us is the universe, while proper flow of that energy is determined by chakras."

"Chakras?"

"Yes. Inside the body, there are seven energy points called chakras, which regulate the flow of the energy in the universe. If one of your energy points is blocked, this may cause you to receive bad signals that your own body is sending you."

"But how would that man know if my chakras are blocked?

"Every energy point is of a different color. Together, they form your aura. The therapist will see their colors."

After what I had heard from the woman waiting in line, I wasn't sure if I was in the right place at all. Anna and I looked into each other's eyes with much skepticism. When I was waiting for my turn, another woman came in. They stroke a quite lengthy conversation. The lady who joined us recapped her story. It turned out that she had cancer. That tumor had devoured ninety percent of her kidneys and, as she put it, if it wasn't for the therapist and his chakra treatment, she wouldn't be able to live and function normally.

That information gave me hope and evoked my imagination.

That's something! I thought.

It was my turn. I was concerned that in that office, I'd be greeted by an African-American with a feather headdress of the Apache leader on his head, a Voodoo doll in one of his hands, and a chicken foot in the other. Meanwhile, to my surprise, sitting behind the desk there was a tall Caucasian male that reminded me of my uncle's friend, the cardiologist. His physical appearance wasn't in any way different to what a doctor practicing conventional medicine typically looks like. The only thing missing was a stethoscope dangling off his neck.

"What brings you two here?" he asked, voicing no objection to me bringing in my security guard.

We told him our story.

"Lie down on the couch, please. Let's take a look at your aura," he said.

I lay down, and the therapist started swinging his hands above my body in a weird way, moving them like a scanner along my body from head to foot.

Without touching me, he stated, "I see that the solar plexus chakra and the sacral chakra are blocked. You also have some issues with the third eye chakra."

"What does it mean?" I asked surprised at hearing all these quaint terms.

"It means that they need to be unblocked, and then your problems will disappear. You'll see. This will bring joy back into your life."

"Help me, please!" I begged him.

For the next fifteen minutes, he was moving his hands above me, acting as if he was detecting bad energy, and then dusting it off into the air by rubbing and clapping his hands.

When it was all done, he asked me, smiling, "Well? How do you feel?"

I felt that he was very convinced that his chakra-unblocking procedure was successful.

"Same," I replied dead serious, looking into his eyes.

"Come on! You're a tough one, aren't you? Let's get you cleaned up and everything will go back to normal. You'll see. Please remain seated! Where's that uncomfortable feeling in your neck? Show me!" the therapist asked me, putting his hands on my neck. He massaged me for a while and asked again, "Well, how's that? Any better?"

In the moment when he started administering a simple massage to my neck, he made me realize that his treatment intending to regulate pathways of energy that comes from the universe apparently didn't cover the key issue of my neck pains. It dawned on me that I shouldn't have come there at all.

The price I had to pay for the twenty-minute-long appointment was equal to that charged for private visits by doctors practicing conventional medicine. I was okay with it, as far as that man really was keeping that severely ill woman alive. To this day, I have no clue how he did that. I did know, however, that I had to keep seeking the solution to my problems elsewhere.

Time passed inexorably quickly and my condition neither improved even a bit nor came back to normal. The prickly sensations inside my head, which up until that point had been only sporadic, started occurring more often and with more intensity. After every instance of feeling as if a needle was being driven deep inside my skull, which hurt like a small thunderstrike and which was preceded by an odd tingling sensation in the back of my head, I felt as if I was disconnected from reality for a moment. It was as if I had drunk several vodka shots all at once and got stupefied in just a second.

"The man got my chakras all messed up," I laughed, managing to not take that entire situation too seriously.

I wasn't happy thought when shortly after my appointment with the chakra therapist I woke up feeling pressure growing inside my head. It didn't come to my mind that it could be a delayed side effect or a positive result of that therapy that started like that. I felt like something inside my skull was about to make it burst, which certainly wasn't anything good. Trying to free myself from that sensation, which began affecting my ears just as unpleasantly, I felt that I needed to equalize pressure by performing the so-called Valsalva maneuver.[7]

---

[7] Valsalva maneuver – one of the methods for assessing the condition of the middle ear that consists in verifying the patency of the Eustachian tube.

Pinching my nose shut with my mouth closed, I started blowing air from my lungs into my nose to make that unpleasant feeling go away. I could feel the air slowly filling my ears, pressing on the membranes of the eardrums. Each of us performed that maneuver at least once as a kid, when some water got inside the ear, when jumping around on one foot wouldn't help get the water out.

Day by day, I was getting more and more irritated. I knew I had to do something about it. I didn't know that the growing pressure was just about to get worse, coupled with the unease in my neck that over time started feeling like a stiff stick. I felt that my state was deteriorating and I knew I had to seek someone's help. I was well aware that I wouldn't get it from Armani nor his colleagues from the outpatient clinic, whom I had been seeing, too, as none of them would make any effort to recall the knowledge they all had learned back in med school. Therefore, I had to take action and find help on my own accord. I recalled the masseuse's words, who made me realize that the spine could cause a broad range of ailments; I decided to follow that path.

I knew I had to find a good physiotherapist who would dedicate more time to me than the masseuse did. Many guys would tell me, "Man! Are you out of your mind?"

I knew that this time, I had to find a male masseur who I knew I had to find a good physiotherapist who would dedicate more time to me than the masseuse did. Many guys would tell me, "Man! Are you out of your mind?"

I knew that this time, I had to find a male masseur who would use his strong hands to simply knead my back, as it was probably where the cause of all my issues was. As the masseuse claimed, I was very tense. Due to all those bothersome, intertwined symptoms, very often I'd ask Anna to massage my back, especially to apply much pressure to the thoracic spine area. Particularly in the evenings, when I felt my ailments aggravating, I'd lie down on the floor and Anna would do her best to help me with all the strength in her small hands. The area I'd ask her to press on was not chosen by accident. Just as I felt a strong need to blow air into my ears to get rid of the pressure, I felt a need to have that specific area of my back pressed on.

In both cases, it very soon became a habit to me, particularly pinching my nose and blowing air into my sinuses, the consequences of which proved dreadful for me shortly afterwards.

The Internet is a powerful tool that can do much harm nowadays, but can also do a lot of good things, too, provided it is used skillfully. A few clicks of the mouse was all it took for me to find a psychotherapist who'd accept self-pay patients. And so, I found myself in the hands of a man who not only did physiotherapy but was also a certified chiropractor.[8] Later that afternoon, I felt the pressure inside my head rising, coupled with a sensation of having a stick for a neck, which was getting increasingly uncomfortable. It was one of those days when I wondered if I should go to hospital or just call an ambulance. However, given my highly ambivalent sentiment for healthcare services and my strong belief that I wasn't dying just yet, I decided to focus on saving my spine.

Knowing all too well that it was late, I made a phone call to the physiotherapist and recapped my issue. Cool and collected, the man listened to me closely and, despite his hectic schedule, he invited me to see him on the same day after his work, so that he could try alleviate my suffering. Up until then, it was the most humanitarian treatment a therapist offered me.

I arrived at Marek's office at ten o'clock. From the very start we hit it off. He was one of those people who you stumble upon in your life and you just know that's a decent human being. As per usual, I gave him a recap on my unamusing story.

Despite the late hour, the physiotherapist calmly listened to me once again, and then asked me to go to the massage parlor. Scanning my physique with his eyes, he concluded that he could see what was probably hypertrophies and that some of my core muscles were relatively poorly developed compared to other groups of muscles.

---

[8] Chiropractic – a field of unconventional medicine; a type of manual therapy.

"I can see already what you've done to yourself with all that training," he said.

According to his swift diagnosis, weight lifting was likely the reason behind my issues. I was very glad that finally someone found the probable cause of why in just moment I started to see light at the end of the tunnel.

The massage administered by Marek didn't take much time; as soon as he put his hands on my back though, I instantaneously felt a difference between his manual therapy and the massage delivered earlier by the female physiotherapist.

"Breathe easy. This might be unpleasant."

Marek detected areas on my back that once kneaded, made me grit my teeth to not cry out in pain.

I knew I had to hold on in order to feel better.

The masseur promised me that.

"You'll feel much better, you'll see." And, indeed, he told the truth.

Having had my body kneaded in all ways possible, I felt relieved.

"It's amazing!" I said.

"Now, for some time, you might feel a little dizzy, but that will pass."

Indeed, I was weak at the knees afterwards, but being optimistic, I hoped to see good results. I made another appointment right away, which was scheduled just a few days later.

Having returned home, I got to bed. Feeling that my neck was much relieved and that the pressure in my head got regulated, I slept better than usual.

On the next day, as soon as I got up, all the receptors in my brain laser-focused on my ailments to see if the massage was of any real benefit to me.

"Yes! It works!" I shouted, surprised, feeling hopeful again. Marek and his manual therapy greatly improved how I felt. However, in order to make the positive effect of the massage last longer, I had to attend ten more sessions.

"Most often, to get the expected results, it takes more than just one treatment session," the physiotherapist said.

"If that's what it takes, so be it," I replied.

I had no objections, as it was the only place so far where I got help and physical relief. The sessions were taking place on a weekly basis. Sadly, my joy didn't last long, because with every massage that was performed after the first one, I didn't feel any improvement. Though the first experience of being massaged by Marek brought me an immense relief, every session that followed was simply ineffective and my problem was getting worse.

The next two months didn't bring any significantly positive results; regardless of it all, I kept believing that I'd finally find what the reason behind my issues was.

Not enjoying life that much, I continued rummaging through the Internet, hoping that one day I'd accurately diagnose my issues. Aside from reading about illnesses, I was googling ideas for proposing in an original way, as the date I planned for the ideal proposal trip was knocking on the door. Though my physical and mental condition was making my life difficult and didn't portend well into the future, I didn't forego my happiness or the desire to bring my relationship with Anna to the next level, which would show her at the same time how much I loved her and how much I cared about her. I was looking into the future hoping everything would work out just fine. I bought a ring with a tiny diamond and scheduled the trip. I got into my car and set off to see my bride-to-be to tell her how happy I was that we'd go on our brief vacation together soon. Later that evening, in pouring rain, I was driving along my favorite route that was linking our homes with a smile on my face despite the weather. Moments like those allowed me to forget about my concerns for a while. On my way, I was wondering how I'd ask Anna for her hand. Suddenly, my vision of a love scene with us, two lovebirds, disappeared into thin air as I saw a man lying on the side of the dark road, close to the same spot where I had an accident one year ago. The elderly man was lying flat on his face with one leg on the asphalt, the other one on the grass. Lights of all the cars passing him by, including mine, flashed on his rain-soaked black jacket, one by one.

For fuck's sake, what's happened? Did no one else spot him before me? Why did no one stop? I wondered.

Passing him by, driven by curiosity, I looked at the man to see how he was doing over there. Driving away, I was peeking at the rearview mirror, hoping someone would surely stop. For as long as the distance allowed me to keep counting the vehicles going behind me into the dark and damp evening, I could see that none of them even slowed down for a moment. Wrestling with my thoughts, I arrived at the intersection where the Franciscan sanctuary was located. I looked at the monastery and then into my own eyes reflected in the rearview mirror.

No, I can't leave him like that! I thought.

With no time to waste, I turned back to get to the spot where the man was lying on the ground. I turned hazard warning lights on and got out of the car into the rain. I quickly rushed to the man lying down on the ground to check if he was alive.

"Hey, sir! Are you alive?"

Fortunately, still lying on the ground, the man replied, "Yeeaah!"

Instantaneously, I realized what had happened.

"You're very drunk, sir. Get up quickly or someone will run you over!"

He raised himself off the wet asphalt road with great difficulty, his legs all wobbly.

"They didn't run me over yesterday, they won't run me over today," he mumbled.

Trying to stop myself from laughing, I offered to give him a ride to his home.

"I live there!" he pointed with his finger to a gate about twenty yards away.

"Well, in that case, walk home!"

I got into my car and, irritated with all the water pouring down my hair, I started the engine.

The drunk man appeared next to my car again, knocking on the window.

"Can I help you?" I asked.

"Hey, big dog, can I borrow a cigarette?"

I looked ahead and, disgusted, drove off, wondering why hadn't I ignored that man, as most of the motorists on that road had. The answer was very simple: my moral code that had been guiding me throughout my life simply wouldn't let me. Though earlier I had put him to a test by passing him by, I felt that I had to go back and I couldn't have done otherwise.

When I was already at Anna's, as usual, I asked her to knead my back. After ten physiotherapy sessions, I still felt the need to get it really well massaged. There were days when I felt a bit better, but still, I didn't stop tensing my neck muscles, time after time. Another ailment made its way on the list; a warm sensation primarily on my face that was really getting to me mainly in the evening, the time of day I'd most often spend hanging out at Anna's. I still hoped that all my afflictions stemmed from my ill back. Neither Anna nor my relatives would leave me in peace.

"We need to go see a doctor!" they'd say.

"Okay, but what kind of a doctor?" I'd ask.

I recalled that I still didn't check the neurologist off the list despite having the referral issued by Armani. Without unnecessary delay, on the very next day, I went to the outpatient clinic to have my referral updated. This time, I saw a female colleague of my PCP's, whom I had seen there on many occasions. Although the medical staff at that outpatient clinic comprised mainly younger doctors and relatively young nurses, that lady was one of the old-school staff members and could easily be taken for Dr. Armani's mother. It was only my hypothesis, though; obviously, these two were not related. However, they both applied an old-fashioned approach in their practice. Each time I went to see the female doctor, she'd ask me if I came to request her to approve a leave letter for school. Clearly, she considered me a faker who frequented their clinic only because he had too much free time on his hands. Since my parents and I were running our own business, which she was aware of, it was logical that a leave letter wouldn't do anything for me. Sadly, each time I saw her, I had to account for being questioned about that. This time, despite her suspicions, she gave me another referral to a neurologist without me having to describe my new issues in detail. She even went one step further and, unrequested, gave me a referral for blood work. I could have the blood test done on the next day at my outpatient clinic. I was positively shocked.

Obviously, I got the blood test done to have some extra information for the neurologist. Now, the only thing left to do was to find the right person who'd finally examine me thoroughly and explain my issues to me once for all. With this approach, I started looking for an experienced neurologist on the Internet. Though I didn't always agree with the theoretical claim "An older doctor is a good doctor", this time, I hoped that a neurologist with impressive seniority would quickly come up with an accurate diagnosis. Although there were many names online, I found it hard to find the right doctor. Eventually, I decided to go with a female neurologist who had many years of experience recommended by Dr. Armani's friend.

"She's very experienced. That woman's a walking encyclopedia. I learn a lot from her when it comes to certain subjects," the PCP said.

Nice! She must be like a hundred years old. Or maybe I misjudged the age of Armani's coworker, I thought, scrutinizing the female physician carefully.

Despite the accolades the internist awarded the medical expert with, I soon realized seeing her wasn't worth the wait, either.

"Enter!" I could hear her shouting through a crack in the door, which was left not entirely closed by her previous patient.

Immediately, this brought to my mind the times of elementary school when I was called at the carpet right after playing some childish prank; upon hearing a knock on the door of his office, the principal would invite me in in the same fashion.

I slowly opened the door a little, like a scared protagonist in a horror movie who heard some suspicious noises coming from the most distant room in the attic. There she was – my last resort.

I did a double take - I could swear that the person in front of me was Dr. Armani's elder colleague from my outpatient clinic.

Is this a joke? I thought.

As soon as I closed the door behind me and approached her desk, I realized that my eyes were wrong; she could easily be an elder sister of the PCP, though.

Shouldn't that lady already be somewhere else on her retirement? I thought.

Not only were they the spitting image of each other, but they both had the same trace of cynicism in their attitudes.

"What brings us here?" she asked using that weird mannerism from the old days that for some reason makes people refer to a single person in plural.

"I have some grave issues, Doctor. Please help me."

"Go on."

"I feel like I'm an astronaut trapped in a heavy spacesuit. I feel myself losing focus and living as if dissociated from reality. When I look at my hands, I get flooded with anxiety because I can no longer tell if they are mine. Talking to you here and now makes me very sweaty, and I have no idea why that is. For some time, I've been having a highly concerning sensation in the neck; a kind of stiffness, like a stick on one side of the neck. This makes me constantly flex the neck muscles, trying to make it go away. In my head, I feel pressure and prickly sensations that are painful and last for a second, sometimes two, preceded by inexplicable tingling in the back of my head; on top of that, quite recently, I've started getting odd, warm sensations that wear me down, particularly in the area of the face."

When I finished my elaborate description, the neurologist slid her glasses down to the tip of her nose with the tip of her finger, and gave me the stink eye.

"What are you so stressed up about, pal, huh?"

"I don't understand," I replied.

Judging me for my young apparition, she asked, "You're having your high school exit exams this year, is that it?"

I could tell right away where she was going with that; I could feel myself slowly getting irritated, as I was well aware how my appointment was about to end.

I told my whole story in detail, but even that didn't spark in the experienced neurologist any willingness to make some effort and find the reason behind my problems. On the contrary; hearing about my episode with antidepressants, she concluded right away where the problem lied.

"Lifting loads is what a crane does, not you," she said, unable to stick to one form of referring to me.

She asked me to stand up and walk to the couch. She performed a series of basic neurological tests to see if I was okay in terms of neurology. After an examination consisting in making me stand on one leg, touch the tip of my nose with my eyes closed, and hitting me on a knee with a small mallet, she concluded that I was a picture of health. Having cast an additional glance on my blood test results, she wrapped it up.

"I see no grounds for recommending any other testing. I think that you should continue seeing a psychiatrist, because I can't help you. I can only suggest some other antidepressant drugs you haven't taken yet."

I didn't know whether to laugh or cry. I never had much respect for doctors, but I also knew that I couldn't let myself explode in a fit of rage.

"I've been there and done that, and I know it does nothing for me," I said, regretfully.

"Perhaps the choice of drugs was inappropriate for you," she remarked.

"What about those prickly sensations in my head and the pressure? What if there's something wrong going on up there?"

She retrieved a blood pressure cuff, put it on my arm, and started measuring.

"Your blood pressure is fine. Physically, nothing's going on up there, but there certainly is something wrong with your head!"

Irritated with that conversation, I knew I stood no chance to win a dispute with this elderly woman who should have retired long ago.

"I ask you... No, I demand that you give me a referral for a head MRI scan!" I raised my voice.

I could feel that she wasn't happy with that, but I managed to persuade her to issue such a referral for me.

"Very well. I'll order a head MRI scan, but in my opinion, it's not necessary," she concluded.

I thanked her and, as usual, not surprised at anything I didn't expect, I went home. The only thing left to do was to go have my head checked.

Waiting for a skull scanning test was not the most pleasant experience. We were all aware that this was where our search came to an end. At least that's what we thought, since of all the medical experts I had the pleasure of meeting in the course of the previous two years, no one suggested anything other than psychotherapy. None of these people even tried to associate my symptoms with any other disease on this earth. After all, a man is just like a car in this sense; if you know nothing about auto repair, you go to a car mechanic and trust that he'd get your car fixed. Although my intuition and even my body were telling me otherwise, I entrusted my fate to medical experts in the exact same way. Either way, back then, the verdict was plain and simple: all my issues were in my head.

There came a day when I was about to unravel the secret and learn the cause of my suffering. We were all very concerned about what the MRI scan results would be; however, I was more concerned about the test itself. I knew that I'd be driven into a narrow chamber inside of which I'd have to remain still for thirty minutes, so that the machine could produce a reliable and accurate image of my brain. And so, we arrived at a medical center, one of the more renown in my city, where you could have various insurance-covered examinations performed, undergo a treatment, or seek a paid consultation with experts without having to wait for an appointment or test results for too long.

The anxiety I felt before being slid inside the MRI scanner was not because I feared this new, completely unknown experience; it was due to the fact that I wasn't the same person I had been a few years earlier, but a completely disheartened young man exhausted with his problems, struggling with a feeling of being trapped inside his athletic body. Throughout the process, I felt derealization and tribulation, feeling as if I was carrying some foreign matter around, ball and chain; it was like having to wear a spacesuit all the time. I knew that once I got slid into the cylinder of the MRI scanner, I'd be trapped twofold, like Matthew McConaughey piloting a spaceship from a cramped cockpit in the blockbuster *Interstellar*. Although my attitude was optimistic, I couldn't help but feel anxiety creeping in on me. I hadn't had any anxiety seizures for long time and, without taking antidepressants, I was doing great; however, inside the very tight, oddly illuminated cylinder of the machine, generating loud sounds when turned on, I could feel the immense anxiety building up inside me while I had to remain perfectly still.

It was the longest thirty minutes of my life. Though the scanning seemed to take ages, like interstellar travel, I didn't have to wait long for the results. Quite quickly, I was handed a CD with the MR image and a radiologist's impression.

The moment when we opened up the envelope with the impression issued by the radiologist from that medical center was undoubtedly one of the least pleasant moments of my life. There are lots of people who, when faced with their potential death following an awful accident, see various beautiful scenes and the most significant memories of their life flashing before their eyes. At least that's what they claim. I never thought if it would be the same for me. In that very moment, when I read the impression pertaining to the MR image, all I could see was just one scene – me kneeling before Anna, handing her the engagement ring, and then the two of us standing before an altar as newlyweds. Lost in the fantasy of the happy, smiling couple smartly dressed for their wedding day, I painted in my mind a picture of myself holding my beautiful bride by her hand; then my body suddenly disappears into thin air like a hologram, my wedding tux falling down on the ground on black Oxfords.

"What is it, Michal? Tell us. Read aloud," my loved ones asked.

"Clear visualization of small (up to three millimeters in diameter) oval changes hyperintense on T2-weighted FLAIR images, and hypointense and isointense on T1-weighted images, situated in the left cerebral peduncle. The MR image requires clinical differentiation between growth alteration and damage to corticospinal tracts on the left side," I read aloud.

In that moment, each of us was living through his or her own personal tragedy. I couldn't decipher the thoughts my parents and Anna were struggling with.

"It'll be okay, you'll see," they wept.

Though we had no certainty if our understanding of the impression was accurate, each of us eventually arrived at the conclusion as to what was behind my complete transformation. And though me reading the impression brought much drama into the lives of my loved ones, there was a part of me that felt greatly relieved and appeased that I finally found the reason for the ailments that had been tormenting me for two years. The constant uncertainty and helplessness that I had been experiencing throughout that long time were more painful to me than the awareness of the fact that I could soon be dead.

After receiving my MRI scan results, I could see my previous neurologist again to check what her response to this would be, and to ask her to interpret the results as an experienced specialist in the field.

"Indeed, you've got something in there. That's not good. It would be better for you if it was anxiety disorder. You have small tumors that will have to be monitored throughout your life. As for now, they're tiny, but you'll have to undergo an MRI scan of the head every six months and we'll keep an eye on them together."

Without suggesting that I start taking antidepressants, the female doctor had nothing more to add, and so she suggested I should schedule a follow-up visit.

"I'm very sorry. A man this young, and already ridden with so many problems. There's nothing more I can do," she concluded.

That's it? How about something like, 'I've made a mistake, I'm sorry'? I thought.

It was hard for me to find the right words to describe my feelings.

Is this how my story ends? I asked myself. I wondered how does it all actually work; a young boy feels bad for a couple of years and, learning all of a sudden that he's got tumors, he hears nothing of substance from an expert. *How come nothing can be done? Can't it be stopped? How's that possible? What's wrong with this world?* I was scratching my head.

Doctors continued to disappoint me and let me down, but my intuition kept on telling me that something was not right and that it couldn't be the end of my adventure with healthcare professionals. I decided to find another neurologist. However, before I did, the day of my previously planned engagement trip arrived.

Although my future and life further down the line were put into question, the only thing I dreamed of was to become my Anna's fiancé. I knew that at that very moment, it was probably not the best idea to take our relationship to the next level, and I felt that it could be somewhat egoistical on my part; however, my hope, positive attitude and, most of all, the power of love I had for my girlfriend allowed me to make up my mind and take the risk; I decided to propose as planned.

November was probably not the best month for mountain hiking, but it was definitely a time when it was less likely to get scorching sun or vast amounts of snow in the lower parts of mountain ranges in Poland. The famous Polish golden fall is one of the most beautiful seasons, with all plants slowly preparing to go to sleep. Before losing their leaves, tree canopies take on red-and-golden hues, and mountain trails indulge hikers with landscapes of green, orange, and yellow foliage. And indeed, a view in these colors welcomed us when we went hiking together, acting as the perfect scenery for the event that was one of the key moments of my life.

I was planning to perform that major act on the top of Kasprowy Wierch. In the past, I had climbed that summit in winter once, and it was one of the best hiking trips of my life. I had no sentiment for mountains or for that one specific summit, for that matter. I simply concluded that it could be very romantic when after ascending the peak, I'd get on one knee and muster the courage to ask one of the key questions.

And so we began our small adventure together. When entering the trail leading to Kasprowy Wierch, I asked a woman selling entry tickets for directions to assure myself that we'd take the right path. The kind lady pointed us to the right trail. Happy, with our faces all lit up, we started walking towards Kasprowy Wierch. It took us only halfway up to realize that we weren't well-prepared for conquering that mountain. We both started feeling discomfort in our feet. My winter boots that had been through a lot started acting out and gradually peeling the skin off of my heels; in turn, Anna realized that her shoes were getting wet too quickly. This didn't stop us from carrying on with our adventure, though.

And yet, at one point, when I started wrestling with my thoughts, the pain of my hurting ankles was getting more and more noticeable, while the occasional prickly sensation in my head wouldn't let me be even on a day that was so important to me. At one point, I felt a very characteristic sharp pain in my groin. Without showing that anything was off I sucked it up and, despite the discomfort I was experiencing, I kept moving on. Like Muhammad Ali would say, "It isn't the mountains ahead to climb that wear you down. It's the pebble in your shoe." Visualizing what awaited me at the summit, I didn't think about bailing out because of the pain – not even for a second.

After a quite lengthy walk, we both started having a feeling that something was not right. When we looked into the distance, to the sides and up, we could spot neither the cableway leading to the summit nor the characteristic building of the Meteorological Observatory that should be visible on the very top of Kasprowy Wierch. We decided to ask some tourists who were passing us by for directions.

"Hey there, how far to Kasprowy?"

"What do you mean, to Kasprowy? You're not going to Kasprowy. That's the trail to Giewont!" one of them replied.

Surprised by how on earth we found ourselves on the trail leading to the Giewont Cross, we looked at each other, smiling.

"How could this happen, Anna?"

"I've no idea."

I was even more surprised than she was, since in the very beginning, I planned to go to Mount Giewont. However, I knew that crossing the last three hundred feet before the summit, where the Cross was located, required climbing a route with steel chains fixed to rocks; as I didn't want out first mountain hiking trip to be that extreme, I chose Mount Kasprowy.

"What shall we do, Anna?" I asked.

"We're not backing out. We keep moving," she said smiling, unaware of what awaited her there.

Reaching the elevation of about 5,675 feet in great pain, I cast a glance at the summit of Mount Giewont, which was less than two hundred yards away from us.

It hurts but you can do it! I told myself.

In that very moment, a very strong gust of wind hit us, scaring Anna, who already had frozen to the core.

"I don't know if I'll make it!" she said.

I didn't object, content in the depths of my soul that Anna felt like going back, too.

"If you don't feel like doing this either, let's call it a day," I suggested.

Seeing us contemplating, some tourists who were passing us by advised us to forego our further trip, as the wind was getting more and more violent.

We both decided to get over with it.

I was slightly disappointed with the situation at hand, as my plan misfired big time.

Oh, that's a shame. Tomorrow, we'll take a cable car to the top of Mount Kasprowy and I'll propose to her there, I thought.

Making my first steps down on our way back, I heard my Anna's saying, "It's a bit of a shame, you know. If you intended to propose to me at the top today, you'd probably be mad with me for getting too scared to go on," she remarked jokingly, laughing in that typical way of hers that always had a good effect on me.

Without speaking a word, I stopped and fell on one knee in front of her. I took my cap off and slowly reached under my jacket for the little red box.

"What are you doing? Stop playing around, get up! I was joking," she was crying one tear after another.

I looked deep into her eyes, showing her the engagement ring.

"Will you be my wife?" I asked in a shaky voice.

"Yes!" she said without hesitation, throwing herself into my arms.

CHAPTER II

How difficult it is to put in words the situation my sweetheart and I found ourselves in! Perhaps we both wanted to forget what was happening there and then; nonetheless, we were looking into the future with hope and optimism, like most of our peers were. Although living in the moment, the longer we were together, the more we could picture ourselves at the altar and, later, holding hands with at least two small kids of our own. Over time, this picture became obscured by the grim, uncertain reality. I was aware of the scale of the problem I was tackling and of what was to become my immediate future, while my anxiety was getting increasingly troublesome.

Sadly, we couldn't enjoy our engagement to the fullest. Sometimes, when talking to our loved ones, it was hard not to mention the bad news, as everyone who cared about me even a little bit deserved to know. However, we decided not to share this sad news with friends and relatives until the cause of all my ailments was pinned down with certainty. Since the female neurologist whose services were covered by my insurance plan didn't make a good impression on me, and I couldn't imagine someone like her handling my health and the tumors that were potentially developing, I decided to go see someone younger who would re-examine my brain scan images and verify the diagnosis.

The key issue aside, from then on, I was wrestling with other matters.

What about training? Can I train? Can I do sports?

Among all the drama, I forgot to ask the neurologist about the part of my life that was obviously the most significant to me at that time.

Despite my bad mood, I had no intention to forgo my passion for training, even at the cost of damaging my health permanently.

"What are you doing? Stop training!" my loved ones were begging me.

I was so irresponsible and consumed by my passion that despite their requests, I didn't give in and continued training. Unfortunately, it didn't take long until I learned I had to give it up regardless, because my issues couldn't be overcome solely with character and strong will.

Although I still tried not to be overly committed to office work at our family business, I always took much pleasure in doing the physical tasks that required much effort. I knew that when it comes to lifting heavy carton boxes, I had to spare my parents that burden and not let them be the ones to do my job. Although work was giving me less and less satisfaction, I had to fulfil my duties - not because I was forced to, but because I knew my dad or my mom, always eager to go ahead and carry loads herself, would do my tasks for me to make it easier for me. So, I wanted to keep helping them for as long as I could.

One day, I recalled the day I proposed to Anna; not because it was a highly important event for both of us, but because I felt the very same unpleasant, immense, sharp pain cutting through my groin like a knife.

"Oh my!" I cried in pain, lifting a box up.

What is that? I asked myself.

Already on the brink of emotional exhaustion, I'd get irritated by any new ailment that came up.

From then on, I started getting that prickly sensation in the groin more and more often. The problem was aggravated to the point that simply moving the right leg when sitting was causing me agony. Although sometimes I'd suddenly cry out in pain, scaring those sitting with me at the table, I didn't take this issue seriously.

"Oh, well, I must've strained something. Surely, it'll pass with time," I told them.

After all, I had bigger problems waiting to be solved. Shortly after our engagement, I was on my way to a paid appointment with a neurosurgeon well-known throughout the country. I went there together with Anna and my mother, who would often accompany me on my trips from one doctor to another. By a twist of fate, without knowing anything about that expert, we encountered him completely on accident during one of our visits at a medical facility. We learned from a medical receptionist that they had an excellent neurosurgeon working there, who at that very moment had two hours of free time, as the patients who had been scheduled cancelled their appointments. We didn't hesitate even for a second, and took advantage of that situation.

"Consider yourself very lucky, because usually, patients have to wait months on end to see him." the receptionist said.

Wow! He must be a House, M.D., or some other medical superstar. Awesome! I thought.

On that late afternoon, fate was indeed on our side. Not only did we happen to have lots of free time that we could spend at the appointment, but on top of that, it turned out that my mom had a CD with my head CT scan results including the interpretation with her.

This time, in order not to avoid confusion, I entered the neurosurgeon's office accompanied by my mom only. Anna decided to wait in the hall.

Although this man didn't look anything close to Dr. House, both my mom and I realized very quickly that the medical receptionist's praise was not just empty words. Despite being tired due to seeing patients throughout the day, the neurosurgeon listened to what I had to say calmly and respectfully. Sitting at the desk in a slightly creased, dark jacket that was too big for his slender figure, he was paying close attention to my words. Leaning back in his chair, he reminded me of drug lord Tony Montana from the film *Scarface* played by the one-and-only Academy Award winner Al Pacino. Holding his head low, the doctor was casting a brief look at me and my arms every now and then with his big sad eyes. I took a glimpse at a clock hanging over his desk and, not accustomed to giving a free-flowing, detailed monologue at a doctor's office, I realized that half an hour had passed already. From time to time, my mom would add some remarks about important issues and events that had taken place over the course of the previous two years that I forgot to mention.

When I concluded my statement, the neurosurgeon said, "Very well. Let's take a look at the CD with your MRI brain scan."

He began analyzing the images of my head MRI scan on his computer. My mom and I were waiting to hear the doctor's opinion.

"Okay. Alright. Now, show me the interpretation. Moron!" he said in a loud voice.

"Pardon?" my mom was flabbergasted.

"Moron! The radiologist who interpreted your brain MRI scan. He misinterpreted it, and it's not the first time that happened. I know that man and I know how often he gets his analyses confused. I believe he should've lost his license long time ago."

Baffled at the neurosurgeon's reaction and his statement, we weren't sure what actually happened.

"What do you mean exactly?" I asked.

"I mean that you're healthy and you have no tumor. I've been opening skulls many times and I know what they look like. I've seen an image identical to that only yesterday. It's not just that the radiologist failed to read your images accurately; I've also found his interpretation to involve some oxymorons, which only points to his lack of knowledge of neurology."

My mom and I were speechless.

"God, that's great! Thank you, Jesus," my mom said. Content with how the appointment went, I couldn't wait to leave the office and tell Anna that I was healthy. While my mom continued to talk with the doctor, I lowered my head, getting lost in my thoughts.

What's happening with me, then? I wondered.

Perhaps someone else in my shoes would jump for joy hearing this news from a good neurosurgeon; however, I still had no reason to celebrate. The more time passed, the more I could feel my health running out on me, just like sand runs out of an hourglass.

Time went by, and 'Pacino' and my mom found common ground. They touched upon several different topics.

Now I know why they have such a high opinion of you, Al, I thought.

It was unquestionably unprecedented to see a doctor dedicate so much time to one patient. Telling us about severe cases of people suffering from cancer, he shared with us an anecdote from his own life. He told us that one time, he and his friends nearly drowned on a yacht that started sinking in open sea; luckily, they were all rescued by the Coast Guard.

"This is why the significant thing is that you're alive," he said.

I had an impression that he was trying to help me by evoking emotions and some other feelings in me, like a psychiatrist would. He cast another glance at my arms.

"You look great. Keep working out. I don't know what do you want from yourself. I wish I looked like you!" he admitted.

Thanks, mom, I thought, nodding softly. I had another déjà vu moment, as the cardiologist had said the same thing earlier.

In reply to our questions about what could be the cause of my problems, he stated, "Seeing you and taking to you, I don't see a person suffering from anxiety or depression. Hence, I don't recommend that you continue stuffing yourself with any drugs that you've been taking up to this point. I think that you should rest and take a short break from working out. It seems to me that it's nothing more than your body feeling tired, insisting to get some rest. This is why I recommend that you take a solid break," he concluded.

My mom and Anna were overjoyed at the course the appointment had taken. They got the information they asked for, which boosted their endorphins. Such a diagnosis from a respected and diligent expert who gifted us with an hour and a half of his time was enough to make my ladies happy. However, they didn't feel what I felt, and they even couldn't have felt that. As for me, I didn't completely agree with the neurosurgeon's opinion, and

I wouldn't have agreed with him even if he was the top neurosurgeon in the entire Europe. My body and my intuition were still telling me that that was not the case, and that my problems were due to something much worse than just fatigue. Soon after, I learned that indeed, they were right.

Then the year two thousand thirteen came along. Winter is the time when people with compromised immunity most often end up ill in bed. For me, that was a standard procedure. It didn't take much for me to get a fever and a sore throat all of a sudden, which would force me to stay in bed for over ten days straight. My immunity was in shambles.

Since a Sports Medicine Center opened up very close to my house, I decided to go there. Not only was this place situated much closer to my home, but also, as the name suggests, it was closer to my heart. I had high hopes that, with due consideration of my passion if not anything else, specialists at the center would take a different approach to treatment than Dr. Armani and his colleagues did.

Initially, it might have seemed that I would get a completely different treatment; however, I didn't see much difference long-term. On the day I visited the Sports Medicine Center, I could feel myself falling prey to a serious illness. I ended up examined by a young female PCP. I was glad. After all those elderly doctors I had visited up until that point, her young blood was like a very much needed breath of fresh air. I also had an opportunity to tell the internist about my ups and downs in detail, hoping she would happen to find a trail overlooked by every other expert that had diagnosed me earlier. Quite soon, I noticed that there were two fundamental differences in how I was handled during the preliminary meeting at the Sports Medicine Center; the first being that the female PCP was much prettier than Dr. Armani, and the other being that the manner in which that lady was trying to solve her patient's issues.

"Let's try give you some vitamins and electrolytes to boost immunity. You need to take it for a few months and then we'll see if there's any improvement."

That's something. Armani, look how it's done, I thought.

Having been given the medication intended to stop the bronchitis that was yet again developing, we proceeded to discuss my daily ailments. I could see that the doctor had a tough nut to crack and that it was difficult for her to come up with anything.

"Cardiology, neurology, physiotherapy, psychiatry... It seems that you've investigated every field possible. I'm not sure where else we could be looking for the cause. For now, let's address your issues related to recurring inflammation," she said.

Neither consoled nor content with my visit at the new clinic, I knew there was nothing I could do other than continue to seek the answer on my own.

Meanwhile, I knew that I would end up bedridden for the next ten days, as usual, and that none of the drugs administered by the young female doctor would make any difference in that regard.

"Keep telling yourself that and you'll be ill forever. Tell yourself, 'I'm fine' and you'll feel better immediately. You'll see," my mom would say.

Maybe, in all actuality, I was attracting bad thoughts like a magnet. Sadly, no attempt at tricking my brain made me feel better even for a while, and as for the illness that would come and knock me out in wintertime, there was no way I could curb the expansion of the virus. The tea my mom and Anna both made me with love lost its healing power, unfortunately; likewise, the medications prescribed by doctors, including the female internist from the Sports Medicine Center, proved ineffective. For this reason, I buried myself back under the duvet to overcome the virus and recover as soon as possible. After just a few days, my temperature reading was over one hundred point four degrees, while my horrible sore throat transformed into a green-and-yellow phlegm that was sluggishly going from the sinuses down the back of my throat. Though it could seem that I was accustomed to staying in bed long-term and that this state was not unknown to me, this time, the discomfort I felt in the neck, the high pressure in my head, and my clogged sinuses combined with runny nose were giving me a rough ride. Tormented by the awful sensation of high pressure inside my head, I did one of the worst things that could come to my mind at that moment, turning my life into an even worse nightmare as a result. Accustomed to doing Valsalva maneuver consisting in blowing the air from the lungs into the sinuses, I pinched my nose with my fingers and I blew.

No, no, no, please! No!

Highly annoyed with myself for what I had just done, I knew that I had made a grave mistake.

In the very same second when I performed that mindless act, I felt as if someone had put stoppers into my ears, but from the inside. Not only was that a horrible physical experience, but it was also accompanied by a sound proving that what I had done was a very bad thing.

I immediately realized that most likely, I had blown the secretion from my sinuses into my ears. At least that's what it seemed like to me. It didn't take long until I felt extremely anxious. Whenever I was swallowing saliva or just blinking, I could feel something odd in my ears getting all tense, making a loud noise resembling a thunder echoing in the sky before an approaching storm. Petrified by the sudden synchronization of my esophagus and eyelids, and by what was happening inside my ears, I felt my heart beating harder and harder.

"Oh my! What have you done?!" I said to myself.

I hoped that it was merely a matter of time, that this horrific complication would disappear together with my inflammation. I tried not to panic and to make it through the worse time. I kept telling myself, "It'll surely pass, it must!"

Then, I recalled that back when I was a seven-year-old child playing usually near a staircase leading to an apartment in an apartment building where I lived, I picked a willow florescence commonly called a catkin. Without giving it much thought, I put it into my nostril and instead of blowing the air out, I inhaled the catkin so that it got stuck inside my nose for some time. Luckily for me, the catkin came out of my nostril with some mucus one time when I got the common cold. I hoped that this time, the course of events would be similar.

Just as unexpectedly as the flue-like disease came, it decided to leave me alone and finally let me regenerate after tormenting my body for two weeks. Unfortunately, this time, the viral inflammation left some marks that I had never dreamed of, which I had been completely oblivious of up until that point.

Over three weeks after the day on which I first felt like I was about to fall ill with some condition, I could finally return to the world of the living, or rather to a state free from fever that allowed me to continue my daily struggle with the ailments I had been tackling for some time. From then on, I had to include on the list of symptoms that wouldn't let me enjoy life a new awful feeling of a foreign object stuck in my ears.

Although I had high hopes that this problem would disappear together with the phlegm and runny nose caused by the inflammation, that was not what happened, sadly. The feeling of my ears being blocked from the inside decided to stay with me for longer. It was as if all the ailments that can affect a man had an innate awareness of their own existence that in some way allowed them to localize the prey and enter its body at a specific moment for a specific period of time.

I felt as if my body was a luxury hotel for guests who not necessarily lived in symbiosis with myself, making it their goal to destroy me and to take me down from within. From then on, aside from moving my neck in all directions to make the discomfort bearable, as it wouldn't leave me be even for a moment, I started moving at random all body parts connected to my esophagus and eyelids in any way. Every time I squinted or closed my eyes, or continued to swallow saliva, I could feel the object that was allegedly inside my ears getting all tense, making the sound much like a massive thunder before a storm. With my eyes closed, I could imagine dark, navy-blue skies indicating that a great windstorm was just around the corner. Terrified by this phenomenon which was inexplicable to me, every day I'd take up a many-hours-long fight, trying to free myself from the nightmare I found myself in. Squinting my eyes repeatedly and swallowing countless times, I managed to separate the movements of my eyelids and the esophagus from the possible foreign object that was generating the awful sound of a storm inside my ears. Blinking or swallowing saliva didn't cause that 'thing' in my ears to become tense, but I realized that from that moment on, I could make 'it' tense, thus generating that horrible sound at will. As soon as I felt that my sinuses and my nose regenerated after the viral inflammation, I impulsively returned to the habit that was the reason why I got problems with my ears in the first place. That was not only because I wanted to reverse the anomaly in my ears using the Valsalva maneuver, but I still felt the need to equalize pressure inside my head in this manner. I lay down on a couch. I knew that it wasn't helping me in any way, and that in fact, it became definitely detrimental. Aware of the fact that I shouldn't be doing this, I had no idea what would be another way to get rid of the sensation of high pressure inside my skull. Sadly, despite pinching my nose and blowing the air into my sinuses and my ears, I couldn't reverse the newly arising issue. I was getting more and more devastated because of the myriad of symptoms that were becoming more and more numerous with every day. The only thing I could do was to try get help at a doctor's office, yet again. It didn't even cross my mind to turn to the outpatient clinic where Armani worked. I knew that had I appeared on their doorstep, I'd be instantly labelled a super-hypochondriac, and that most certainly, they wouldn't be able to help me. I also knew that I exhausted my limit for referrals to medical experts that I could get at that clinic, as the staff was getting annoyed with me for some reason, without even trying to prove to me that it wasn't the case.

Therefore, I went to see the female internist at the Sports Medicine Center again and, without getting overly stressed out, asked her for help. By that time, I was already used to the idea that the PCP would probably not be able to solve my problem; to my surprise, she had objections against referring me to a laryngologist whose area of expertise covers treating conditions of the throat and the ears. Having heard what I had done, she only confirmed to me that my hypothetical diagnosis was true; I had in fact pushed some purulent secretion into my ears by performing the Valsalva maneuver. Without going into the details, the doctor took my pressure.

"I have no idea why do you keep feeling high pressure inside. Your pressure is normal."

I was clueless, too, but this wasn't the answer I expected medical professionals to give me. I still lived in hope that one day, I'd hear her or any other doctor say, "I know! I know, and here's what we're going to do about it."

During a check-up following my most recent inflammation, which I turned up for a little later than I should have, the PCP peeked inside my throat.

"It's bad. You've developed a peritonsillar abscess. Please keep an eye on it and, better yet, show it to the laryngologist during your upcoming appointment."

"An abscess?" I asked.

"Yes. That happens sometimes, especially to patients who often suffer from tonsillitis. It is likely that you'll have to have your tonsils removed soon," she wrapped it up.

My tonsils? Removed?! Now that's just great! I thought.

I got referred to a laryngologist and I ran home quick. There, I rushed to the bathroom to see what the doctor was talking about. In disbelief, I took a look deep inside my esophagus below the tonsils. I noticed a small, protruding bubble with some redness, which was the size of a pinky nail. Terrified by the recent, not thoroughly accurate diagnosis made by the radiologist who diagnosed me with brain tumors, for a moment I reexperienced the same feeling. Yet again, my imagination started painting negative images of metastatic cancer.

That must be what hypochondriacs are like, I thought.

The sound generated by my continuous struggle with the inconvenient feeling inside my ears, which was much like dramatic melody of a storm approaching, significantly aggravated the state of mind I was in at that exact moment. For a while, everything started falling together again into one catastrophic whole inside my head.

Were you wrong, Al? I asked myself, looking at the reflection of my mouth in the mirror, blaming the neurosurgeon for the mistake.

I assumed that if I paid to see a good specialist, the female internist would probably refer me to the first laryngologist at hand. This was the impression I got, for instance, after seeing the experienced neurologist. Therefore, I decided to rummage through the Internet and this time, rely on peoples' reviews. I came across a rapidly growing website that allows you to browse through online users' reviews about experts in various medical fields whom they had an appointment with. Having entered a specific phrase, I saw a list of numerous laryngologists, with the one who had the most positive reviews on the very top, obviously. The number one was standing out with his enormous advantage of a multitude of positive reviews left by his patients. Every doctor on the list had at least a few, but the leader of this ranking had about two hundreds. Naturally, I was aware of the fact that such reviews or comments could be fabricated and not entirely reliable. However, I decided to verify that and I made an appointment with the medical specialist with the most positive reviews of the online community. I very much hoped that this doctor was in fact the great professional all his patients described him to be on the Internet; I didn't expect though that meeting him would become forever imprinted on my memory.

Back when I did the Valsalva maneuver while having inflammation, I wasn't aware that aside from the fact that most likely I blew the secretion up into my ears, there was a highly suspicious process that occurred, triggering a recurring wave of cumbersome, disgusting, gnawing sensations inside my ears. Despite all the ailments I was learning to live with on a daily basis, in moments when I wasn't busy trying to solve how to get rid of them, I was trying to live an ordinary life, like every other human being. I've always been a funny guy who drew much pleasure from singing his favorite artists' songs. I really liked shouting under the shower and, most of all, singing along to Bryan Adams or Jon Bon Jovi when driving. One day, when I was singing behind the wheel, feeling as if I was on my way to get auditioned for *The Voice of Poland*, my life changed completely, and a few more pounds were added to the overall weight of all the problems that I already had on my shoulders. Suddenly, I felt weird tension in my right ear, followed by a slight change in the pressure; this caused an awful sound that I heard on the right side of my head, similar to the distorted sound that a speaker at full volume makes. Initially, I thought that the passenger door speaker died and that I'd have to have it replaced. That would have been awesome for me. Sadly, when making other sounds while singing along, I soon realized that the distinct sound of a broken speaker was coming from (or rather taking place) inside my right ear. That experience, which was nothing short of horrible, was yet another reason for a mental breakdown, which I was heading towards. This wasn't the only tragic surprise, though; another one awaited me on the very same day. Having returned home, highly focused on what was happening inside my ears, I started examining the events that had taken place on my way home. Terrified, I realized how bad an idea it was on my part to blow the air up into my ears while having a flu-like inflammation. When I got into my room, where acoustics and soundproofing worked completely different than inside a car, I could experience that sensation from a completely different angle. To some extent, the sound of music coming from the car speakers had been drowning out the sound emitted in my right ear, neutralizing concurrent physical sensations. It wasn't until I found myself behind closed doors that I realized how 'screwed' I was. In moments when I was reaching a high pitch while singing songs or when I was hearing a hoover roaring, it was as if an invisible fly appeared in my right ear, not only 'buzzing' like crazy but also moving inside and I could feel that I had it inside me. To me, this awfully annoying sensation resembled most closely the sound typical of a broken speaker. What's worse, in the evening on the same day, I got even more devastated. Although the 'fly' in my right ear ruined my mental state in no time, the bright side of that unfortune was that it appeared only with high-pitch sounds and, sporadically, during phone calls. The worst complication didn't come until the evening though, when I realized that there was something moving inside my left ear, instantly exasperating me and driving me into an even more depressed state. I still didn't know what it was, but it started reacting to nearly every sound that was coming from my surroundings, which would then exacerbate the sensation of having some alien object rubbing on the internal walls of my ear. Every sound coming from my mouth, every click of a ballpoint pen, every sound made by a flip-flop shuffling against the floor, and every bark of a dog became unbearable to me, though all these sounds were insignificant to other people. I could compare that sensation to a ball inside a chamber in an ordinary plastic whistle, moved around by a flow of air when you blow it; the ball disrupts the airflow, thus generating vibrations that make a trilling sound. The 'ball' inside my left ear wasn't generating any sounds, that's for sure; however, with every sound coming from the external world, it was pushed around my left ear chamber, causing an annoying sound of rubbing against the chamber walls.

These highly irrational sensations of purely physical nature that were inexplicable to me, manifesting inside my head in the area of my ears, would be enough to make every healthy, adult man who never experienced any health difficulties start panicking and losing his mind. Though I was very close to do so, somehow my experiences, both previous and those I was still tackling on a daily basis, taught me that whatever doesn't kill me makes me stronger, allowing me to move forward in my uphill climb. This time, I started looking for help from a laryngology expert who had the best reviews on the Internet.

I hoped that the two hundred positive comments under the laryngologist's name didn't come from thin air. I booked my first appointment online instead of via phone. I got into my car, googled my destination – the address of the doctor's office, and set off. I was glad, since the visit was to take place near a route that I knew very well, as it led to Anna's.

"Head north! In six hundred feet turn right," the pleasant voice of the navigation app specified the direction I should take. Having turned off the route I had taken multiple times into a side street, I soon realized that something was probably not right. When I was almost there according to the navigation app, I was driving past empty fields, tree stands, and woodlands.

"Your destination is on your left," the navigation app concluded.

In front of me, there was a deserted old barn made of planks, barely held together, standing in an open field. It was the only building at that specific address.

What's going on? I can't believe it, I thought.

Already tired with all my health issues and terrified because of what was happening with my ears, I was ready to get out of the car and see the doctor even if the appointment was to take place inside the barn, and the doctor had straw sticking out of his ragged pants; I couldn't be bothered. I imagined that the medical specialist with the most positive comments must have received these reviews for the beauty of the natural setting where he was seeing his patients or, perhaps, he got some of them from people who felt bad he couldn't afford a better location for his office. I wished I had had the time to read through all those comments. Without hesitating any longer, I called the head office in front of which I theoretically parked my car.

"Good morning! Nice venue you have here! Is the doctor at his office already? Or did he go fetch some water from the well?" I jested.

The voice on the other side went dead silent.

"I don't get it," the medical receptionist said.

As it turned out, I was indeed on the right street and at the right address, but, unfortunately for me, in the wrong town and even in a different province than the one where the laryngologist was seeing his patients.

Fantastic! I thought. The kind receptionist broke into profuse apologies for the error that had crept into the system, and hung up on me.

Disgruntled and discouraged by the fact that I wasted so much time waiting for that appointment, I returned home to reflect on what to do next.

A few hours later, I got an unexpected call. It was the laryngologist himself – the one I didn't have the pleasure of meeting in person. He apologized profusely for the situation and expressed his appreciation for my understanding.

With a distinct image of medical experts already formed in my mind, I was positively surprised at the doctor's attitude and I truly started regretting that our appointment had not come to fruition. I also came to understand where did some of those flattering comments come from. With a modest range of possibilities to choose from, exercising more caution when using the Internet, I decided to book a visit with the laryngologist suggested by my PCP.

A doctor is a doctor, I concluded.

Despite the differences in the range of skills I observed among the medical professionals I met with, I still believed that given that they all specialized in the same field, they all should have the same knowledge. For this reason, with no other objections, I wanted to see any laryngologist as soon as possible to have my most recent issues diagnosed.

Who knows, maybe that's the right direction – to have all the remaining symptoms checked? I thought.

Unfortunately, on the day I was about to have an appointment with the laryngologist covered by my health insurance, I was soon informed that the reason behind most of the symptoms I came in with had hardly anything to do with laryngology. I realized that giving the specialist a recap on my entire medical history was not necessarily a good idea. Upon hearing the reason for my visit, the fairly young and highly attractive laryngologist blinked at me. Her eyes were very similar to those of my Anna's and almost as pretty. Many men would simply forget why they came to see her. Unlike them, I was focused on all my immense suffering, and could see only one thing that her eyes were telling me, "Oh, this will be a tough nut to crack." When the doctor learned what was happening to my ears, she was unable to make a diagnosis; clearly, she had never come across a similar case. Having a multitude of problems that I was impatient to get rid of, I was open to taking any opportunity to discuss them with a doctor. I was well aware that a laryngologist couldn't do much when it comes to my other ailments, but I felt a strong need to tell each doctor about everything regardless, hoping that one of them would stumble upon an idea, or perhaps even recommend me that I should see one of their colleagues. Unfortunately for me, the laryngologist had no colleagues among doctors who could help me, nor did she have any knowledge that would allow her to make my laryngological symptoms go away. Moreover, upon hearing my honest description and my entire medical history including, among others, the appointment with the psychiatrist, she subtly withdrew herself and took a somewhat more distanced approach to me.

"Let's deal with your ears first, shall we?" she suggested.

I could feel that she was completely oblivious as to what could have happened, but I kept urging her for an explanation, nonetheless.

"What's happened to me, doctor?"

"Perhaps the generated pressure was too high indeed, and you've pushed the secretion to the eustachian tubes, thus clogging the canal that regulates pressure in the ears," she replied in a serious tone.

"What tubes?" I asked.

"Eustachian tubes. You can't do that, you can't do that! You mustn't! I'll come up with something in just a minute."

I felt like a small boy who misbehaved. I felt that I had to trust her; maybe it wasn't as bad as it seemed to me.

"I'll prescribe an anti-allergic and anti-inflammatory nasal spray that will help you clean the tubes. Keep applying it for one month straight."

Giving some extra thought to my ears, she added something that for a second woke my heart up from a nap, making it speed up.

"I wonder if you're not starting to develop hearing loss issues by any chance."

I was stunned.

With no more methods that could potentially solve my ear problems at hand, the expert started diagnosing my throat. Having put a headlight on her blonde head, she dazzled me with a warm yellowish light, and put a wooden tongue blade deep into my throat.

"In general, you have chronic pharyngitis," she noticed.

"What's that?"

"It makes you prone to getting bronchitis and tonsillitis more often."

"What should I do then?"

"Take care of yourself and your immunity, and avoid drafts."

Great! Yet again, the magical immunity no one seems to have any exact tips for, I thought.

It seemed to me that all doctors who mention the legendary immunity were like virgins constantly babbling about sex while knowing absolutely nothing about it.

"And what about my abscess?" I asked.

"You have more like a cyst, and not an abscess. It's nothing serious, don't worry about it. It'll go away on its own with time."

I told her about my tumor-related concerns. She quickly corrected me, informing me that it certainly was no cancer and that I had nothing to fear. As for my ears, however, she decided that I should undergo a free hearing test and tympanometry[9] to determine the obstruction of my eustachian tubes, which would then allow her to take further steps to diagnose me.

A hearing test? But my hearing's good. Too good, actually, I thought.

From the very beginning of that appointment, I had a feeling that this expert wasn't sure which test she ought to administer, but I had to agree with her suggestions and wait for the results, regardless. There was nothing else I could do but start testing the prescribed spray for a month and wait for the next visit.

"I'll see you in thirty days. Until that time, please do a hearing test and stick to the spray therapy."

I had no other option but to follow her recommendations and medicate myself with the drugs she prescribed, hoping that they'd

---

[9] Tympanometry – anon-invasive method for evaluating the middle ear.

make my problem go away. Throughout the next month, I was living in hope that the spray would do the trick.

After my appointment with the laryngologist, I started giving more thought to why did she recommend me to test my hearing. The more I pondered on it, the more anxious I made myself feel.

Is it really that I've hurt myself by blowing the air up into my ears? Maybe it was a coincidence and the truth is, I'm going deaf? Is that why all these tests? I thought.

My fear wasn't unwarranted. All these 'paranormal' sensations that wouldn't let me be fueled my concerns. This was not the sole reason to be afraid, though, and being afraid was what made my imaginative mind come up with the worst scenarios.

Since I was born in a family afflicted by various ear-related ailments for generations, I feared the worse - the mentioned hearing loss. In her golden years, in order to hear better, my late grandma had to wear hearing aids. She despised them. Her daughter, my aunt, in her young years started suffering from a horrific condition called tinnitus that would keep tormenting her to no end; she would always hear countless odd sounds generated by her body. Not to mention my gran's siblings who were hearing-impaired in the winter of their lives. Aware of my relatives' ailments and of sharing the same genes, I felt disheartened after seeing the laryngologist. I knew, however, that I was much younger than any of my relatives were when they got struck by these maladies, and I firmly believed that it was impossible that on top of all that I had to endure, hearing loss would become yet another of my problems. Nonetheless, my relentless imagination and persistent stress were ruining my mental health, giving me no space to breathe between all the suspicions made by medical experts. I still didn't fully recover after the immense fear instilled by the radiologist and the neurologist, and now, there was high likelihood that I was developing hearing loss – a dreadful uncertainty I had to wrestle with for a whole month.

Time was passing by inevitably, and my life was turning into a nightmare that was getting worse and worse, from one day to the next. Ever since I can remember, I loved watching movies whose main protagonists were affected by some life tragedy or a lifechanging situation, not necessarily a good one. As most other film buffs, I always looked forward to a happy ending. I didn't think, though, that I could experience such an immense, unwanted change in real life; a change that doesn't last only one hundred and twenty minutes like it does on the screen, unfortunately.

After all, from the time when I started exercising and challenging myself at the gym, I felt indestructible. I was giving that "nothing will break me" vibe. Although inside, I still had a deep hope for a swift happy ending to my story, I had to remain patient, as it seemed that my problems were only about to begin.

Having undergone the examination and the treatment with aerosol steroids, one of the longest months of my life ended when I rushed to attend my second appointment with the medical expert. As it turned out, my hearing test results were excellent, so the doctor shifted her focus to the obstruction of eustachian tubes.

"Your hearing is good, so we have to seek the cause elsewhere," she said.

Feeling increasingly overwhelmed by all the sensations that my body had been experiencing on a daily basis, I didn't even have the strength or the will to comment on how easy it was for her to make such a striking impact on these last days of my life. Now, changing her theory and diagnosis in just a blink of an eye, as if it was a vinyl record, she turned a completely different music on, and my emotions started calming down to the rhythm.

"How is it, did the spray do the job?" she asked me lightheartedly.

"Sadly, it didn't; it seems it's even worse, doctor," I said.

With nothing more to add, the doctor scheduled my next appointment preceded by tympanometry, which was scheduled one hour before our next meeting, that is, the third one.

"Then please take the spray for one month more and I'll see you in three months at my office in the hospital," she wrapped it up.

In this situation, no one would be content with the fact there was still no answer as to what was happening in my ears, for I had to wait even longer than I expected to be further diagnosed.

Driven by the ailments whose presence was getting more and more noticeable in my life from one day to the next, I couldn't just wait idly. I knew I had to act and that I couldn't waste time waiting for the spray to magically start working. Therefore, I decided to take the risk and, despite my previous failure, rummage through the internet again in search of a laryngology expert who would be the female doctor's senior in terms of his rank and experience. This is how I found a laryngology professor who had positive reviews from his patients. That physician not only held more titles, but was also twice the age of the young female specialist. Although my attitude towards doctors in old age was still ambivalent, I was glad that this time, I stumbled upon a top-rank laryngologist whose specialty, as it turned out, was otology.[10] Since I had never had the pleasure of meeting a medical expert who had this many titles, I believed that, being an ear expert with a *professor* before his name, he'd solve my problems. However, I soon realized that an academic degree doesn't always go hand in hand with infallibility, omniscience, and experience in a given field.

Although back in college, I did have some professors who were performing various occupations ad each of them looked like a regular Joe working in a warehouse or at a gas station, I'd always associate a medical professor with a tiny, balding man with a huge nose. I imagined a small charismatic figure with a voluminous gray mustache concealing his entire mouth, distorting his every word. My imaginary scientist would always wear too large glasses with thick eyepieces that made his eyes look several times bigger, his oversized white lab coat fitting him like his elder brother's clothes would. Maybe I was too eager to meet a doctor who'd look like a crazy scientist I knew from American movies, who'd know the answers to everything. Maybe I believed that all these stories and characters were modelled on real-life ones. I can't recall that, but one thing is certain: the professor I went to with high hopes for getting help looked nothing like a medi-

---

[10] Otology – a branch of otolaryngology that deals with diagnosing and treating medical conditions of the ear.

cal doctor holding many titles; what's more, he didn't have any charisma that would make him stand out. Somewhat reminiscent of the long-dead movie star Lee Marvin, the elderly, gray-haired man invited me into his office with a swift motion of his hand, letting me know that he was in a great hurry. He asked me to take a sit in an armchair that looked like the one at the dentist's. I sat there comfortably, about to start my monologue, as I'd always done before. In one moment, he put a damper on it.

"Please, tell me, what's bringing you to me, sir?" the professor said.

"I'm trying, you cut me off," I replied.

With his vast experience, the professor probably sensed that I'd like to talk and perhaps tell him more that he was willing to listen to, so he asked me about the specifics. I soon realized that I won't get the chance to tell everything that recently affected my life and how my health was changing. For this reason, I decided to start on a different note.

"Something's bad going on with my ears, professor. Please help me."

Having given him a recap of the whole thing in just a few sentences, including what was happening with my ears, I was glad to hear that Professor Lee Marvin would perform a quick test. He took a small flashlight that was reminiscent of a silver ballpoint pen and flashed the light into my ears, peeking and examining my auricula. Then, using a wooden spatula, he took a look into my throat.

"I don't see anything here, young man! Everything's fine. You say something's moving in there?!" he asked.

"Yeah, it's moving and all, you know what it's like, when something's up between the teeth, causing discomfort?" I replied, referring once again to my auricular experience.

"It'll pass. It happens sometimes, I think you have to wait a few weeks and it will all pass. Is there anything else?"

I was astonished by how quickly the professor completed the test, an examination that wasn't any different from that performed by the first internist at hand, somewhat disappointed and aware that there's no point counting on his help.

"Yes, there's something more," I replied. "What should I do with the cyst inside my throat?"

"A cyst? What cyst?" he asked, surprised.

"Well, you did look inside my mouth," I chipped in, just as baffled.

"I didn't notice any. Please open it again."

I wasn't surprised that an academic cannot determine what was the reason behind the internal symptoms in my ears by just looking at my auricula. The structure of the inner ear that I knew back from school simply wouldn't allow that. However, I was surprised that the physician didn't notice the cyst on my tonsil, the size of which was close to that of the ring finger nail and was still growing.

"It's really there," the renowned laryngologist said, without even showing that he did slip up. "Please don't be concerned about that either, it'll disappear in a few weeks along with the ear issues that are troubling you."

Looking at my body and my face, which on the one hand was sparsely covered with regular-sized moles, the doctor's attention was drawn to one particular situated on my neck that was slightly bigger than the others.

"Please don't meddle your thoughts with your ears or the cyst, young man. I'm more concerned with the mole on your neck."

Surprised by the laryngologist's comment, who stepped beyond the scope of his field of expertise, I said, " I don't fully get it. What do you mean?"

"That mole looks to me like an early form of cancer. Please go test it. On my part, that's all, " he concluded.

The visit at the professor's was one of the quickest I had the privilege to experience. Though it only took five minutes, it was the longest and the most expensive five minutes in my entire journey towards explaining the cause of my ailments. In my disappointed, disillusioned eyes, the academic, like the arrogant pick-pocketer from my high school years, got the two hundred *zlotys* he earned in no time; in turn, I still had to struggle with the lack of any answer to the questions that were haunting me.

Despite the slip-up he had made by failing to notice the 'ball' that was slowly taking more and more space inside my throat month by month, his diagnosis made me feel more at ease. I hoped that a specialist as renowned as he surely wouldn't be mistaken.

Already accustomed to bad news that I used to get from medical experts, at first I wasn't concerned by the mole the laryngologist mentioned about.

I had a feeling that the doctor, who was already in old age, simply decided to mention the mole to keep his face, so that he could give me any diagnosis. Shortly afterwards, I decided to verify his thesis.

It is easy to work out that after each meeting with medical staff we were all losing our sanity. Just as bad I did, my loved ones wanted me to finally feel good and find someone who'd answer most of the questions that were affecting us all. Every time I sought help and answers, I'd get none at all or, alternatively, I'd get the worst suggestions and suspicions that were destroying us all mentally from within. Despite the fact that each time every medical expert was proven wrong in his or her diagnosis, every expert opinion or evaluation was destructive enough to leave a long-lasting mark on my family members and myself. It is said that time heals all wounds. I think that it all depends on a given situation. In my case, each passing day undoubtedly taught me patience and humility. Instead of treating my wounds, the physicians I was in contact with were simply adding fuel to the fire with their erroneous diagnoses, leaving us all with extra problems and no clue as to what was happening.

"What if that man is right? Maybe all my issues really do stem from moles? Does it mean that I can have a cancer?!" thoughts of this sort wouldn't leave me be.

Roughly at the same time, my sister could learn firsthand how difficult it was in the 21st century to obtain an accurate, reliable diagnosis. She also experienced a nightmare that healthcare professionals can easily put anyone in. Though we were very different and we didn't agree in all matters at all times, we shared the same passion. We both loved sports and forcing our bodies to do physical effort. Unlike me, Paulina was an enthusiast of aerobics. Although the nature of these exercises was not as invasive as strength training that I was involved in, my sister started feeling strong pain in the lumbar spine area, which could be attributed to her physical activity.

Seeing on my example, if anything, how difficult and time-consuming it is to get a thorough and accurate diagnosis, she decided not to wait any longer and rush to get help from health professionals. Just as I had, she started seeing one doctor after another. Sent away empty-handed, with no accurate diagnosis, she wondered from one internist and orthopedist to another to eventually come across what would seem a competent female neurologist who immediately referred her for an x-ray of the spine. However, she soon was left disenchanted when, having read the x-ray image of my sister's spine, the medical specialist concluded that the image showed no pathological changes that could cause the pain she was experiencing. She didn't suggest any other, more thorough form of examination and failed to recommend further treatment right at the very beginning.

"Can't we do some more detailed MRI scans? I'm really in awful pain, doctor," Paulina said.

"Doing MRI scans is pointless in your case, because x-ray imaging is also very accurate and I see no need to do so. I think that your lifestyle and the stress that affects us all can be the reason behind your ailments," the female doctor concluded.

My sister got some muscle relaxants that were said to help her ease the pain she was struggling with. After the visit, with her lower back still aching, she immediately went to a drug store to purchase the medications she was prescribed. A kind clerk that my sister would often speak to asked her, "Paulina, have you taken a longer break from work?"

"I haven't, why?"

"The drugs you were prescribed are powerful and addictive antidepressants, and usually, most people who take them sleep much longer."

"Antidepressants? How come?" Paulina asked, flabbergasted.

My sister was gravely embarrassed. She decided to not wait any longer and have the MRI scan done despite having to pay for it. To obtain a reliable result, she asked for a contrast[11] MRI, which was more expensive than the regular one.

Employees advised her having more expensive testing done, stressing that a contrast agent is administered only when a radiologist or a neurologist is unable to accurately read a previously generated image.

"It makes no sense, really. If you have anything down there, it will surely be visible without contrast. We administer it very rarely," one of the employees tried to calm my sister down and persuade her to ditch that idea.

Despite the fact that it was a private facility, such testing required getting in line, too.

There came a day when Paulina was about to learn what the reason behind her pain in the lumbar spine was. Unfortunately, she didn't expect it to be one of the worst days of her life. The day when she'd start asking herself "What next?", "Why me?"

Just like me, she had to face her thoughts, take a step on the borderline between life and death and rearrange it all in her head; and all that because of one sentence the radiologist said.

"Paulina, I'm very sorry, but I've found several diffused neoplastic foci in your spine area. This is no good news for you, but in order to confirm my diagnosis, we need to have you tested again by giving you an intravenous contrast agent. I'll see you in two weeks," the radiologist said.

Regardless of all the drama my sister and everyone close to her had to go through, not only until the second test result was confirmed, but living with the awareness that we both were wrestling with something that shouldn't happen to young people like the two of us at all, Paulina was continuously haunted by yet another issue.

---

[11] Contrast – also called a contrast agent; a chemical substance used in diagnostic radiography for performing examinations such as an MRI scan.

"I get that you'll cover the cost of the next contrast-enhanced testing?" she asked, reminding that she had requested such testing be done the first time, having bad feeling about it.

"Unfortunately not, miss. You have to cover the costs for the second testing and the intravenous contrast," a medical receptionist informed her.

The two weeks spent on waiting for the additional diagnosis of my sister's lumbar spine only added to the tragedy we had been all experiencing for a longer time. Having learned that we must be patient, we were waiting for the same situation to happen all over again, overwhelmed by helplessness. Meanwhile, I managed to get an appointment with a surgical oncologist who would check my moles, particularly the one on my neck that made the professor very concerned. As it turned out, having examined my moles meticulously, the oncologist concluded I had no reason to be concerned and that none of them had to be removed or put under special observation. One load off my mind.

There came the day we all had been waiting for, although this time, after doing the highly costly testing again, Paulina had to wait for the result and the radiologist's interpretation of the image for a week. The day she received the result made us realize once again the great extent to which a single incompetent individual can affect others' lives. Yet again, we were all going through a déjà vu. It turned out that the person who interpreted my sister's first image took a shadow cast by internal organs for tumors, thus giving my sister the longest three weeks of her life. The newly performed contrast-enhanced test showed hernia that was responsible for the pain my sister had been struggling with for a longer period of time. With this information, Paulina got back to her neurologist and showed her the result, telling her solely how big a mistake she had made to assume that she was experiencing the pain due to ubiquitous stress. The expert didn't even show for one moment that she was ashamed.

We're living in a world where suffering of every older man is supposed to be something natural. Though malaise, discomfort, or pain among the elderly can have many reasons, the answer and the suggestion of the healthcare staff is usually very simple – old age. I couldn't comprehend why when it comes to young people fighting various issues medical doctors who had taken the Hippocratic Oath would only see issues with mental health and stress which according to them in many cases is the main or sometimes the sole reason for health problems among the youth.

Hippocrates would turn in his grave! I thought.

The key idea underlying the Hippocratic Oath is obviously *Primum non nocere*, that is, "first, do no harm". The Oath also states that each doctor shall help those in need without accepting any payment from the ill. Nowadays, not accepting any remuneration from the ill for some reason would be impossible but the key message of the code should be a priority to every medical practitioner. My experience throughout the recent years showed that healthcare staff lacked knowledge, competence; what is most important, I noticed a tendency to diagnose patients with mental illnesses. I often had a feeling that many doctors missed their calling. My case or the example of my sister show how easy it is to do harm to a young person, albeit not physical but primarily mental.

Although for years, the wording of the ancient oath was transformed and developed in line with contemporary standards, which doesn't change the fact that until this day, every doctor vows to counteract suffering, prevent diseases, always strive to expand their medical knowledge and, most of all, guard their dignity and not to tarnish it in any way. The way I see it, the experts I had contact with did nothing to ease my suffering and their notorious recommendations of psychiatric treatment made not only towards me due to their lack of ideas and proper knowledge, they were tarnishing their dignity and the title of a doctor repeatedly, as I could see myself while continuing to look for the reasons behind my deteriorating health.

Nothing brings as much joy as finding the reason behind your pain or ailment that has been tormenting you for a longer time. Paulina succeeded although it wasn't easy. As soon as she was diagnosed with hernia, she was subjected to rehabilitation therapy. In my case, all the symptoms were still one great unknown; to make things worse, fate took away my last source of endorphins and what was still making me enjoy life to some extent.

For some time I had a feeling that the lack of motivation to continue my passion was not entirely due to feeling low in general because of inexplicable symptoms that had been tormenting my body each day. My family and healthcare employees were trying to convince me that I was exhausted or stressed out. I felt that it was imply impossible and that something bas was slowly annihilating me. Despite the suffering I had experienced and the fact that my training sessions got significantly less intense, thus not giving me the usual drive to undertake further action and up the ante, my self-discipline and routine wouldn't allow me to forego physical activity completely. The fondness for strength training that I had developed over the previous several years became an essential part of my life, without which I couldn't imagine neither the present nor the future. Somewhere in my subconsciousness I hoped that I'd keep lifting heavy weights until the end of my days, and continue to build my physique to no end. That was the plan. As one of the best fighters in the history of boxing, the legendary Mike Tyson used to say, "Everyone has a plan until they get punched in the mouth." Although I tried my best, there came a day I involuntarily got out of sync with my gym routine; the day I got 'hit' so bad I couldn't do anything about it.

Like any other great effort, I began that one from a short yet intense warmup. None of my present training routines was like the one before. Watching my body reflected in the mirror evoked inside me a train of thoughts inexplicably difficult to put in words. They took on the form of questions such as, "How come I'm alive?", "What am I living for?" Getting down to training on a bench serving for lifting a barbell above my chest, I felt even more discomfort than before. The pressure I was struggling with filled my head; sitting and slowly leaning my torso backwards to take the proper reclining position on the bench, I felt as if I was submersing my head under water, like a masked diver descending undersea. Hearing my characteristic mode of breathing, as if I was indeed diving wearing a mask, I got exceptionally concerned. Seeing nothing but the white ceiling and my hands on the shiny barbell, I felt uneasy; it didn't feel like my extremities were mine. I became even more overwhelmed. Regardless of it all, I continued the training. Having completed my session, I realized that I was getting swept off my feet by a feeling I had never experienced. Suddenly, my head got flooded with an odd sensation of being squeezed, as if there was a steel ring closing in on my forehead. It was as if the upper part of my head started going numb, while my forehead felt as if one of the cast iron weights of a dozen pounds that were fitted on the barbell got stuck to it. The discomfort in my neck that forced me to constantly move it around in all directions became even more noticeable, thus adding to the bothering sensation of high pressure and tightness in the area that connects the spinal cord to the medulla. I was experiencing the least pleasant sensations in that very spot. The feeling of having a steel ring closing in on my head and the very subjective feeling of utter discomfort in my neck stupefied my brain, rendering it unable to focus and completely confused for a few days. The only thing I was thinking of was to lie down on the side and place a cushion folded into a cube under my neck so that having identified the right spot I could get some relief by pressing on it. Thinking that it might have been a one-time experience, I repeated the training routine a couple of days later. Sadly, it turned out that from that moment on, every instance of doing some physical effort was ending up the same way, usually costing me seventy-two hours of some inexplicable extra intense suffering. I started linking these two sensations with an excessive load that I initially mistaken for the cause of my new ailments. Despite the torture I was going through, my ego and strong training routine wouldn't allow me to even think of ditching weightlifting. I hoped that if nothing else, I could just keep up the results I had worked for over the years by using my own body weight. Unfortunately, as it turned out, every time I did even ten reps of regular pushups, these horrible sensations would strike twofold.

It was only then that it could be said that I started getting a neurosis everyone were so eager to diagnose me with from the very beginning. I was unable to do any physical effort anymore, as it usually exacerbated my symptoms. With each day, I was closer to a mental breakdown. The absence of any opportunity to engage in my passion of many years was taking a toll. From a young, strong person who dedicated each and every free moment to keep his body busy and do physical exercises engaging nearly all the furniture in the house, I was slowly turning into a train wreck. From that moment on, the chairs I had been using for pushups at any possible moment spent in the kitchen, for instance, when waiting for a meal to be served, became merely something to sit on. The pull-up bar I used to 'hone' my back muscles on turned into a shirt hanger, whereas the entire strength training equipment I had at home found itself in the attic, gathering dust.

"Baby I want you like the roses want the rain, You know I need you like a poet needs the pain. And I would give anything..." These are the words one of my favorite music artists Jon Bon Jovi addressed to a woman in one of his songs. At that stage of my life, such a proclamation of love for my fiancée would very rarely come out of my mouth. Anna felt she couldn't win with my passion I got lost in to think about anything else than my suffering, which I needed back then like a man needs water to live. She, in turn, needed me, and hence, the lyrics penned by the artist were the most accurate reflection of the state she found herself in. Although I repeatedly swore to her that I'd stop lifting weights, since that, too, was considered a potential cause of my issues, I never kept my word. Although I despise lies like probably no one else does now, I was lying to Anna. Since my boyhood, I've been taught that it was something a man mustn't do and I'd always been overly truthful; however, to satisfy my desire, I lied for the first time. I couldn't just ditch my passion overnight. I knew that there was nothing my fiancée wanted more than to stop me from hurting myself even more. I promised her I'd stop weightlifting only if she managed to lift a barbell of two hundred and twenty pounds even a little while on her back. Aware of how big a load that was and knowing cases of bulky buddies who lacked the strength to do anything more than to lift a barbell that heavy only a couple of inches up from its rack, I made a deal with Anna that was a despicable ploy. I was convinced that my petite girlfriends of a hundred pounds couldn't lift a weigh that heavy with her willowy arms even for a fraction of an inch. That would be simply impossible.

"If you manage to even yank these two hundred and twenty pounds a little, I promise I'll stop," I said.

"Very well!" Anna replied with an unusual glint in her eyes, as if she knew she could handle that.

She lied down on the bench under the two-hundred-and-twenty-pound-heavy barbell. Having watched me doing that exercise many times, she positioned her body accordingly and proceeded to undergo a test that was about to jeopardize my training. With extraordinary faith, self-denial, and a request hidden deep in her heart that I wouldn't fulfil with no sacrifice on her part, Anna momentarily did the impossible, lifting the load over one inch over the rack. I was stunned.

"Here you go. Now you must keep your word," she said.

With no idea what to say and still believing that what I had just seen didn't happen, I managed to mumble, "That's what it looks like."

Either way, I was unable to keep my word and continued to exercise. My weekly training routine, which I had been practicing for years, was stronger than me. I wasn't addicted to physical effort, but I was certainly close to becoming addicted. However, there came a time when I had to pay for not keeping up my promise I had made to my sweetheart. My body decided for me, and I regretted that I wasn't the one to make that decision on the day I promised her to change.

I had to accept my condition and have faith that I'd soon find the cause of the symptoms that were ruining me. And yet, I couldn't stand that at our company, my dad was doing all the heavy lifting for me. Seeing him and my mom carrying heavy packages, I was simply ashamed of myself. Feeling as if I was handicapped, embarrassed by my helplessness and the awareness of what the consequences of doing any physical effort would be, I was slowly driven into a mental breakdown.

Lifting goods at our family business wasn't the only duty I was supposed to do. There was also mental work and customer service. The time I had previously largely spent weightlifting could now be dedicated to putting more effort at the company. Although I was trying my best, the results weren't always good. My physical condition and, for some time, also my mental condition were making it all tremendously hard for me, pulling the rug from under me every day. I couldn't handle my own self, I couldn't handle trivial tasks many of which could be solved in a matter of minutes, but took me several hours to do so. Although my dad, who was working with me, tried to understand what I felt, he also expected the job to be well done, yet he had to correct it himself after me. Our discussions and exchange of opinions often ended in a fight, my annoyance bringing up inexplicable aggression within me, which was making me throw a plate at dinner or simply punch what was within my reach at a given moment. I have never hurt any of my loved ones, but often after meeting a wall, my hands needed a few days to regenerate.

"What does the other one's face look like?" a doctor at a hospital asked me once when diagnosing my hand.

"There was no 'other one'," I replied shortly, having neither no idea for nor a desire to engage in a needless conversation with him, assuming that he wouldn't be able to help me.

"Yeah, sure!" he smirked.

I didn't know what was happening to me, but I could feel it was yet another symptom in the entire chain of my issues. Never before had I been explosive, let alone never had I given vent to my anger in such a way. Over time, I started losing control over myself too easily. More and more often, I'd get irritated with ordinary everyday situations that I had handled perfectly until that point. Deserving none of my increasingly often explosions that were oftentimes a form of shifting bad energy onto her, Anna was taking it all on her delicate chin, suppressing her negative feelings, hoping she'd soon get her old partner back.

Sadly, the stronger these forces inexplicable to us all were pulling me down to the bottom, the less I was able to handle the emotions and the stress that undoubtedly stemmed from the symptoms that were showing up more and more intense. I was even more aware that I was turning into someone else than I used to be. With the entire burden of bad sensations that were like a pesky shadow following me around at all times, it didn't take much to fill my body to the brim with aggression that I had never known before.

This is the picture of my personality, suddenly overtaken by the 'demon' of anger in just a matter of minutes, that my mom could experience on the day we went together for a private appointment with an expert in orthopedics.

Finally, there came a day when the visit I was awaiting for quite a long time was about to take place and I was going to learn what was going on with my groin, the painful pins in which wouldn't leave me be. Before we arrived at the meeting with the experienced surgeon who was recommended to us, well known in the medical and orthopedical circles, we stopped at a hypermarket for some minor groceries. I parked the car on the parking lot by the store. I always try do that most meticulously, so that the vehicle fits between white lines marked on the paved surface. Ever since I can remember, I've always been a reasonable person whose actions were largely well thought-out before I performed them. Since childhood, I've been guided by the principle, "Before you do something, think about others," and thus I've never been creating a reality that would be convenient for me.

For this reason, a thing as mundane as parking the car by the store, for instance, had to be done most precisely, so that I didn't take up another driver's space. Sadly, with every next day, I could feel the level of my reason declining. I was getting more and more tired and unstable. Imbalanced, easily distracted by anything, I found the key aspects of my personality were slowly disappearing. On that day, a breath of fresh air in my mind allowed me to park my vehicle perfectly, ideally in the middle between the marked lines. At the very same time, on the next spot to my left, a silver-and-gold Honda Civic drove up.

As soon as the car stopped by the store, the woman behind the wheel turned the engine off. The passenger seat was occupied by another female with long blonde locks, wearing characteristic angular, disproportionally big glasses. Seeing the women inside the car enjoying themselves, as their reactions and loud giggles suggested, I restrained from opening my door first. I imagined our front doors high-fiving each other, and so I momentarily stopped myself from acting on impulse. My intuition didn't fail me this time, either. At that very moment, the woman decided to swiftly get out of her car and, paying no attention to my vehicle, pushed her door full open absentmindedly, banging it hard into my left side. I'd get that whole situation if the lady apologized to me for her carelessness, having realized she caused damage unintentionally. After all, things like that happen all the time at various parking lots. One time, a man who was in fact moving his car backwards on the same parking lot in heavy rain that obscured vision for both of us, didn't stop until he touched my door. Fortunately for me, having done not a single scratch, he stepped out and apologized for what he had done. It could have happened to everyone. Sadly, in this case, the circumstances were completely different, showing me how malicious a person can be. Hoping that the woman would unstuck her door from mine and step out of the car, at least acting all terrified or shocked by what she had done, I experienced one of the biggest flabbergasting moments of my life. When the paint job on each of our vehicles got smashed together, the women were still laughing boisterously. Even the pretty blonde, who to me seemed to look a bit like Cameron Diaz with her hair all curly, shut her door and, looking deep into my eyes, gave me a bright, white smile to then head towards the store as if nothing happened.

"Did you see that? That's freaking nuts! No, no, no. That just can't be," embarrassed, slowly growing more and more angry, I knew I had to do something about it.

I left the car and quickly followed the women.

"Hey! Hey! Women!" I shouted.

They stopped and turned my way. Their smiles and bubbly, joyful demeanor vanished into thin air, their faces in a pout that said, "Beat it, man!".

"You hit me with your door," I said in a loud voice.

"So what?" she replied.

If my bite force expressed in pounds was equal to that of wild animals, I'd crush my teeth to pieces.

"What do you mean, 'so what'? Is that how you always open the door, damaging others' property?"

Having clearly no desire to listen to my monologue and feeling completely no responsibility for what she had done, the woman swiftly retrieved a wallet and pulled out a fifty-*zloty* bill.

"Okay, man, take it and get lost," she held her hand with the money towards me.

"You must be kidding me!" I replied, looking at her with pity.

"God in Heavens! Don't bother," she and her friend turned away and rushed towards the store.

"Give yourself a break, son. There's no point letting people with no brains get your back up. You've pointed out her mistake, she must feel stupid already," my mom said.

In my old days, I'd certainly let it go, or maybe get infected with their bubbliness that was surely the air inside their car. However, on that day, I felt I couldn't overcome my annoyance. I was being punished by my own body on a daily basis; my annoyance level was at 90 percent already, and the situation at hand made it go ten percent up. That was enough to make me demand justice ardently and ruthlessly. And so, enraged, I rushed to the store and, having found the women in-between alleys, I didn't let it go.

"Get off me, man," the blonde said, just as angry.

"You fucking hit my car, woman, and you can't even say sorry!" completely irritated with the situation, I cursed in a loud voice to stress the seriousness of it all and emphasize my grave embarrassment.

Yet again, she retrieved a fifty-*zloty* bill, as if she had a predetermined price for damaging others' vehicles on a regular basis.

"Take it and get lost!" she repeated.

A few people gathered around us, watching the entire incident and our fight.

"I don't want your money! I won't leave until you apologize."

"We won't apologize for anything! What a snob!" the blonde's friend, the driver, chipped in.

Feeling that I was tackling a really difficult case, I started giving up slowly.

"Let it go, son. You see what kind of people they are," my mom added.

Suddenly, a bulky tall man appeared among the onlookers, who turned out to be an employee of the store and the blonde's acquaintance. Having no clue about how all this quarrel started, which must have looked comically from the outside perspective, he decided to play the hero.

"Leave the ladies alone, youngster, and beat it, or I'll throw you out," he said, touching my chest with his index finger.

Despite my discontinued training, my body still looked as if I came back from the gym that morning, making me more bold. I was aware that the guy was twice my weight, but overtaken by aggression, I felt extremely self-confident.

"Touch me one more time!" I snapped. Forgetting about the women who damaged by car in an instant, I added angrily, "Bro, I'm waiting for you outside the store!"

Having let the women off the hook, I left my somewhat shocked mom at the store and went outside. The hero didn't turn up. Maybe that was for the better, as he was two times bigger than me, so it could've ended not pretty for me, and, after all, we were in a hurry to see the orthopedist. One of the onlookers turned up, though. It was an elderly gentleman, hunched and gray-haired, who found me after I left the store.

"Let it go, young man! You'll have worse situations than that in your life. No point wasting strength on brainless people. Better use it for something else. Maybe you'll need it soon," he said as if he knew me well and walked away, leaving me in thoughts.

Although my mom agreed I was right, I knew she was highly concerned about my attitude, extreme stubbornness and fierceness. Never before had she witnessed me acting like that. Having cooled off a bit and calmed my emotions down, we headed to meet the surgeon. Throughout our way, I could see the face of the woman who damaged my front door before my eyes.

Where do I know her from? I wondered, knowing that I had dealt with her somewhere else.

As fate would have it, we managed to get to the orthopedist's office at the scheduled time. We were prepared that the hour a patient is scheduled for is not always the exact time when the appointment with a doctor starts. Usually, the specified time is a starting point and a longer wait in line may be involved. And so was the case this time. After an hour spent in the waiting room, we entered the doctor's office. Though many physicians could find it odd that a young, fit, quite good-looking adult man comes to see a doctor accompanied by his mom, to me, it was completely meaningless. Aware of how absentminded I can get and how blocking my lack of focus can be, I was glad my mom had no objections to come with me. It was very important to her that she could present and describe the symptoms that were tormenting me most reliably to everyone who could help me. I was very grateful for her company and assistance.

Aside from the obvious knowledge aimed at helping patients, I judged the class of medical doctors not only by their manners towards the patient, but primarily by the way they respected his time, since specialists would often make little of it. On that day, once again, we fell prey to our time being downplayed highly untactfully, which let us know that it was us who were not respecting the doctor's time, and, what's worse, we were wasting it.

"How can I help you?" the elderly man asked us.

Still hoping that age goes hand in hand with knowledge and rich experience that might be the key to the several-year-long mystery of my issues, we accepted the offer of an acquaintance who recommended that doctor to us as one of the most prominent orthopedists. Bearing a cross of unexplained sensations that were changing my life, we believed all this time that finally, we'd meet someone who'd dedicate a little more time to me, and transform himself into the detective we all wanted so badly. Feeling the utter hopelessness of the situation and, most of all, helplessness, each time my loved ones and I were fooling ourselves that some of the experts in various medical fields I was seeing would dig out in the archives of his knowledge some information, even back from the time of his Ph.D. studies and specialization, that would somehow give me the right direction. Unfortunately, most of them didn't even want to try and reply in any way. The answer was one and the same, every time: "I'm an expert in this field, and if you have a sore throat, please go see a laryngologist." During that visit, for a second my mom and I felt that for the first time, there finally was someone who knew just the right person from the medical circle who'd be able to help me.

"I have a great problem, doctor. I don't know where to start," I said.

"Preferably start from where it hurts you."

And so I did, providing a detailed, several-sentence-long description of the sensation of painful pins in my groin.

"When I move my leg, very often I feel as if someone was putting a knife in my groin! I'm afraid to crouch because when I get up, I never know when this horrible pain will strike me. I try not to sit in the way you do, because I know how it ends."

At the very moment I stopped, my highly concerned mom chipped in, "But tell the doctor what else is constantly bothering you. Maybe the doctor will help us and know where we should go. Please, sir."

Fearing that the orthopedist would look at me like the other physicians who suggested psychiatric treatment had, I decided not to tell everything from the beginning to the end. I decided to simply mention other symptoms that I was having every day.

"For some time now, I can't handle physical effort, as each time, it makes me disconnected from reality, unable to focus, my head gets all numb and so heavy I struggle to keep it up. I feel great discomfort in my neck, which make me constantly try get rid of it and move it around in all directions. The acute, prickly pain in my groin that reminds me of a pin aside, I suffer from occasional prickly sensations also in my head, which distracts me momentarily. I'm extremely worn out, and the sight of my hands alone seems strange to me. When I'm talking to you, something very bad makes each sound that comes out my mouth cause an alien object to move inside my ears, or at least that's how I feel it. That's just some of my ailments. Today, I come to you mainly with the groin. I am aware that being an orthopedist, it is possible that you're unable to help me. However, if you know another expert specializing in a different field, we'd be very grateful."

For a moment, I had a feeling the orthopedist dozed off while listening to my nagging, as sitting with his legs crossed, he didn't even move a bit. This was evidenced by white light reflected on his polished black shoe up in the air, which I was keeping my eye on throughout that time. With his arms crossed on the chest, his head slightly tilted forward, I assumed the doctor fell asleep.

"I can help you!" he said suddenly in a louder voice, lifting his tilted head up towards me.

Glad to hear that, my mom and I looked at each other, smiling, with much hope. Our eyes instantly went bright at that good news. We looked at the doctor, waiting what he'd suggest.

"Vis-à-vis my office, there's a door. Behind it, there's my good friend. We both work at the Military Medical Academy. He's a great professional who works with many soldiers who have various conditions, such as phantom pain. Judging from your physique and symptoms, I can tell there's much in common. My friend is an excellent psychiatrist and I think he'll certainly help you," he said. Casting a glance at his watch, he rapidly got up off his chair and added, "Forgive me, but I can't help you. On your way out, please let the next person in line in," he concluded.

Slightly numb, tired, and deconcentrated, I was already accustomed to receiving no help from doctors and to their standard way of sending me away to a "man whisperers". I saw through the orthopedist's intentions and rushed to the exit. This time, however, it was my mom who got driven over the edge. Certainly the incident by the store had filled her cup of negative emotions, and the surgeon's behavior filled it to the brim, making her snap under the growing pressure.

"You're being ridiculous!" she said in a loud voice. "We've waited over an hour only to leave after five minutes without you giving any diagnosis of my son's problem with the groin? Sure, it's better to claim everything's up in the young man's head! Does my son look like a soldier to you? We won't leave until you look at his leg!" she added.

I looked at my mom and thought, *Nice, mom!*

Somewhat confused, the orthopedist said, "Alright then. Calm down, lady. I'll examine your son's groin."

He told me to lie down on the couch and then he approached me. He was placing his palms on my groins, trying to sense with his fingers if there was anything wrong that could have affected my sensations. Then, having lifted my legs, he was moving them to see in which specific moment I was feeling the pain. Unfortunately for me, during that test the pain didn't appear even once.

"You're fine. You're a healthy young man. I think you just need to work on your head. Your groins are alright, there's nothing more I can do for you. I really can't give you more of my time; there are other patients waiting," he wrapped it up.

Sadly, that was what most of our visits with medical doctors were like, and I was still looking up to them for help with much hope for success. We all realized quite late that for some reason, I was at a disadvantage. Perhaps it was my fit body and the appearance of an average healthy man that didn't let doctors think things could be different than their gut told them. Or maybe I was just gravely unlucky, and ended up seeing morons and not true descendants of Hippocrates? Perhaps that's just how it was meant to be, and I was walking a path that I was destined to take? "Remember, son, that everything in this world happens for a reason," my mom would say. "Maybe there's a reason why you have to suffer so much," she'd add. My mom's words were not evident to me; after all, back then, they weren't evident to her, either.

We were all asking ourselves hundreds of questions notoriously. What was happening to me? Why are they referring me to a psychiatrist? Why there's no help anywhere? Be it Dr. Armani or other internists I was seeing again with some new symptoms after some time passed, they all considered me a cry-baby and a hypochondriac who made it his goal to pay frequent visits at an out-patient clinic asking for any tests possible. Quite often yet reluctantly, they'd give me referrals for basic blood and urine tests the results of which were very good every single time. It was yet another proof and, at the same time, a reason why I was treated like an individual who was feeling sorry about his uneventful life, desperately looking to diagnose himself with diseases and visiting medical clinics as a hobby.

Being increasingly more aware and educated, as I was online at all times, I asked PCPs for more comprehensive blood tests that would determine the level of some vitamins or elements in my body, which if low would suggest a deficiency and probably some diseases I was developing, or maybe could just serve as the reason behind some of the symptoms I had been struggling with every day. The more often I visited my internists with yet another suspicion arising from playing the role of a detective by necessity, the stronger I felt about their negative approach to my case. I even had to demand a blood test as seemingly mundane as erythrocyte sedimentation rate (ESR). Having seen the large cyst bulking inside my throat, every medical doctor should immediately order such a test; at least that's what I believed. Sadly, I couldn't get all the blood tests that could help me solve that extraordinary, painful mystery done at the regional clinic. As doctors informed me, not all of them were covered by the national health insurance program. As usually, what's relatively inexpensive can be offered to people, but the more expensive things you have to buy yourself. And so, there was nothing else I could do but get expensive tests done, covering the costs myself at private laboratories. There were moments when I regretted having spent several hundred *zlotys* for doctors who were comparing me to wartime heroes suffering loss of legs or undergoing persistent, post-traumatic stress. In moments like these I wondered who needs a psychiatrist more, me or them? After all, I could spend the money I had paid for private appointments that brought me no good on costly blood tests otherwise not covered by medical insurance in my country despite my health insurance contributions settled on a monthly basis.

I was still asking myself questions, why it is me who has to act and seek the reasons behind my disease? The answer to this question was very simple – because only I knew that I had one.

One of the hardest tests I had to go through in my life so far was the role of a healthy boy I had to keep playing every day. Carrying the burden of all the negative ailments on my back was not easy. Though I wasn't capable of sharing my suffering with others and everything I felt was highly subjective and only mine, sometimes, over time, some "errors in my system" could be observed. My exhausted face aside, which was showing my pain repeatedly, when talking with me you could notice that I'd leave out some words or say oxymorons. "It's raining on my rain," I told my friend while pointing at a bicycle that was getting all wet in the rain. I also said "I've mistake a mistake" instead of, "I've made a mistake".

Surely everyone happens to mix up words like that from time to time. In my case, however, this had never occurred before, but now, it became a permanent element of my speech. It was a sign that something really bad was developing inside my body. More and more often, I'd leave out not only words but also subjects I was addressing. That, too, happens to all of us – "What was I talking about?" Each of us happened to forget the topic in a conversation on many occasions. I also started steering more and more away from having dialogues with people, as for some reason thoughts that were waiting for their turn and for being mentioned by me were vanishing from my head all too often. As long as I could, despite it all, I wanted to keep participating in the life I knew from before my horror show. Nonetheless, it seemed to me that my family and friends didn't understand me thoroughly and considered me either a hypochondriac or a guy who found a new way for a living and made constant nagging and pitying himself the goal of his life.

If high-profile people from medical circles thought in this way, why others wouldn't have the exact same attitude towards me? I thought.

"Get down to work," "Find some other hobby, the world does not revolve around the gym," "Oh, is something bothering Michal again?" "Do something with your life! You have a fiancée!" "You said A, you now say B," the last one being a reference to my postponed wedding with Anna. On many occasions, I heard sarcastic comments from my loved ones. Some of my family members went one step further suggesting this would leave me free to 'ethically' leave Anna in a sly way if I had no other idea how to part ways with her. Although they had absolutely no clue what was going on with me, and they were putting forward false hypotheses, they were very close. The increasingly bothersome symptoms, the uncertainty, and that awareness of the worst that doctors managed to accustom me to, it all made me beg Anna to rearrange her life with someone else who'd give her everything I couldn't.

"Leave, please! Forget about everything, forget about me," I told her.

But Anna didn't forego her faith and dreams that a healthy life by my side was still possible.

"Don't even say that! I love you and I'm not leaving! We can make it! We'll overcome this together, whatever it is!" she said.

Sadly, I was aware that something very bad was going on with my body. Something that wasn't only slowly attacking different parts of my body, but also started getting more noticeable and malicious in my head.

We couldn't imagine a better engagement period that this, I thought.

I could feel my state deteriorating day by day, while the awareness that with time I was developing new, more exhausting ailments I couldn't stop in any way was destroying me even more. And so I didn't have to wait long for more symptoms checking in in a short time, forcing me to adopt bigger and bigger restrictions in my daily life.

The female internist from the Sports Medicine Center near my place, who didn't treat only young fit people, slowly began declaring me the patient of the year. Before me, that title was held by an eighty-seven-year-old man named Jan, an asthmatic with Parkinson's disease, who had already had two heart attacks. The elderly man simply stood no chance with me, as I became a more frequent visitor at the center than he was. Many times, leaning against a wall in a hallway or sitting on small, characteristic chairs installed along a hallway in front of doctors' offices, out of boredom, patients played a somewhat popular game of "find an element that does not fit the rest." Usually, I was the 'element' that didn't fit the background, each time boasting a colorful array of elderly people who were seeing their doctors regularly. Listening to them sharing remarks on their ailments, I couldn't imagine myself in fifty years.

If I could exchange such remarks on my health with these old folks now, does it mean that once I'm their age, I'll talk about parachute jumping or the sports records I broke? I pondered.

It wasn't only the PCP from the Sports Medicine Center who could award me with such titles.

Dr. Armani and his coworkers, due to seeing me frequently, began thinking about implementing a promotional appointment scheme, such as "Visit us twice a week, and you'll get Emergen-C for free to each prescription issued!" Obviously, no promotions for patients have taken place at any outpatient clinic and that is rather unlikely to ever happen – I was just joking.

My peculiar sense of humor, though not always well received by everyone, was one of my few traits I didn't manage to change until this day, no matter what. Regardless of how many times I was in pain, I could always find also the good aspects of life and a reason to laugh. After all, I had good friends I could always count on, and vice versa. At least that's what it seemed to me. I had never wondered what do my buddies like in me and why do they keep in touch. Does anyone? Perhaps that was because of my peculiar sense of humor that hit the mark on many occasions? I don't know.

I had high hopes that the way I made people laugh was not the only reason. I trusted that they considered me something more than just a clown to spend some time with to fill a gap in-between daily life chores. That was what I was doing; I wasn't hanging out with them to get something out of it. I simply love sharing my time with my friends. Each of my buddies with whom we had been hanging out since we were twelve had his own way of being. We'd never judge one another or criticize our actions, though we knew we all had shortcomings. One of us was habitually late and never arrived on time. Another one hated wearing shorts and dressed in black all the time, even if a heat of over ninety degrees was pouring down from the sky. Yet another one would abuse alcohol and yet another one had a thing for marihuana. Tomek had his vices, too, but he saw them in a completely different light from his perspective. To me, Tomek's biggest flaw was simply his infrequent presence.

What was my flaw? The guys often mentioned I struggled with finding my way outdoors, but also in general. They all knew I was quite lazy and often heard me saying, "I don't feel like doing that." Was that a flaw o mine? I don't know. If I had to choose, I'd probably say I was just falling ill all too often. Regardless of our shortcomings, I couldn't imagine a life without my buddies. Though two of us had already left abroad and we were seeing one another very rarely, I had high hopes that our ways would never be parted.

"I'd stick my neck out for my friends. I think we'd go to the ends of the earth for one another," Is said once when conversing with Anna's mom.

"May God let it be so! I hope you're right, but life's cruel, and one day, you can find yourself surprised," she replied, taking due account of her bad experiences.

"I know what you're talking about, but with us, it's different," I claimed.

The time of carelessness, school, and studies went by in a snap of fingers we barely even noticed. One by one, we all slowly entered the key stages of our lives: a stable job, engagement, marriage. Franek was the first to get in the front firing line and decided to marry his sweetheart. I was ecstatic at the prospect of spending time with my buddies at one of the most important events in every man's life – a good friend's bachelor party. Sadly, as fate would have it, instead of getting prepared for a fun trip with my friends, I had to attend a routine visit at Dr. Armani's office. A flu-like state that overtook me at an inappropriate time, as usual, was no surprise to me.

Why is it happening? I asked my fate.

Seeing me depressed, Anna said, "Get dressed! We'll drop by for a moment.":

Thanks to my sweetheart, despite my high fever, I could take part in my buddy's party at least for a while. It was very important to me. However, I had no clue that with another infirmity episode I'd develop yet another, terrifying condition that would prevent me from continuing relationships with my friends in the way I used to up until that point. Regardless of how much I wanted it and how much effort I put in, I was simply unable to maintain social life. I didn't realize, though, that I was about to lose it altogether soon.

The sensation of being locked inside my own shell is horrifying even when you talk about it or hear about it. For an athletic individual who had been highly aware of his physique and capabilities for almost half of his life, it is all the more troublesome. The spacesuit I was wearing permanently was making my daily life difficult. It didn't make me feel heavier, but I could always feel the weight of my problem on my shoulders. All the previous symptoms started merging into one to form the ultimate disease, ideal in its role, intended to ruin my life as it was.

Although I'd never dreamed of it and had no plan to conquest the Milky Way, as fate would have it, without many years of training for the job of an astronaut, I could feel like one of them. From then on, there was a filter superimposed on the glass visor of my helmet, filled with an extraordinarily subjective and bothersome sense of pressure, altering my perspective on what I could see. It was as if I found myself on a different, alien planet, or as if our terrestrial atmosphere was getting filled with optical phenomena previously unknown to me. My brain was not putting illusions or hallucinations in my way; I did though take repeatedly the sight of distant landscapes for a mirage the presence of which I couldn't feel at all, as if the information sent by eyes to my brain was corrupt. Though I loved drawing since being a little kid, I've never been interested in arts or painting. It could've changed back then, since the symptoms I was developing from one year to the next could undoubtedly be considered a style that was one of the most intriguing for the human eye, namely, surrealism. Who knows? Perhaps I could paint it, but what for?

Would symptoms of a suffering endured by a young boy be of interest to anyone if put down on canvas? Maybe this way others would become interested and understand what I felt, I wondered.

I was looking at my dad's beloved garden, where I'd spend a lot of time in, unable to comprehend why things were the way they were. Like members of my family I grew up with, and among which I used to chase my beloved dog around for fourteen years, the green arborvitaes, junipers, spruces and pines were constantly growing and bulking, pleasing us all with their charm. That year, they became completely alien to me. Small, yellowish garden lights that were illuminating many years of my dad's labor and effort in the evenings became unreal to me overnight. The picture that was reaching my brain was causing me discomfort. Each time I'd go out to the garden I felt like I had never been there before, and the glowing lights were evoking a sense that they didn't really physically exist.

"My view on your case hasn't changed. I still think that ailments of this sort in young people, and not exclusively, have their roots in mental conditions. I don't know how to help you, all the more that your blood test results are great. If I'm not the only person who claims this, I think you should continue your mental treatment," Dr. Armani told me.

When I was leaving the outpatient clinic and Dr. Armani's office, whom I saw for a check-up after yet another episode of flu-like bronchitis, I caught a glimpse of a female employee of that medical facility, someone who had annoyed me greatly not that long ago. I rubbed my eyes, flabbergasted.

I can't believe it! The blonde! Now I know why she seemed familiar! I thought.

"A drowning man will clutch at a straw" – many sayings can make a man reflect and seek their hidden meaning. But none of them was able to speak to my imagination as strongly as that one. Perhaps that is because the pain was frequenting my life all too often, of which I was well aware and could visualize it perfectly. For some time, I also noticed that my threshold for pain became lower than ever. It didn't take much for me to experience it more intensely than I used to. My life got turned upside down on nearly all levels of the body and the soul. Even in my worst nightmares, I didn't imagine something that horrible could happen to me. If it didn't concern me, I'd say, "Cheer up! After all, it's twenty-first century! Quantum computers, the Great Hadron Collider, people sending rovers to Mars! There's must be a drug for your problems!"

Sadly, the reality of a twenty-something living in the twenty-first century proved much more brutal than it could seem. Never in my life I'd think that I'll find myself in a place with no exit, a trap with no escape, a state where there's no help, and where empathy of ordinary Joes is as precious as gold. I didn't give up; I knew there must be an exit somewhere and that I had to find it.

Unquestionably though, I was drowning in a sea of inexplicable experiences that were taking away the best years of my life. I could only watch my good friend getting married and visualize myself and Anna in their shoes. Sadly, I knew that at that moment, our plans could not be put to work. Perhaps, being a man raised in Christian faith, it was a mistake on my part to seek help in various odd places, but back then, I wasn't aware of that. I didn't know that ramifications could affect my life further down the line to a greater or lesser extent. I was clinging to anything that could bring me relief even for a moment.

"Hey, how about seeing Ewa?" one of my good friends suggested.

"Who?" I asked.

"I have a number of a woman who once gave me a massage. She fixed a few of our acquaintances. Maybe she could help you, too? I've heard she has healed spine issues in many people."

"Definitely. Thanks, I'll consider contacting her."

Still believing that my life was probably in shambles because of my spine, I concluded it could be the right path towards finding the origin of my problems.

"You know what? I've got nothing to lose! Give me her number," I said.

When he was about to pass me a card with her telephone number on, he stopped for a moment and added, "Just don't look into her eyes!"

"What do you mean 'don't look'?" I asked.

"There's something weird about them. They scared me; you'll see for yourself," he finished with a smile.

If my buddy was all shivering at the look of a woman, I knew she was either very attractive or really terrifying. I thought the guy was demonizing her, but in fact, I had no clue whom I was about to see.

He surely did intrigue me with that line a lot, and so I decided to learn what it was all about firsthand. Although I had already gone through a failed chakra therapy, I could recall every word said on that day by the woman who deeply believed in the miraculous power of such non-conventional methods.

Maybe that road's really worth taking? I thought. If conventional diagnosing methods failed me and I still got no help from doctors, why not take a chance? Maybe the lady with a terrifying gaze would help me?

I decided not to put that decision off for too long and so I went to see mysterious Ewa. There was nothing weird about the voice I heard in my phone when calling her for the first time. It was quite pleasant and womanly.

The guy's crazy, I thought about my buddy.

And so I made an appointment, took Anna with me, and we went to see the masseuse. The woman was said to run a professional studio downtown, but she invited us over to her private apartment. We didn't find it troublesome at all and I had no objections. Ewa lived in an old tenement building downtown that didn't make a good impression from the very start. The dark, unkempt, pre-war staircase undoubtedly had a horror-like feel to it, adding to the climate of terror imposed by our friend, evoking unpleasant feelings. The apartment we were heading to was situated on the top floor, and the decades-old, time-worn wooden stairs that were creaking under the weight of our feet exacerbated our fear with very step up to the very top.

We made it to her door. We looked at each other and smiled, which showed we shared the curiosity that was eating us from the inside from the time we got the masseuse's number. I knocked on the door.

With the climate and the emotions that we were experiencing at that moment, the only thing missing was some music score from Hollywood horror movies I loved to watch among other genres to make the picture complete. Everyone who saw an American horror even once is surely familiar with a popular scene where a dark door slowly opens making a squeaking noise that matches the rhythm of well-chosen music intended to hype up the tension and feed your imagination, and out of that door, something jumps out on you and scares you. The last time I felt this way was when I was opening the door to the elderly female neurologist's office, which left a mark on my memory for a long time. Therefore, I couldn't wait to see what the mysterious women's eyes looked like. Impatient, we waited until she opened the door to her apartment. We saw a petite female. Anna and I quickly realized how suggestive to others' stories a human brain can be. Ewa was not a monster that we expected her to be, but I didn't find her charming, either. Her somewhat poor physique could be a proof that she wasn't meeting people too often or that it was simply the way she lived. It wasn't only me who instantaneously noticed her sticky, unclean, dark-cherry hair put in a messy ponytail. To provide a better description of Ewa's appearance, I could compare her to Meryl Streep known from the movies who neglected her looks, though that would be inaccurate. If I were to put some more effort in, I'd point to Willem Dafoe dressed up as a lady when playing an FBI agent in the action movie *The Boondock Saints*. His peculiar features are very alike the masseuse's looks, which were nothing but unconventional, albeit a female version. And the mystical eyes my buddy warned me not to stare in most seriously. There really was something wrong with them; I could venture to claim that they weren't fully natural. The very pale color of the iris that was merging with the shade of the whites was giving a feeling that they were one, as if Ewa didn't have any. Thus, staring into the woman's eyes, we were convinced that all she had was tiny pupils situated in eyeballs, much like a cat does. Although her appearance could scare away many who were passing her by in the dark gate of the tenement building, we quickly realized that "the devil is not so black as he is painted."

Before we could make ourselves comfortable, we had to pass through a very dark, untidy hall that didn't let any sunlight in, which once again could cause some mental discomfort. What caught our eyes instantly was some jagged wallpaper coming off the wall here and there, clearly with no one to fix it. We were invited to the living room which also gave no substantial proof that there might be something wrong with the lady. Although you could get the feel of the early 1980s, we weren't discouraged by that. I even believe that in today's crazy world abundant in electronics and cutting-edge technology, nostalgic, old, vintage furnishings like those have some unique charm to them. Ewa's room, which wasn't well-lit either, was filled with timeless pieces of furniture. An old wooden table, a foldable sofa, a book case with a TV set with a kinescope, which was a rare sight – it all added to the ambiance; however, what stressed this climate the most was a thick, retro, wool carpet with a typical pattern of that era, covering nearly the entire room floor. It is said that this type of old-school house furnishings have a soul. Though you can't always grasp it or feel it, on that day, it all had a mystical effect on us. Perhaps it was the intense odor of cigarettes the owner of the apartment was definitely smoking all too often, or perhaps the dark furniture that were making the obscurity even greater. There were no decoration in the room that could make that place look more sophisticated and welcoming. The only decoration, if that's the right way to put it, was a tiny vial with some substance in it, sitting on a bare, dark tabletop.

We took our seats on a couch whose springs made themselves noticeable under our buttocks.

"Very well, let's start from the beginning," the woman said, smiling.

Though not particularly pretty, she was extremely likeable. The way she was speaking made everything else that could be otherwise considered atypical or revolting simply meaningless. She dedicated much time to listen to my story. Hearing about the attitude healthcare services had adopted to my case, she concluded that she fully understood and that she had to deal with that on many occasions. She also informed us that in the circles of her 'patients' and friends there were many doctors who were coming to her not only for advice on how to treat difficult cases they couldn't handle, but also themselves. As her words seemed thoroughly reliable, considering the former stories of my friend about the people she healed, we were smitten by the thought we finally encountered someone who could help me.

Having heard about cases of incurable conditions she managed to heal many people from, infertile couples who got pregnant after a few visits, or disabled people who couldn't move without crutches or a wheelchair, whom she gave back normal life and the use of their legs, we were hypnotized by the hope that seemed within our reach.

"Please lie down on the floor," the masseuse said.

Sitting on the couch, I was wondering when she'd bring in a frame or a massage bed, or would she invite me into another room where she administers treatment. To our surprise, she only took out a small colorful towel that she then spread on the carpet by the table, asking me to take off my shirt and lie down.

That's a hell of a start, I thought.

The woman informed me that she was going to put a special massage oil on me and then she took the vile off the table, and started rubbing its content on my back. The scent that went up my nostrils was reminiscent of a regular camphor oil my mom used to rub on my temples many times when I had a headache as a small boy. With the previous experience I obtained while visiting physiotherapists I was seeing, I expected a typical massage intended to relax the muscles of my spine and I thought that nothing would surprise me in life – up until that moment.

Continuing to converse with Anna and sharing with her stories related to diseases and health, Ewa was touching and circling around each vertebra of my spine using very light touch of two fingers. At some of them, she would stop for a longer moment and I could feel them relocating or going into the position they were supposed to be in. This was evidenced by a characteristic sound of cartilage that was being pressed in. Once that odd massage of the vertebrae was over, she proceeded to rubbing my loins, which took some time and caused me a very pleasant, warm sensation. Still chatting with my fiancée, she asked me to switch from lying on my belly to lying on my back.

Likewise, during her conversation with Ewa, Anna was intoxicated by her extraordinary stories about impossible instances of healing that had taken place in that seemingly ordinary room. Although she wasn't in pain due to sensations as complex and horrible as I was experiencing, she took the opportunity to ask the lady if she could also help her solve her own problems she had been struggling with for years. As nearly all of us do, she, too, had some lesser or greater ailments or worries that were troubling her on a daily basis.

"What's the matter, honey?" the woman asked.

Anna informed the astonishing masseuse that many years ago, her legs were very slim, but for some unknown reason, they started turning bandy in the recent years. In my eyes, my sweetheart's legs were the slimmest in the world and I've always been telling her that. And indeed, everyone who started focusing their attention on Anna's petite legs, especially her knees, would notice some disproportion happening there, which for most people would be completely meaningless. Many of us would attribute that to my fiancée's very low fat tissue, as she was a very slim woman. In turn, she herself felt much discomfort and her intuition was telling her something bad must've happened in her life, possibly causing that big (in Anna's eyes) deformity. This was backed by the fact that a few years earlier, she was having repeated pains in the knees that preceded the said disproportion.

"You need to take large doses of collagen supplements. I think a collagen deficit might be the cause of your issue," Ewa said.

Continuing the massage, now by slightly pressing my belly, she started informing me of the condition of my internal organs.

"You need to take care of your spleen. The rest seems alright. That's all."

"Can I show you one more thing?" Anna asked.

Although any doctor who provides private medical treatment to his patients wouldn't like the fact that a person accompanying the patient is asking questions about her ailments, for we had been in that situation, too, Ewa showed no sign that she had any objections. On the contrary, she engaged in a discussion with Anna most eagerly and I had a feeling it was me who came there to keep company. I was glad that both of us could benefit from that situation, especially that seeing the mysterious masseuse cost us one-seventh of the usual price charged by doctors for private appointments. Anna felt very comfortable talking with her and up until then, I hadn't seen her that honest and open, sharing her complexes with a person who was a stranger to us. It was as if Ewa was inspiring great trust, making it possible for us to tell her everything.

"Sure, tell me what else is bothering you, my child," she replied.

"Please take a look at my tongue. Could you do something about this?"

Anna noticed long time ago that her tongue was a bit different to those most people had. She had a fissured tongue with numerous grooves on the surface.

Suddenly, the doorbell went ringing.

"We'll do something about that, too, my dear, but next time. I must say goodbye now; we'll fix you up, dear, don't worry," she said to me. "There's another person I have to see now."

On our way home, Anna and I were very excited at how that appointment went. Despite some visual shortcomings and the lady's somewhat unpleasant, untidy appearance, we were impressed not only by the stories she told us but also by her unconventional knowledge that she offered. Though I didn't hear her proclaiming any diagnosis, I was enchanted by the abundance of positive aspects and driven by the prospect of possible healing. No medical doctor we had visited did that great of an impression on us. The very fact that the masseuse could sense if there was something bad going on with any of my organs inside my stomach by touching me alone made me somewhat excited and eager to return for another appointment as soon as possible. Anna's feelings were the same. For the first time, we felt that there really was a hope I'd recover; we both believed that lady cat-eye had otherworldly abilities. Sadly, due to her schedule already booked by nearly two hundred patients she was allegedly seeing during the week, we couldn't return for another session as soon as we wanted. Amidst all the stories the therapist told us, only the number of individuals in need whom she was seeing on a weekly basis seemed quite implausible to me. I decided not to make a mountain out of a molehill, though, hopeful that she'll help us.

Meanwhile, the date of my next appointment with the female laryngologist was just around the corner. Before I went to see her for the third time, however, I decided to educate myself on the subject of the ear. I wanted to know what could be the cause of sensations as horrific as those I was experiencing in my ears, sucking my personality dry of the last drops of good humor. Rummaging the Internet looking for the answer to all my concerns had become one of my main activities. Despite the fruitless attempts and no traces found that would be consistent with my symptoms even a little bit, I was following online forums and news websites relentlessly. Although sitting in front of a computer monitor wasn't enjoyable due to my sensation of derealization, and the effort I had to put in to fully focus my mind was squeezing all the energy out of me, I didn't give up. As if that wasn't enough, each sound of a letter typed on a keyboard was making that something in my left ear move inside in most unimaginably annoying ways.

"How am I supposed to live?!" I cried with my head directed up to heavens.

Penetrating all Polish websites, I still couldn't find anything that would somehow put me on the right track, aside from a forum where several people were struggling with similar ailments and, like me, they were unsure were such sensations originate from. Some claimed they sustained an injury in the head, while others claimed the reason was in a terribly loud bang made by a closet falling down on the floor. There were also individuals for whom waking up in the morning, a usual, natural thing, became the last pleasant wake up in their lives for some inexplicable reasons. Joining the virtual group, I hoped that together we could solve our problem or find someone who could help us. Back then, there were only a few of us; we could be counted on both hands. The similar ear-related symptoms aside, which were tormenting us all, we found a common ground – lack of knowledge among most experts each of us was seeing.

Fortunately for me, my grasp of English allowed me to expand the scope of my search to include foreign websites. There, choosing the right words to depict what was happening inside my ears, I managed to come across a condition called the Tensor Tympani Syndrome[12] or the Middle Ear Myoclonus.[13] In both these cases, all troublesome sensations are caused by a disfunction of muscles of the middle ear. As it turned out, the Eustachian tube aside, hearing of which I said something like, "Damn, how did that Eustachi guy fit in there?", there are much smaller elements of the body responsible for the proper functioning of the ear. Delving deeper into such content in English, I learned that

---

[12] TTS – also known as the tensor tympani myoclonus.
[13] MEM – a syndrome that is a form of tinnitus.

my symptoms within the ears were most likely attributable to the smallest muscles in the human body that are situated in the ears, namely, the tensor tympani and the stapedius. Despite their petite size usually expressed in a fraction of an inch, they both serve a very important role by regulating the frequency of the sounds coming in to the ear so that they do no harm.

Following this trail, I came across foreign forums where people were sharing their stories. The tragedy of other people struggling with various issues related to their ears, the fact that they were all trying to find help by using the Internet as a tool to solve many of their problems, I managed to determine the most reliable clue and the possible reason behind my sensations.

I soon realized what was the origin of the horrible sound reminiscent of a thunderstorm and what was the thing I could move inside my ears. As it tuned out, many of us have various supernatural abilities hidden and not necessarily useful in daily life. Some can roll their tongues, other can touch the tip of their noses with their tongues. There are individuals who can make their eyebrows 'dance', while some others can manipulate very tiny muscles inside their ears since childhood to generate the sound of a thunder. Ever since I can remember, I've never had any problem rolling my tongue, whereas the ability to make thunder sounds inside my ears was completely new to me. I learned that that sound was most likely produced by the second smallest muscle in the body – the tensor tympani. Obviously, there would be no problem if at the age of twenty-something I learned overnight that I could 'create music' using my muscles or simply add some accords to the rhythm of my favorite songs.

Sadly, this ability, which I could use only to produce scores for horror films, triggered by me doing the Valsalva maneuver at the least favorable moment, came along with extremely annoying and unnatural sensations that were murdering me every day, possibly called the middle ear myoclonus, that is, a sudden muscle contractions.

As it turned out, I wasn't alone in this world. There were a few of us in my country; perhaps the others simply hadn't gone online yet. Each of us was looking for help relentlessly. Having contacted laryngologists, I was often convinced that some must've been cheating at their finals, while I could imagine others wearing shirts stating, I LOVE NEPOTISM, always under a white gown.

Maybe I was too strict in how I approached it all. A doctor is still just a human, after all. Not everyone is a know-it-all," I wondered.

There are some boundaries, though, that should not be crossed, for as the Medical Code of Ethics puts it in the Hippocratic Oath, "To defend the dignity of the medical profession and not tarnish it." Doctors should rise to the challenge and not give anyone a reason for making any allegations. A physician who diagnosed one person from our small group of receivers of extraterrestrial ear-related sensations left all my previous experiences far behind.

"Please, help me, doctor!" the suffering woman said to the laryngologist.

"I'll do my best. What's happened?" the doctor replied.

"I'm suffering from muscle contractions inside my ears, please do something about it! I beg you!"

"My dear, there are no muscles inside the ears. Perhaps a draft gave you a cold?" he concluded.

Though anecdotes of this sort sound like a joke, they were sadly real and on many occasions I could learn that firsthand.

Using the incredible tool that the Internet is, I managed to reach a group of people struggling with similar ear-related issues around the world. Many of them were listing their experienced on the forum pertaining to "Hypersensitivity to sound", while others shared their knowledge in a group suffering from tinnitus, while yet other ones were describing the sensation of having a broken speaker inside or a foreign body tossing and turning inside the middle ear. I could momentarily join the group of sufferers of at least two of these phenomena, completely abnormal and unimaginable for a regular Joe.

Although the nightmare I was going through as regards my ears had just begun, I could already earn the foretaste of what could happen to me down the line. "Please, help, I beg you," a desperate female wrote, requesting assistance for her husband whose ears were in much pain. "I've already replaced all metal cutlery with plastic, that's all I can do for him," she begged.

"Don't spend so much time reading things online! Most of it is baloney!" my mom would tell me time after time in an attempt to protect me from harm. She didn't realize though that so much of what was written there was true and similar to the experiences I was going through, which soon became an inseparable part of my life.

Driving to the hospital to see the young female laryngologist for the third time, I was armed with the knowledge that didn't make me more content, though. My mom's warnings were not just empty words. Despite the knowledge from the Internet, that wasn't necessarily consistent with the truth and with what I was going through, my stress levels continued to grow, unfortunately. The information that TTS or MEM affect one person in a hundred thousand didn't make me optimistic, and neither it made me more hopeful for a swift and easy resolution of my problem. Although up until that point no one had diagnosed me an ear dysfunction, I knew that there was nothing else that could cause these sensations. Spending hours online reading articles and websites dedicated to various conditions of the ear, I felt like I was a student again, but at a medical academy instead of a college; I realized that most likely, I diagnosed my issue myself.

Maybe I'll become a doctor? I thought jokingly.

I had no reason to be happy, but some part of me was glad that at least I managed to do that. In truth, the other symptoms could be linked to any disease in the world, all of which were passing me by according to experts, aside from one – neurosis.

Having all that knowledge, I was heading to the hospital with a different mindset. Nonetheless, the awareness that treating TTS or MEM doesn't involve administering a nasal spray, but usually a difficult, meticulous surgery, was causing me even more anxiety. For that reason, I still hoped that I was wrong and that the laryngologist with her extensive knowledge would surely find a different solution.

There, at the hospital, I had tympanometry performed, and then I had to stand in line, which I didn't account for. I hoped that waiting three months for the third meeting with the expert was just enough, but I was wrong. I got invited to a hospital and my imagination went wild. Not in a bad sense, but in the sense that there was likely a more extensive range of diagnostic tests that the female doctor could use, which she didn't have at hand back at the poorly equipped office where she was seeing her patients on a regular basis. Aside from the time when I was undergoing an additional hearing test and having my Eustachian tubes checked for a clog, which was performed in a separate room, I thought while standing in line, *Surely she has some awesome equipment behind those doors that she'll use to fix my ears.*

Concerned, I only wondered why the female doctor had referred me for a hearing test earlier and now, a woman who was operating the appliance at the hospital tested me again. Utterly stressed out and uncertain, I entered the office upon being called. I saw the attractive laryngologist accompanied by three much younger girls.

Oh. This is nice, I thought.

All four of them were dressed in regular white hospital gowns. I swiftly realized that the young girls were students who were in the course of their internships, watching closely the authority figure that my doctor undoubtedly was.

Naturally, I had no problem with the fact that the interns were going to participate in my appointment, thus gaining experience and acquiring the necessary knowledge. However, I didn't realize that having waited three months for help and for my issues to get resolved, I'd had to face one of the least expected surprises I had ever had in my contact with healthcare staff.

"Take a seat, please" the laryngologist said.

Indeed, the seat looked more like a piece of professional equipment than the one she had back at her office.

"What brings you to me?" she asked.

Three months is unquestionably long enough for some small wounds to heal. Some would even claim that ninety days is all it takes to fall in love again. Others yet need eighty days to go around the globe, and use the remaining ten to rest after the journey is over. But to forget a patient with an extremely rare condition manifested in his ears, who was told to wait quarter of a year for some reason – there clearly must be something wrong with that?

"You don't remember me? I've seen you twice already, doctor! The woman downstairs tested my hearing, for the second time. Retaking a hearing test, is there any point doing that?" I asked.

"Oh, right. I remember now. Okay, okay. And how do you feel?" she asked, taking a glance at my tympanogram.

"My cyst on the tonsil has grown bigger, and my ears are even more annoying than before," I replied.

"Your test results are great. What do you make of it, girls?" she said, looking deep into the students' eyes.

At that point, my intuition was telling me something was not quite right.

"Perhaps something's going on with the Eustachian tube, doctor?" one of the students replied, jotting something down in her notebook, thus making the exact same diagnosis I had heard a few months earlier.

"And what do you think?" she asked the other two.

"I guess so, doctor, we think the same," they chipped in.

"Right. Right. That's what it seems to me, too," the expert added, informing us that she'd get back soon and leaving us alone in the office for a while.

Sitting in the armchair, gazing at the timid faces of the girls who sent some smiles my way while taking notes, I smiled back, hoping that the doctor would be back soon to take up a serious discussion with me, as a doctor should. After several minutes, the specialist returned to the office. Having my head swiftly turned from one woman to another while they were replying to their supervisor's questions, I had a feeling that I was part of some hidden camera TV series, and that in just a moment, one of my friends would jump out from behind a curtain that was separating the couch along with a cameraman, informing me that I got pranked in a grand style.

"Well, girls, what else do you think?" she asked them again, standing in front of me.

Seeing that the young students ran out of new ideas, she added, "Sir, your results are okay. I'll prescribe you a different nasal spray and I'll see you in a month. As for the cyst, please don't touch it for now. Let the next person in," she concluded.

Feeling as if I was a guinea pig, shocked by what just happened, I knew there was no point even touching on the subject the expert and her supervisees probably never heard of in their lives. I even had a feeling that the woman didn't even know who I was, and she was poor at acting. Thinking how much time I wasted waiting for the visit at the hospital that was supposed to hopefully change my situation, which was far from perfect, I was petrified and disenchanted, and not for the first or the last time, either.

Every cloud has a silver lining; at least I was confident about one thing – the retaken hearing test yielded excellent results and I had no reason to fear anymore. I knew, though, that putting a spray inside my nose on a regular basis wouldn't fix the issue, and there was nothing more the female doctor could offer me. I had to roll the dice and wait until I meet someone reliable with a calling who would know anything about my ear-related condition.

The only person who was doing her job with a smile on her face was Ewa. Although the astonishing masseuse held neither titles nor a scientific degree that would come right after her last name, I considered her more competent for that profession than many medical doctors. Her expertise that she wholeheartedly wanted to share coupled with her smile that never withered made me put all my hopes for a full recovery in her.

Ewa's appearance and the place where she was seeing her patients would cause more than one person to question her. Despite the stories about people leaving their crutches behind, which would give many sceptics a good laugh, I felt that she could help me.

On the day when I was about to meet the masseuse again, Anna couldn't accompany me – she was studying and fulfilling her other chores. She wasn't always available to keep me company during my appointments with doctors, as she had other important things to do. This was understandable to me, naturally.

Despite Ewa being highly likeable, I felt some anxiety and discomfort at the thought that I was about to go to her alone. Perhaps it was by virtue of her weird eyes, atypical for a regular man, or perhaps, as most matters I was handling by myself downtown, it became difficult for me and I needed another person's support. Therefore, I asked my mom, who had already grown accustomed to keeping me company at medical appointments, to come see the unusual healer with me.

"God, where did you bring me to?" she asked, going up the creaking, old, wooden stairs in one of the tenement buildings in Lodz, fearing they would fall to pieces instantaneously.

"No worries, I'm sure you'll be delighted, just as we were. She really knows a lot and she's helped many people. I can feel she'll help me, you'll see," I said.

Climbing up the top floor, we noticed that the door to Ewa's apartment were wide open. This time, there was no one who'd greet us at the door.

"Come in!" she shouted from the living room, where she was administering her massages.

At the very beginning, our nostrils felt an intense smell of cigarettes that fed into my mom's imagination even more. Her look was telling me one thing: "Have you lost your mind? To whose place have you brought me to?"

My mom and I decided to leave our coats and boots back in the very dark hall, and then went to the room where we were about to get surprised.

Still wearing the same clothes, just as unkempt, the woman greeted us cordially. What made her look different than during the last visit was her smile, now different, and the lack of a shine in her eyes, which previously showed how joyful she was.

Maybe she's having a bad day? I thought.

Ewa offered my mom a cup of tea, which she hadn't done when receiving me accompanied by my fiancé. My mom declined, since she was somewhat repulsed by the very location and Ewa's appearance, her hair looking as if it hadn't been washed since our last visit.

"No, thank you," she replied.

"Very well. Let's get down to business."

As usual, she took a vial with oil off the dark tabletop and asked me to lie down on the floor. Aware of my mom's preferences when it comes to aesthetics, I knew that what she was about to see would terrify her to no end. Ewa placed the same towel I had been lying on the first time on the carpet and told me to lie down. Seeing the horror and disgust in my mom's eyes, most likely having the same thoughts, I was afraid to ask if all the massage clients were sharing the same piece of cloth. However, I tried not to focus on such trivial matters. I knew what I came for. Hearing doctors proclaiming that I should be seeking help solely in antidepressants and psychotherapy, a place like that one was giving me hope for a better tomorrow, regardless. I didn't meet a doctor who would show me a light in the tunnel; on the contrary, with every visit, their disparaging attitude to my case, their lack of knowledge and incompetence were making me closer to losing my mind and returning to the psychiatrist. I didn't want to let them all win. I knew that all my symptoms had their source elsewhere and that it definitely wasn't my head; for this reason, I had much hope that the healer would help me.

Just like Anna, my mom engaged in a dispute with Ewa. The difference was massive, though. The warm, pleasant conversation Anna had with the masseuse could be compared to a chat between two good friends who had known each other for years and are overjoyed for any reason.

In the course of that conversation, lying on the carpet, I could feel that there was no chemistry between the two women. Aware that I was looking for help anywhere possible, my mom was still concerned that I could simply get conned and hurt even worse. It wasn't as much about the money, as it was about giving a false hope, something many conmen are trading as if it were stolen goods. Seeing the way in which the healer was performing the massage, she became even more suspicious.

"What an odd way to give a massage!" she remarked, staring at the woman's hand with which she was pressing one vertebra after another again, shifting them to the right location.

I don't know if the lady sensed my mom's irony that slightly elevated her blood pressure, or maybe she didn't even identify it accurately; however, she began engaging in the discussion with even more zeal without losing her peace.

"That's the only way I can help him. Trust me, please," she replied.

Carrying on with administering the massage using circular motions and pressing selected vertebrae of my spine, she was telling us about the secrets of her technique. Suddenly, her hand halted and she threw a question at my mom.

"Can I ask you a question now?"

"Sure, go ahead," my mom replied.

"The girl that came with him the previous time, is she your daughter?" she asked.

All of a sudden, I felt as if I was completely absent. I had had the very same feeling at the moment when Anna and lady cat-eye were having an unusually nice dialogue. This time, however, I was feeling as if I really were not there, and Ewa, giving no consideration to the fact I was lying there under her hands, asked a totally weird question. Thinking that perhaps I misheard due to lying on the floor, I was waiting for my mom to reply to see how the conversation would go on.

She knew we're engaged! I must've misheard her, I pondered.

"No, Anna is my son's fiancée," she replied.

"Oh, that's good, very good!"

"I don't understand," my mom was surprised.

"And you allow something like this?" the lady asked in a bizarre way, her voice somewhat louder.

"what are you talking about?"

Lying down on my belly, I was listening closely to the women's conversation flabbergasted, waiting for how they'd expand further on the subject that had already made me a little anxious and uneasy.

"If my son brought a girl like her to my home, I'd send her right out the door!" she added.

Neither my mom nor I could believe what we had just heard. The spell that Ewa had on me broke instantaneously like a bursting soap bubble, turning in a matter of a second into unspeakable disgust and anger that wanted to slowly take control over me. My reason was telling me that I wasn't in the best position to allow myself to react to such words in any way. Pressing my vertebrae, the woman was basically sitting right on my back. Fearing that she might chose to maliciously mishandle one or two vertebrae, I decided to remain silent and let my mom continue the discussion herself.

"But what are you even talking about?" my mom asked again.

"That girl, she's very sick!" Ewa said most seriously, as if she knew something more than we did. "Ditch her, please, while you still can!"

"Even if that child was sick, do you think she doesn't deserve love?" my mom asked.

"If my son brought a girl like her, I'd throw her out and that's that!" the woman emphasized, frowning.

I couldn't believe what I just heard, especially given that Anna had shared her most intimate complexes with her. I was stunned; when the lady took her hands off of my body, I got up, got dressed, and started walking towards the door. I left her the money for the treatment and, remaining silent, let her know that I was deeply disappointed.

When we were about to leave her apartment, she stopped us for a moment.

"Come back to me with your girlfriend! I'll cure her for you," she concluded, having no shame or tact in this entire situation.

Never again have I set one foot at Ewa's apartment. Anna listened to our story about what had happened in disbelief.

Although to me, it was a grave disappointment, for the chance to have my problems resolved sailed away like a ship beyond the horizon, once again, I didn't give up and I still hoped to find a solution soon. Knowing from her experience that appointments like that not always bring positive results, my mom started worrying a lot. She has always taken people like that lady for grifters selling bull to their victims to make money off their suffering. However, the words of lady cat-eye made a mark on my mom's heart that was much deeper than any other before, leaving an air of uncertainty. From then on, she wasn't concerned only by my health, but also Anna's.

The meeting with the mysterious healer blew up in all our faces. Though throughout my life, my mom had been warning me of various forms of danger, evil people in particular, I still ventured different places looking for help. I didn't consider Ewa an evil person and I haven't taken her for one until this day; however, without a doubt, on that day, my mom and I both experienced a weird aura that had a detrimental effect on us all. Although Anna wouldn't show that the healer's words got to her even a little bit, I knew that she was profoundly affected by them. Both she and my mom are the type of people who believe in esotericism.

Horoscopes and dream dictionaries pertaining to hidden evets and prophecies were nothing new to them. Having a thing for astrology, they always believed that all things were somehow interconnected, and that everything happened for a reason. Although Ewa didn't have a crystal ball on her table, a deck of cards or a black cat, my mom couldn't forget her words. In turn, for some time, I stopped believing anything. I happened to go to church, walk around a pole or a ladder, or honk at a black cat so that it wouldn't cross the road in front of me, but it was all completely meaningless to me.

Maybe had I honked during my first solo car ride, the black kitty would still be alive, and I would still be healthy? I wondered.

After what I had recently experienced at the hands of medical staff and others, I had neither the strength nor a desire to continue seeing these physicians. Though my intuition was still telling me they were wrong and that I mustn't give up, my heart was sinking and I was getting closer and closer to retaking the only path that most of the doctors determined for me.

"Come on, don't break down!" Tomek told me when he stopped by during his visit to Poland. "I've met someone who might be able to help you!"

"I know those 'someones' of yours all too well already," I replied sarcastically, referring to my most recent appointment, likewise, with a person recommended by a friend.

"Don't worry, there's nothing to be afraid of here! I've met a lady doctor who's not a Pole; she came to Poland from China long time ago, and aside from conventional treatment methods, she also uses some 'magical' herbs that she has already cured many people with. Even cases of cancer that went into remission, they say. Give her a try! What do you have to lose?"

Fearing another disappointment, I didn't want to step in the same river again.

Since in this case, time had already healed my wounds, I decided that despite it all, I'd go with the friend out of town to meet the Chinese medic. In a sense, I was no stranger to Asian medicine. On many occasions, I used various Chinese herbs to remedy headache, which I rubbed on my temples; I had also eaten the health-boosting Korean root called ginseng my friends brought me from Korea. However, I'd never had the pleasure of talking to an Asian with a medical degree, which persuaded me to go on this meeting.

Given the haunting image of the crumbling stairs leading to the apartment of the cat-eyed masseuse, I could imagine a tent or a hut the Chinese doctor would see me in. To my surprise, Tomek parked his car by a building that looked like a regular outpatient clinic.

"I told you we were going to see a doctor!" Tomek said smiling, as he always did.

Always charismatic with a great sense of humor, Tomek was a person with whom I could feel healthy even just for a moment. His smile never faded. Whatever bad thing was going on, he could find a way out of that situation, always seeing the positive sides in an all-black script.

"Why are you worrying so much? At least you don't have to work a lot!" he'd say jokingly.

He was right; I've never been a person desperate to find a job, and now, even if I really wanted to, I was simply unable to function as I used to. In order to change that and go back to normal, I had to keep trying everything fate was putting in my way.

We entered a clean and well-kept building that wasn't any different to a standard medical facility. Though we had an appointment for a specific time, as usual, I had to wait for my turn to be called among other people waiting in line.

"Next person, please!" a young woman said from behind a half-open door, definitely Polish-born.

Having entered the room, I saw a tiny, petite Asian woman, certainly of old age.

"Have a seat," she said in Polish, slightly distorting syllables in a charming way typical of Asians.

Without inquiring me about the problem I came to her with, she asked me to open my mouth and show her my tongue. Then, she grabbed me by the wrist. She started pressing the spot where pulse is often checked in with her thumb.

"You're very stressed!" she said.

That wasn't anything unusual for me; for some time now, my each visit at any doctor's was beginning with an elevated heart rate. It was surely because I felt that everyone I turned for help to was considering me a hypochondriac. At the very start, I already had concerns about whether it was even a good idea to go there.

"You're suffering from anxiety. I can see the feal within you," she added, finding virtually nothing else.

"Feal?" I asked.

"Feal, feal, fear... fear!" she repeatedly corrected herself.

"Oh, fear!"

"I'll give you just the right herbs and you'll come in sometime later," she wrapped it up, requesting the young woman sitting next to her that she gets a choice of herbs appropriate for me prepared.

The girl approached a white cabinet and, having rummaged drawers filled with different small bags, she brought a few that were right for me. The Asian lady told me the price for the selection of herbs and asked if I was okay with it. Although the cost of the appointment including the herbs was similar to that of a several-minute-long conversation with most professors of medicine, I decided to take the risk and purchase the herbs.

Meeting the Asian didn't change much in my new life. Though she didn't make a great impression on me, since the list of my ailments was much longer than just the anxiety and fear she mentioned, it was enough to shift my mindset again. The way in which the Chinese woman identified one of my problems were quite spectacular and I had never seen anything like it before. And yet, I was disappointed, as she was unable to determine the other conditions that were tormenting me.

Perhaps they all were right, after all? I wondered.

The diagnosis put forward by the female doctor who combined conventional and unconventional methods made me ponder again if my intuition wasn't leading me astray.

What if my feelings are misleading me? Maybe other symptoms, aside from the visible cyst inside my throat, are only figments of my imagination, and there is nothing more than anxiety that generates it all? I thought.

I started taking the herbs that the Chinese recommended; however, over time, as usual, instead of improving, my symptoms were getting even more severe. Yet again, the anxiety that was there every day, unlike other symptoms, started giving me sporadic seizures of panic that once again was emerging in the least expected moments. This time, already having that enriching, awful experience, I got quite good at stopping that speeding train of odd, panic-inducing thoughts.

It was a day that preceded my final decision to resume psychiatric treatment. For a long time now, my dearest friend, my dog, was struggling with a disease, likewise. Puma was a sweet, tiny bitch of eleven pounds whom we all loved, and whom I had spent half of my life with so far. Growing with her by my side in one household, I considered her nothing less of a member of our family. Everyone who saw her fell in love with her at first sight. The connection I had with my dog was often the cause of Anna's jealousy.

"You love her more than me," she'd say.

Who knows, maybe that was true, indeed? Maybe I loved her more than everybody else? Puma was the only one who could listen to me and she never let me know that she had to be right.

When she was fourteen years old, she contracted pyometra that attacked her by surprise. Sadly, she had to undergo a surgery that didn't go as we hoped it would. I'll never forget the moment when the veterinary surgeon handed us her dead body. On that day, I felt as if my entire list of worries got extended to include yet another symptom I couldn't put in words. My thoughts were a tango of two different feelings dancing together – profound grief and anger.

With no chance for getting any help from doctors practicing medicine outside the scope of psychiatry, I had to put my trust in them again and go back for help to someone who'd fix my head. It wasn't an easy task.

I was born in times when every medical expert who had no clue how to help a patient used the offload technique, handing him over to psychologists and psychiatrists. By boosting in this way the economic situation of their colleagues who practice that specific field, they make it so that people who do that job don't have to make any effort to advertise themselves.

That's a great business, I thought.

The Internet, which I used most often, was abundant in contact details of people advertising as human mind experts.

Once I overcome this, I'll give much thought to taking up studies again, I contemplated.

As usual, basing my choice on positive online reviews about doctors of psychiatry and their experience, I came across a very likeable man.

"We'll choose just the right medication for you. You'll see for yourself; soon we'll both laugh at it all," he told me with great optimism.

Many would probably be very content with such an attitude towards my whole situation. The prospect of forgetting about it all and reliving that nightmare solely when sharing frightening stories to friends around a campfire, or to grandchildren when I'm old, was much to my liking. Unfortunately, even when in a dead-end situation with nothing else to count on, there was still a part of me saying, "Don't do this, man, that's not the way."

"Let's not waste any more time", "We administer meds at once", perhaps these lines work on people who really have mental issues and feel that only a psychiatrist would help them.

Maybe when they know that their problem stems from life events, experiences, complexes, but they continue to hide it on the outside nonetheless, they look forward to and accept such an approach taken by a doctor, I thought. My situation was completely opposite. In desperation, I was trying to believe in what everyone else around me told me, though deep in my heart I knew that the truth was different.

When I was telling my story to the human mind expert, yet again I felt like I was taking part in a hidden camera show, and my reaction to the specialist's behavior was recorded for an episode of a comedy series broadcast on Sundays. In my view, the man sitting in front of me undoubtedly suffered from a mental condition himself; I had no clue how to behave and, most of all, I didn't know what I should be looking at. Sitting in front of me at an office who, as per usual, failed to fit my perfect model for such a venue, staring at me and listening closely to my lengthy story, like a little boy, he was picking his nose constantly throughout that time. It dawned on me that that doctor could do that obsessively at every session we were about to have. Since I knew a person who struggled with such a problem greatly from childhood to adulthood, I decided to forego further appointments and look for someone else.

How is that man supposed to help me if he himself has a problem? I kept asking myself.

Knowing that I could continue pharmacotherapy under the eye of any other specialist, I decided to take the risk and see how the drug I hadn't tried yet works.

Who knows? Maybe I will laugh at all the bad things that happened to me, I thought.

Movies in a broad sense that we all watch from our childhood years, often leaves in each of us a picture of what we would like the world to be like every day, sometimes making an impression on our senses and feelings that is just too strong. The trick is not to shoot any movie, but to show a story and acting in such a way that makes us fall to our knees laughing or unable to stop a river of tears. That's a challenge. Before I got to be a part of scenes that seemed taken right from a movie set of a top-shelf horror, which I was just about to experience, I had to face more new emotions and feelings that were flocking to me like tourists on a journey seeking accommodation. I've always been a sensitive person for whom it didn't take much to tune in to a protagonist's suffering. Pictures known worldwide such as *Titanic*, *The Lion King* or *Legends of the Fall* could make me shed more than one tear. Whatever was happening to me, it was taking away all my human emotions and reactions. Movie scenes that used to make my eyes a little bit watery, if nothing else, suddenly stopped touching me in any way. Maybe for this reason, watching the psychiatrist penetrating his nostrils deep didn't give me a laughing fit.

There came a time when I finally came across, as it would seem, the right human whisperer. That man was seeing his patients in his detached house. His office was the first that had much in common with the images I was accustomed to from the movies.

That's it! I thought.

A meticulously clean beige carpet, two slightly rocking chairs we sat on facing each other at a small distance – that's just part of the ideal conversation room that I held tightly to in my imagination. An enormous bookcase with shelves filled with volumes from the floor up to the ceiling, no African deities that would distract the patient and steer his attention away from an unintelligent therapist – that was exactly what I expected. In the room half-dimmed by curtains, which was also significant, I felt like I finally found myself in the place that was right for me. But still, that wasn't what I had been after all this time. Fearing yet another failure, I didn't know what I could expect from that specialist. To my surprise, the psychiatrist's very first words made me feel hopeful. Though the doctor's age was surely close to my dad's, he boldly started the conversation.

"At my office, there are rules to abide by: I call you by your first name, and if you wish, you can call me by my first name, too. If I don't like something about your conduct, I tell you that, and if you, too, find in me something that doesn't fit your convictions, you tell me straight as it is! If we have to smack each other, we do that, and then we continue talking. Is that clear!?"

With his huge, thick mustaches that brought to my mind an older version of famous actor Tom Selleck, the psychiatrist won over my trust with his professional attitude.

Way to go, Tom, I thought.

Wishing to tell the therapist how I got there as briefly as possible and to begin my standard monologue that would describe my symptoms, I was shot down instantaneously.

"Stop, stop, stop! I'm not interested what is wrong with you! I want to know why!" Tom said in a loud voice.

I knew where he was going with this: like any psychiatrist should, he wanted to learn more about me to then somewhere along the way identify the reason behind my issues, perfectly hidden in a collage of events from my past, which he would then put together like a jigsaw puzzle. And so I started seeing him because, the charm of his office aside, he was standing out with his exceptional intelligence and solid approach to my case.

I started going back in my mind to one of my diagnosis that I put forward myself using the Internet, which was to some extent very consistent with my symptoms.

"Perhaps it is depersonalization or derealization?" I asked him, pointing at two conditions that are quite typical of metal disorders.

"Depersonalization and derealization are what most medical students have when attending lectures. Don't talk yourself into having conditions you don't have!" he said.

His intelligence combined with a sane sense of humor was convincing me that I couldn't have chosen better. The therapist also replaced my medicine with the one that certainly helped me alleviate my first symptom , that is, anxiety, which had been tormenting me and attacking me in sneaky ways. He suggested that I should start taking again the substance that was giving me the desired result. And so I did; I started taking the antidepressants that were prescribed for me earlier.

CHAPTER
III

"Time flies, doesn't it?" my parents used to say at every New Year's Eve that reminded us all we were getting older, and also when celebrating my twenty-sixth birthday in 2013. Before we all even knew it, the thirteen was replaced by a fourteen. Three years passed since my first panic attack that triggered a wave of terrible sensations one by one, like a perfectly arranged set of dominoes that got toppled and couldn't be stopped, the ultimate goal being to strike down the last standing piece that still holds. My sensations were still the same, whereas my body and mind, like an angel and a devil sitting on my shoulders, were whispering in my ears, "What are you doing? Keep seeing the psychiatrist! Only there you'll find the solution!" and "That's not the way! You'll never overcome it by doing that!" Once again, I listened to my body; contrary to what you might expect, it was in much more pain than my head, which had to put up with so much. I felt that if I didn't follow the voice of my intuition, it would end very bad for me. However, before I made that decision, there was a struggle of thoughts inside my head; no one on the battlefield except for me and the words of my opponents, who in truth wanted the best for me.

When I closed my eyes, I could see a field of green grass covered here and there with dark sand; they were all standing in a row, clad in silver armor, talking to me one by one, blinding me with the sunlight reflected by their shiny torsos.

"I believe you should continue your psychiatric treatment," Dr. Armani said.

"Get off that Internet! You're exhausted! It's all because of the weightlifting!" my mom and Anna were shouting.

"I told you, you drink too little vodka!" Tomek said.

"Maybe he doesn't want to be with Anna anymore and he's faking it?" some relative chipped in in the background.

"Poor you! How can we help you?" my sisters were asking me.

"Go get a job!" yelled a buddy of mine.

"I don't see a person suffering from neurosis and depression. Don't stuff yourself with all these drugs!" the neurosurgeon who looked like Al Pacino added.

"My pal psychiatrist is waiting for you!" the orthopedist concluded.

Among them all, I could see my dad, unarmored, who, just like me, didn't know what to do and didn't tell me where I should go.

"If you want, I'll take you anywhere," he'd always say.

Already accustomed to the constant struggle to overcome adversities that had no intention to back down, I had to face my thoughts every single day. My parents would always tell me words I'll remember till the end of my days, "If there's no one you can count on, always count on yourself."

I knew that only I was the master of my fate and that the responsibility for my state further down the line and all the decisions I take lies with me. Before the new year started, yet again, I forewent seeing the psychiatrist who'd seem perfectly tailored to my preferences. Although despite a few sessions that served as an introduction to the psychoanalysis, the psychotherapy as such was not commenced, I didn't regret spending those several hours with Selleck. However, I knew that in the future, I might regret that I didn't use that time for carrying out an investigation that would lead me right to the next 'crime scene' of the unidentified suspect who was eating me up from the inside. He, too, knew that in reality, every end result, not only that of a therapy, depends on ourselves and accepted my decision with much respect. I think that at the moment when he heard me describing my ailments, he wasn't really sure if the issue was in my head, but his experience and professional approach didn't let him show that.

I was back to taking Seronil again, which had a redemptive power of tuning my anxiety down; however, it couldn't affect the many other of my symptoms in any way and, what was worse, it had no power to stop that speeding train with cars full of despair and suffering. Yet another nightmare of my 'ideal' young life that only proved to me that I made the right decision by foregoing attempts to fix my head and choosing to seek further instead.

One day, when going downstairs in the house I was living in from the second floor to the first floor, I stopped, focusing my vision in front of me. Suddenly, I realized that I didn't know how I got to the place I was standing in. I could compare that sensation to the commonly known blackout induced by alcohol overdose. I've never been a person who had a thing for liquor and for the most part of my life, particularly the part I dedicated to sports, I was avoiding drinking. Tomek would repeatedly throw a fuss as I didn't agree at all times that any occasion is a good occasion to get a drink. This doesn't change the fact that back as a teenager, I'd often try keep up with my buddies who could consume much more than I could, which usually ended up in catastrophically for me. One of such memorable evenings was a party organized by our two high schools when we finished half the program. Tomek, the rest of our friends and I, we all definitely had too much. To this day, I can only recall fragments of that night at different locations where either I woke up or I am woken up by my buddies. I'd never suspect that there will come a time when I'd be drunk day by day without having any contact with alcohol; worse yet, that I'd start losing a sense of time and reality like a teenager who's partying hard.

That sensation got more and more frequent. Obviously, I never happened to have to pull myself off the floor or some completely unknown places, or open my eyes at the movies or a hypermarket and wonder how I got there. I did, however, lose my sense of time repeatedly at shorter distances. It was as if I forgot that a while ago I was upstairs at my home, on my way down to get a cup of tea. Like any new symptom, this one started wreaking havoc in my life, too.

There were days that with all the symptoms I had to fight on a daily basis, one of them was more severe, thus causing me to focus less on the other ones. This was making my research very difficult; concentrating what was left of my attention on one ailment, intending to find people with a similar issue on the Internet, if nowhere else, suddenly, I'd get attacked by a second one and a third one that followed suit, outperforming one another in that marathon of my subjective suffering, causing me to lose track of what I was supposed to be looking for. Although the phase of psychiatric treatment was over and I considered that case closed, my loved ones opposed my decision. Some of them believed that I was making a mistake, only making it more evident to Dr. Armani and his female friends from the outpatient clinic that I was an exceptionally odd case of a hypochondriac that they had diagnosed, who every now and then asks for prescriptions for more antidepressants, yet always discontinues that kind of therapy. Given the newly emerged symptom and the fact that the other ailments didn't subside even in the slightest, I realized that there was no point to continue poisoning my body with happy pills that I had given a second chance. The awareness that my anxiety and fear that to some extent were neutralized by the pills could be a symptom of some disease that is responsible for the rest of my issues only gave me more strength to look further and to not give up without taking Seronil anymore.

The optional conditions I could identify my case as were plenty, and often my suspicions were ruled out by the information that I found online pertaining to the nature of various diseases and their symptoms; thus, a given disease entity had to be put away, and I continued my search. The blood tests that I was doing repeatedly every several months each year at Dr. Armani's office or at private laboratories gave perfect results every single time, as they should in the case of a young, strong man.

"You're as healthy as a horse!" the doctors I met with would tell me, recommended by either my relatives or friends.

More and more often, I was losing not only the sense of time and reality, but also what remained of my faith in people working as those who are supposed to help the infirm. Looking relentlessly for the one who'd help me eliminate even just one of my afflictions, I read, rummaged, traveled the country far and wide. Despite my previous experience with individuals using unconventional methods, which weren't always positive, I didn't stop from trying every other possible way to get help. Though you could think that something was pulling me that way, since I had chosen that path many times before, I still felt that I simply had no other choice but to take it.

More and more often, the group of people I sought to be rescued by included, among others, osteopaths, healers practicing naturopathy[14] or bioenergy therapists. They all offered their help highly convinced that their specific methods would surely help me. And so I took their herbs, had my head massaged with essential oils, my ears waxed, and I also brought home watts of bio-energy that was supposed to heal me. It all proved futile against my maladies.

From a young boy who was just enjoying his life, spending his every free moment sculpting his physique and meeting with his friends, I turned into a wreck and a shadow of my own self who started avoiding the world he was living in. Not only did I stop socializing, but also began neglecting all of my duties that I should've been doing. Like a dog with a tail between its legs, I was looking for my place in my room, asking everyone around me to just leave me alone. Aside from getting more and more dedicated to reading online content to find the reason behind my issues, I wasn't doing anything creative, and the safe space I found in my room became the place I wouldn't even leave often. More and more often, I'd stuff the void previously filled by my beloved dog with watching several full-length movies a day, which turned into an essential part of my daily routine. Very of-

---

[14] Naturopath – a person who practices non-conventional medicine who uses natural methods such as physical therapy, herbal therapy and diet.

ten my dad would join me to keep me company. Only in this way I could keep participating in social life in some sense. Though usually, what was on the screen was far different from the reality and often was twisting the truth, to which Hollywood had already accustomed me throughout the years, it was still more real than what was affecting me and what was still growing within me. One of the best-known American authors and an unquestionable master in the horror genre whose novels were repeatedly made into film adaptations Stephen King said, "Nightmares exist outside of logic, and there's little fun to be had inn explanations; they're antithetical to the poetry of fear." In my subjective, real-life horror, it was me who was the victim, asking everyone, "Why?", and just like in most horror movies, there was no answer. My nightmare was definitely beyond all logic, evoking a feeling in me that Dr. Armani and the entire healthcare service simply see no sense in making even the smallest effort to help me.

My loved ones were convinced that I got struck by depression and that despite it all, I should resume psychiatric treatment. This was evidenced by, if nothing else, me weeping and pillows wet with tears, which rendered my relatives helpless and sad. But they didn't realize how bad I wanted to be part of anything and do anything else than be locked in my own room. Sadly, I just couldn't.

Spending more and more time at the crib, each week I was counting down the days from Monday to Friday, waiting for the arrival of my fiancée, who was visiting me on the weekends. Many times, having the choice to pass that time in any enticing way with her friends, Anna would always pick lying with me and staring at the ceiling with me instead, imagining that we're lying on a beach somewhere or on a green meadow, watching birds in the sky, or snow-white clouds billowing and changing their shapes, reminding us of better days. I didn't have imagination as vivid as Anna's; in fact, I didn't have any at all. Lying like that, I'd stare incessantly at my – yet completely alien – hands lifted in front of me; Anna, despite her horror that would always creep on her in moments like these, peeking at me from aside with tears in her eyes, deeply believed that soon everything would be fine.

There were days when I felt a spike of energy and a will to live, which would evoke within me a great need for snuggling with my woman, whom I missed every day despite the six years of our relationship. I'd get into the car and drive to Anna's. All the members of her household were well aware that something wrong was going on with me and they didn't mind that Anna and I were spending most of the time in the exact same way, lying and pondering what would happen with us further down the line. It was a tough time when it wasn't only me who was suffering due to the loss of my beloved dog. Over the previous couple of years, Anna got very closely attached to Puma, too, considering her a companion of hers. I'll never forget the day when we both experienced the presence of our tiny family member.

Lying on Anna's bed, which was situated at a slanted wall in her room, we were both mourning Puma's passing, recalling the best moments we spent with her. Looking at the opposite wall, onto which a skylight would always cast reflected light, I saw the tiny snout of my dead dog. The ears sticking out, incredibly proportionate to the rest and the slim snout in the form of a shadow were obscured by a couple of slats of the blinds in the window. It was as if our beloved doggie was peeking through the window, her shadow cast on the completely smooth wall.

Aware that things hadn't been the best for me lately, I thought I was going crazy. However, before I managed to tap my fiancée's shoulder and tell her what I was seeing, she figured it out herself and, staring and paralyzed by what she was seeing, she went silent for a while. We both couldn't believe our eyes. Anna's room was at the very top of her family house, and the skylight installed in the slanted plane of the roof could only project shadows of clouds passing across the sky. After a brief moment, the silhouette of Puma peeking through the window simply disappeared, leaving nothing but a ray of sunlight. Although I wasn't fully convinced that an afterlife can exist there somewhere, I realized that on that other side, the friend closest to my heart could've found her new home.

If a human can live in this hell on earth, why wouldn't it be better somewhere else? I wondered.

Although in the era of smartphones and the commonplace habit of texting, my human friends, as I've always called them, were sending me texts like, "You coming?" or "At 4, you know the place!", I'd ask myself repeatedly why wouldn't they respond in any way to my quite atypical and, for some time now, too frequent replies. Was I losing them, too? "I can't, I don't feel very well!" I'd text them back repetitiously.

Although there were days when I really didn't feel like doing anything and no force could make me interact with my friends in any way, I was hurt by the fact that none of them had the idea to visit me and ask what was going on with me. Not only was I disappointed by their attitude, but I also started gravely doubting our friendship. I had a very similar feeling at the elementary school when one of my nine-year-old colleagues decided for no reason to bully me in front of other boys and girls, pushing me back repeatedly so that I fall to the amusement of the peers around us. At some point, I felt that I couldn't handle it any longer. I got up, I raised my arms forward like a nine-year-old Mike Tyson, clenched my small fists and threw a straight right perfectly at the nose of the classmate who was attacking me again. Suddenly, the school bell rang like a gong on a ring, saving my opponent and proclaiming to us all that it was time to begin the next class. Then, everything around us two went dead silent. The boy who was harassing me froze when he was standing like a sculpture, a stream of blood flowing down from his nose. Once the pain reached his head, he realized what happened and, terrified, rushed back to the classroom, leaving me and the other students. At some point, I felt as if I got hit in the face, too, as most of them, all enjoying the sight of me being pushed around, suddenly turned away from me scowling, as if I was a dangerous aggressor who hurt the other one so badly for no reason.

Among the kids who momentarily turned their backs on me there were several classmates who were very dear to me. Left by myself in the hall with the first lesson like that in my life, confused, I was staring only at the light resisting the classroom door that was closing behind the last female student with a colorful backpack.

I had been having a similar feeling for some time. I felt abandoned, like back when I was a nine-year-old boy unable to comprehend why his dearest buddies would turn their backs on him. I had a feeling that my friends resented me, that I was avoiding them for some reason. Sadly, it was I who needed support, which I didn't get from them.

Following the ups and downs of various people often when rummaging the Internet, I saw photos that that my acquaintance shared on a social media platform. The guy was studying at the same college I had. Back when we were seeing each other around the halls or sharing a desk at lectures, he was in excellent shape, had many friends and was exuding energy, getting wild at night clubs. One day, he didn't show up for our classes and no one knew what happened. Two years after his disappearance, at a lecture, someone turned on a projector that cast an image on a white screen. We saw our colleague sitting in a wheelchair with his parents standing by his side, asking for support. We were all stunned! The silhouette of the boy we remembered from just a few years ago looked almost nothing like that person. Only the same face, still smiling, revealed it was him.

Years later, going through photos that he had shared, I noticed that nothing about him changed aside from a wheelchair, which became his daily life. What I found beautiful and thought-provoking were photos of his friends, still the same people; with him sitting in the wheelchair, they were claiming the dancefloor as if nothing ever happened, as if his new life didn't bother them the least. Because why would it?

The only person from our pack that I could count on was Tomek. Though there was about a thousand miles between us, he never forgot what a cellphone is for, and whenever he visited the country, he'd always check on me.

"Alright, if you don't want to go out, we're staying in together," he said.

Tomek always stood out from the crowd and everyone who met him liked him a lot. Most of all, he also had some feelings he was stifling deep inside. We have always been a bit alike, and we could always find a common language; perhaps that was owing to the date of birth, as we were born only several hours apart. In childhood, we bonded over our love for a Japanese cartoon that many young boys watched most passionately. To us, *Dragon Ball* was everything. We got obsessed with watching the ups and downs of its protagonists, and maybe even adopted them as role models for life that we weren't even aware of. Though all our parents could see on the TV screens was fighting and violence that their children were gazing at, they didn't realize we were consuming extremely important guidelines on how to live as a human that the cartoon was instilling in us. Brotherhood for better or for worse, protecting the weak, sacrificing your life for the family, cooperation – these are but a few of those positive aspects that *Dragon Ball* imprinted on us. Although we were all following the ups and downs of our heroes, I had a feeling that only Tomek and I were doing that with understanding. Tomek was the only person aside from my closest family who had to listen to and see me crying due to my helplessness and huge desire to get healthy again and resume training.

"No worries, we can do it! You'll train, alright, you'll see! But you have to go meet people or you'll go insane! Leave the room, come with me, leave that comfort zone of yours!"

Although Tomek could only imagine what I felt, he had no idea about the hell I was going through and about what was going on inside of me. No one could feel that. I was dreaming of turning my room or any other place on Earth my comfort zone that he mentioned. Unfortunately, every time I cried, I couldn't run away from my suffering.

I was neither crippled nor a disabled person in a wheelchair, who'd probably have less required of him. I was a twenty-six-year-old man whom the world couldn't understand. Fit and better looking than most people in that age group raised on hamburgers and hot-dogs, a young individual with my issues was taken for a madman and a cheat everywhere he went. No one realized that inside that young body, some horrific, destructive process was taking place, and I couldn't stop it. My dad, who was over sixty, was in a better shape than I was.

My other buddies surely must've thought the same. There were days when they caught a glimpse of me downtown, unaware that most likely, I was on my way back from (or on my way to) yet another location from my 'hope list' I was about to check out.

I came across one of such places when reading an old newspaper that happened to get into my hands. Scanning one page after another, I stumbled upon an article about an extraordinary healer from the Philippines who had already healed hundreds with his supernatural power. I've always been a realist with a sceptic approach to such phenomena; however, back when I'd give everything for a moment of relief, all the principles and models I had adopted in the course of the previous, healthy part of my life, were rendered basically meaningless. If someone told me, "Start eating only grass and tree bark, and you'll recover," I probably would. I didn't happen to hear of or simply read about unusual paranormal abilities all too often. I believe that most likely, I wouldn't even have noticed a headline like that had I been fully healthy. The very headline alone, coupled with one of main subheadings made me grab my phone in a second. The headline reading, "The Mystery of Philippine Healers: The Last Resort", and the two words in the article that followed, were perfectly consistent with my situation, as if the author was addressing me directly. "When doctors turn out powerless, people succumb to despair and panic. They seek rescue at any price and come across healers... one of the best-known being the Philippine healers."

My doctors didn't even lift a finger. And when they're powerless, they send people off to a psychiatrist, I thought.

What caught my attention the most in that article was the testimonies of convalescents grateful to the healer. These people shared their experiences and their current state of health after appointments. The mysterious Philippine doctor caused cancer, pain of all kinds or neuroses to simply disappear.

After what I read, I knew I wouldn't wait long. I had to make the call and book an appointment. And so I did. I learned that the healer comes to my country from time to time, which made me even more glad.

I wouldn't be myself if I didn't look on the Internet for some more information, since the newspaper dedicated only one page to that topic. The things I learned made my desire to meet the Philippine doctor go through the roof. It weren't only articles but also short videos posted online showing utterly illogical treatments performed by Philippine healers on the sick that boosted my imagination even more, causing me to recall the taste of hope that I had been slowly forgetting. Watching how the Philippine healers open human bodies up without the presence of an anesthesiologist and with no proper equipment, using their bare hands only and causing their patients no complications and, primarily, no pain, I knew that I could finally recover. Someway, these extraordinary doctors were putting themselves in a trance, evoking around their hands bioenergy that allowed them to separate innervated human tissues without causing pain. Perhaps it was just an illusion. It made me believe that I really do see a blood-covered wound that a healer retrieves dead tissue from, saving someone from cancer. Nonetheless, that was enough to make me believe.

After all, if it was CGI, I could tell! I've watched so many movies! I thought.

On the day I was supposed to see the extraordinary Asian doctor, I was very excited and somewhat stressed up at the same time, since with the images of treatments still before my eyes, I wasn't prepared for what would possibly happen to me. As usual, I took my security with me, that is, Anna and my mom, who accompanied me during my atypical appointments.

Already accustomed to seeing various places and people that I had visited, I was expecting something profoundly detached from the reality we live in. I expected that the meeting with the healer would take place in some tenement building, an old school or some utility building. This was exactly what happened. The Filipino was seeing his patients in one of the old districts in my city. Happy that we didn't have to go many miles, we arrived an hour before the scheduled appointment to make sure that we're on time. When we got there, not all of the information published online turned out to be true. In an old single-story building there was only a female receptionist and several people aside from us. On the one hand, I was glad that there was no enormous line of people desperate to get the Asian man to help them with his mysterious practices, but on the other hand, I didn't account for a compete turn of events. I hoped that the people lined up there would confirm all the miracles described in the newspaper and other media.

After a relatively short time, the receptionist asked me to enter the office where the Philippine healer was seeing the infirm. The woman informed me that all details concerning my appointment would be provided to her on paper, asking me to not be worried about anything. I got these pointers and entered the office to meet the doctor. Although I had already seen several Philippine healers on photos published online, the physique of the one I met brought to my mind undeniably the image of one of my favorite athletes and the living boxing legend, a Filipino named Manny Pacquiao.

At the very beginning, I came to understand what the sheets of paper the Asian was providing the receptionist with were for. Having no grasp of Polish, the Philippine doctor asked me using gestures of his hands to lie down on a bed similar to those used by physiotherapists. Luckily for me, my command of English allowed me to communicate with the reticent foreigner, who wasn't all that inclined to listen why I came to see him. He asked me to lie down on the bed, close my eyes, and regardless of what was happening, not open them until I heard him telling me to do specifically that. With all the images from the Internet in my mind that I had consumed prior to coming there, I was convinced that most likely, I was about to undergo an extraordinary surgery I shouldn't be watching due to all the blood. I could feel the Asian medic covering my eyes preventively with some pads, the sensation on my skin reminiscent of regular cotton pads. At that moment, my anxiety hit in. Significantly agitated, I was listening closely to myself, focusing all my attention on each instance my body was being touched. The only thing I could feel and hear was as if the Asian man was inhaling large amounts of air and then releasing all the content of his lungs right in my face. After several maneuvers like these, Manny took the pads off my eyes, probably soaked them in water, and then started cleaning my eyelids with them gently a couple of times.

When it wall all over, he asked me to open my eyes and handed me a white sheet of paper. Before I read what was written on it, I inspected my body closely, looking for even one drop of blood. There was no mark on my body that could prove that the kind of treatment the Philippine medics are famous for had been carried out. After these several minutes spent on his bed, as usual, I didn't feel anything that could evidence in any way that the doctor began the healing process.

"Is there a chance that my ailments would soon pass?" I asked, mentioning some of them again.

"Don't think too much about that! It will be fine, believe it!"

With the condition in my ears deteriorating, tormenting me each day to a whole new level, I asked, "Well, what do you think about my ears? Can you help me?"

"Don't think about that. You think too much! Drink a lot of water."

It quickly dawned on me that whatever the Asian had done when I had my eyes closed, other elements of his practice weren't far from those applied by his Polish-born predecessors I had seen earlier. The rule, "Don't think about that" was used repeatedly by many doctors trying to do their job while unable to help. Though I found the Asian man, in his attempt to influence my psyche by repeating that phrase very much alike the archetype of an Asian master known from the movies, passing his wisdom on to his disciple, I knew that it wasn't right for me. I've always drank lots of water because of my training, if nothing else, and sadly, H_2O wasn't a silver bullet that would make all my problems go away. The fact remains that it was the first time anyone from the group of individuals seeking to help others suggested adding more water to my diet, the deficit of which often proved the cause of many human ailments, after all.

Why did the doctors I've had the pleasure to see never suggest that? I wondered.

I realized that it wasn't necessarily the case that some paranormal treatment had taken place, and that the Filipino who looked much alike the boxing legend started looking more like a regular naturopath, who wrote on a sheet of paper, among others, "Lots of water".

"When can I see you again?" I asked.

"I'm leaving for the Philippines now, but I'll be back in three months," he replied. "My colleague will be here sooner, in one month's time, so you can see him instead," he added.

On this rather pessimistic note, he ended his conversation with me and made it known to me that waiting for him was virtually pointless, since just as well as he did, his colleague could blow air in my face and recommend that I think less, too. Perhaps I wasn't meant to come across a true Philippine healer because he'd arrive in one month's time, or maybe I really had to try better and think about my issues less. Sadly, that wasn't an option; time was running out and all my symptoms were getting more severe, manifesting their destructive power even harder. My ongoing struggle with my ear problems that wouldn't stop was taking away my last bits of strength and the will to live.

As per usual, winter was making my life more difficult. Common cold or frequent instances of more serious bronchitis in the course of which the condition of my ears got more than worse, became my routine. The Valsalva maneuver during that memorable bronchitis episode not only caused horrific changes in my middle ears but also made each time I simply blew my nose into a tissue end up in my ears getting all filled up with air. Inflammations that followed, as a result of which I suffered from a terrible case of runny nose, became a great enemy of my ears. After all, I myself let air in on many occasions when performing the Valsalva maneuver notoriously, as it was the only way I could feel relief if nothing then only for a moment, and stop the muscle that was likely moving inside. That release of yet another secretion into my ears when I had common cold and inflammations only made the situation worse.

Since over time, I was losing my mind probably due to the vibration generated by the tiniest muscles in the human body, while the size of the cyst on my tonsil was starting to resemble the size of the human thumbnail, I managed to book a private appointment with a head of a laryngology department who had recently performed a surgery consisting in the excision of polyps from Anna's sinuses. Considering our most recent experiences involving healthcare staff, it might seem that my fiancée would have to face a great unknown of what the contact with the head of the department would be like. As it turned out, she had no objections regarding his approach. The doctor, praised by many patients who came to see him also from other parts of the country, proved flawless, and my Anna, both before and right after her surgery, had nothing against me seeing that respected and renowned physician, too. She was encouraging me to do so herself.

"How about you go see the Head of the Laryngology Department? He's said to be a great professional. Mind that he solved my problem in no time, with no complications!" Anna told me.

"Why not? Very well. I'll go see him!" I said.

Though in the past, I'd put off any medical appointment to no end, and my mom would have to drag me there by my hand, this time, I didn't resist. Every offer of help and every opportunity to have my problems solved were as precious as gold. And so, I booked an appointment with yet another laryngologist on my list.

For some time, I hadn't been affected in any negative way by having to wait for a long time to see an expert. My biological clock lost its track of what a healthy man's routine should be like, such as, getting up every morning with a positive attitude, ready to tackle everyday tasks and reach his goals for the day. Unlike everyone I knew, I was unable to set any target for myself anymore that would allow me to become a better, more experienced young man. I had more obstacles in my way than I wanted, and I had to keep overcoming them every day, yet they kept on coming at me twofold. My only goal that I set for myself for every monotonous day was to survive until the nightfall, which allowed me to escape my suffering into dreams, hoping that the next day, I'd wake up healthy.

The night on which I experienced one of the most petrifying symptoms became the worst night in my life so far. Though daytime and my bed were bringing me relief of some sort, this time, the case was different. Many times, I'd wake up at night, like we all do, either because of the very human need to go to the toilet or to have some water. However, for some time, waking up that night made me too afraid to even close my eyes.

"God!" I'd cry out repeatedly to the Lord, not thinking about him even a bit, and at that moment, likewise.

What's happening? Help! Help me! I yelled in my mind in the moment of despair. Yes, thinking was all I could do!

I yelled, I begged, I wept, but no one could hear me. Each time I tried, my mouth wouldn't even open. I couldn't move even a fraction of an inch. I wanted it so bad, and I tried so hard, but sadly, all in vain. I was lying in my bed like a dead man in a coffin. The only think that made me different was my full awareness of the situation I was in. For some reason, my eyes were open, allowing me to register everything that was going on around me. The moonlight was shining into my room through a window, illuminating furniture and the ceiling. Though the nightmare lasted just a couple of minutes, back in that moment, to me, it was eternity, filled by an awful sound of heavy machinery on duty.

Where is this horrible noise coming from? I wondered.

My subjective eternity eventually gave up, allowing me to regain control over my body again.

I jumped out of the bed for a while to get some fresh air after having my entire body paralyzed in an extremely tormenting, inexplicable way. Feeling awfully exhausted and worn out, I fell asleep again.

I woke up early in the morning. I knew that what had happened was not just a dream or a figment of my imagination. I knew that I had been afflicted by something horrible and I instantly went to see Dr. Armani. Unfortunately, he was absent. His colleague, an elderly female doctor I knew very well, tried to help me. She reminded me of British actress Maggie Smith, known for her quite intriguing and serious facial features, among others.

As soon as I got there, I realized that I could just as well go see a stomatologist or the butcher my mom used to buy meat from, and ask them for advice. I tried to describe to the elderly doctor the fear that had consumed me that night, rendering my body completely inert; looking at me in a way that suggested I was at the wrong office, she simply didn't know what to tell me.

Left to my own devices, as usual, I had nothing else to turn to except for the Internet. I didn't need much time to learn what probably had happened last night.

Sleep paralysis!? That's great! Anything else? I thought.

It turned out that most likely, I had been afflicted with sleep paralysis that manifests in a temporary loss of muscular tension while being fully conscious. It's nothing more than a neurological conditions consisting in the brain waking up sooner than the body does. This state can be caused by persistent emotional stress that I had been experiencing to no end. However, I knew that I mustn't be scared, as sleeping was my only remedy throughout the day. Luckily for me, it was the first and the last time when I experienced something that horrible. And yet, the events of that night made me even more certain that the thing I was struggling with had no intention to back down and was just getting started.

There came a day when I went to see the renowned expert in laryngology who earned himself the position of the head of laryngology department at a local hospital.

The doctor didn't stand out from those I had seen previously in any exceptional manner. Like any other physician seeing his patients during private appointments for big money, he looked nothing like public healthcare staff. Dressed in regular clothes, far from handsome and severely balding, with glasses on his nose, the guy greeted me from behind a desk he was sitting at.

Tired with having to tell my story to every doctor I encountered, as if presupposing that he wouldn't be able to help me either, I decided to not get into the specifics.

"I come to see you as advised by my fiancée, whom you have operated on recently."

"I know. Anna told me a thing or two during her follow-up appointment."

"Did she?" I asked, genuinely surprised.

"How can I help you?" he asked.

Describing to him in detail my ear-related ailments, particularly that they were getting more severe, and showing to the expert the cyst that was still growing on my tonsil, I hoped that maybe just a small part of my unstoppable nightmare would end.

"At first, there was that yanking sensation only in the left ear, but now, I can feel something similar in the right one, too. When I wake up, it feels as like there's a flag in my right ear that changes location like in a blowing wind. My cyst gets bigger and bigger, and I think I should have it removed. No one can tell me if that's what I should do. Can I book a date for a surgery with you?"

"Young man, I'm not sure if that cyst needs to me removed, and even if it does, I won't do it," the Head of the Department said.

"I don't fully understand?"

"I'm afraid that if I remove that cyst, you'll come up with and find some new problems and complications to come see me again, and I don't need that," he concluded.

Acting stupid, I smiled and thanked him for the appointment, which in fact cost me just as much as a fine dinner for four at a decent restaurant. I wasn't the same person who'd probably tell the oh-so-wonderful physician what I thought of him anymore. I was easily taking each new disparaging remark with my chin up, stifling grief and anger deep inside of me, walking away with my tail between my legs.

Although my loved ones were repeatedly affected by my frequent fits of anger, I noticed that it wasn't always there when it was required.

"Did you tell the Head of the Department something I don't know about?" I asked Anna.

"I only mentioned some of your problems with your ears, the cyst, but I think something about your anxiety might've slipped, too," she said.

In that one moment, it all started making sense.

The world I was discovering as a young, ill person, was something completely absurd to me. I wanted to go back in time so bad, to not be born at all. Situations like the one with the Department Head that I had experienced were only making the hopelessness of it all clearer to me. I'd never imagined my twenties would look like that. Even if I thought about any disease that could hit me, I would never believe that situations like that one can happen and that it is so hard to obtain medical assistance.

For most of my adult life, I had been struggling with heavy weights at the gym. And yet, they were nothing compared to the burden I had to carry around on my shoulders, which I had to grow accustomed to. The healthcare services were making that weight heavier and heavier, making the actual weights as light as rose petals in comparison.

After the 'fruitful' meeting with the laryngologist, the faith that I vested in healthcare professionals withered. Shortly afterwards, one man made me regain it.

As any other season in Poland, winter is beautiful in its own way, but it also has come drawbacks that gave me some hard time on many occasions. Like all other ailments, the frequent prickly sensation in my groin wouldn't leave me be, and ice-covered sidewalks on frosty winter days became a sort of an obstacle to me. Everyone who ever had the pleasure of taking a walk when it's even just a little freezing outside knows the feeling of his legs suddenly informing him they lost control over the rudder of the body. If you don't react by balancing it properly, it will all end bad. At the moment when my legs sent this information to my brain, an attempt to stop my right extremity right where it was ended up in a horrible pain that cut through the groin. Although it was an exceptionally painful ailment, I could easily say that it was the least annoying of all I was tackling. However, the problem was gradually exacerbated from the moment I realized my leg had made several attempt to get out of the joint socket, causing me massive amounts of pain. It was as if the bolts that keep the leg in place, properly secured, got loose, thus allowing the leg to occasionally shift its position to a one that was unnatural. Each time it did, I thought I tripped on a curb or a large stone lying on the sidewalk. At the point when I realized there was nothing lying in front of me, I knew my problem was even bigger than I thought.

Already skilled at seeking out doctors online, I was well aware that there was nothing else I could do but sit in front of the computer again and choose an expert who could help me. I stumbled upon a man who could easily compete with the laryngologist I ultimately didn't manage to see when it comes to the number of positive comments from patients. Considering the orthopedist was one of the top on the list in terms of good reviews, he seemed the right person to me. As it turned out, he was seeing his patients at private appointments at a sports-oriented center the objective of which was helping people who do all kinds of sports. Although I didn't have much to do with sports anymore, I hoped that it could be the right place for me. This time, I wasn't disappointed.

Each medical appointment involved waiting for a long time, regardless of whether it was a service covered by your insurance plan or a paid private visit at a doctor's office. Nonetheless, it was worth waiting. There came a day I learned what was the cause of my problem, and thus I regained my faith in doctors. For the first time, I didn't label a physician as a member of the dabblers club, as he simply didn't deserve it.

As usual, Anna and I notices a difference between a specialist who does his job with joy and dedication, and a one who seems to be stuck on his chair like a chewing gum, waiting for the last minutes of his day at work by staring at the clock in his office.

Walking his female patient to the door, the doctor opened it and then, lowering his head in courtesy, smiled and thanked the woman for the appointment. It was a picture we hadn't the pleasure of seeing in ages. Judging from the man's work ethics that we noticed instantaneously, I knew I was about to have a positive experience at his office.

And as usual, my brain started playing by automatically drawing out similarities that would fit a face of some famous person I knew from the movies I watched to the doctor's features. Maybe that was just what I did, being a movie maniac, or maybe it was because lately, I wasn't doing anything aside from following the ups and downs of fictional characters for several hours straight. Perhaps it was my perception of the world that started to deteriorate on top of it all, resulting in a physiological error of that sort. I don't know.

The doctor, who looked like American actor and comedian Michael Rapaport, had an incredible sense of humor. Seeing two young people who weren't really sending him any bright smiles, he momentarily adjusted his behavior to our age group. Walking past his chair like a teenager who's a-okay, he sat on the top of his desk. He referred to us without using any formal 'sirs' and 'misses', maintaining a refined, professional attitude.

"Now tell me what happened." he said.

I was already physically and emotionally exhausted; for this reason, with every time I had to tell the same story, I was getting more embarrassed and stressed up. Nonetheless, one more time, I shared my story in detail. This time, with Anna accompanying me, I didn't care how the doctor reacts to my overall history. Each new physician heard my story enriched with the most recent symptoms, thus making my monologue longer, sucking out more energy out of me, often making me feel uneasy.

"Slow down! Don't get all tense! I'm listening to you. Easy!" he said.

Having listened to my monologue (I stammered a little due to the growing stress I had been feeling around doctors for some time), Dr. Rapaport said, "I've understood everything and I'm very sorry for you. The one thing I don't get is, why have you come to ME? I'm only an orthopedist."

"We've come to you mainly because of my fiancé's groin, and since we desperately need help and there's no place where we could get any, we tell every doctor we see what's been bothering him, regardless of their field of expertise. Perhaps you have any ideas what we could do," Anna said.

To our surprise, the man didn't mention even one time that my problem likely lies in my psyche; on the contrary, he got up, started walking around his office like Sherlock Holmes, thinking about illnesses that could affect my present state. Sadly, he ruled out everything that came to his mind automatically, since in his opinion, some of my symptoms and previous test results, such as blood tests, were not consistent with specific disease entities that at that time came to his mind.

"Damn it, I've no idea, I really don't know how to help you two. Lie down on the bed, I'll check your leg," he said.

I lied down on an orthopedical bed and the doctor started diagnosing my groin. While performing the same maneuvers with my legs on his command that the renowned surgeon had asked me to do, too, among others, this time, I felt pain and let him know it.

"Auch! That's exactly where it hurts so much!" I yelled.

Pressing in the right spots with his fingers, the orthopedist turned to me, "I can't help you when it comes to your other problems, but I do know what's wrong with your groin. Do you play soccer?"

"No."

Having heard my reply, the expert got lost in his thoughts for a while.

"Did you train legs, too?"

"No, I was one of the guys who always skip leg days. Back in high school, I was training taekwondo, where you practically use only your legs. I was very flexible."

"And here's probably the result. I think you have a disorder we call enthesopathy. To verify that, I need you to have an ultrasound done. Please come back to me with the results," he concluded.

He walked us to the door to ask another patient in.

"Wait!" he said to us when I already had one foot out in the hall. "Have an additional ultrasound of your carotids done. I think this type of test can also give you answers, and these neck-related issues suggest that something might be wrong up there."

"Thank you for help," I said.

Anna and I were happy that we finally found a doctor who was willing to think for a minute, which turned our ideas about healthcare services upside down, instilled by the physicians we had been meeting so far, and in a sense save the tarnished honor of his fellow doctors.

Before leaving the facility, I already signed up for the two tests which I then had done as soon as possible.

Shortly afterwards, it turned out that my blood vessels, particularly the arteries and veins in the neck area, were in perfect condition, whereas the test results for my groin were a whole different story.

"Scarring of the pubic attachment in the adductor longus on the right side. Derangement of the fibrillar architecture of the attachment attaching the tendon to the pubic bone, with no post-hemorrhagic deposits. Irregular contour of the bone at the site of the attachment, enthesopathic changes," we read the results together.

"What do you think about it?" I asked the doctor, visiting him with Anna a few weeks later.

"Just as I thought! You have the so-called enthesopathy of the adductor longus, which most often is caused by excessive physical strain. We are often dealing with enthesopathy when the cartilages responsible for connecting tendons with the bone get damaged. Are you sure you don't play soccer? That disorder usually afflicts soccer players. Now, you need to be doing resistance exercises for the leg or sign up for physiotherapy. Cryotherapy would be okay for you, too."

I didn't play soccer and I also knew I never put my lower parts under excessive pressure. For most of my years, I was focused on honing my upper part. Despite the fact I had trained the Korean martial art in high school, I couldn't believe that just like that, after all these years, my leg and groin suddenly started playing me like that. I was convinced that there was some specific reason behind it all the traces of which no one had identified yet, but I was following them relentlessly. I knew that for the moment, I'd put his good guidance aside.

"As for the rest, my pal, you're not an orthopedic case. I'm sorry but I can do nothing more for you. But there's someone who could have a look at you."

For a second I hesitated, uncertain if I wasn't too quick to hold that man in high regard.

Oh, the show's about to begin! He'll probably send me off to his buddy's workshop to get some screws tightened up in my head, I thought.

"My colleague is an excellent neurologist. She's known for her perseverance and she always gets down to the very core of a problem. I think you should go see her. Cheer up! I'll be okay," he wrapped it up.

I relaxed. I expected the standard procedure, but yet again, the doctor surprised me in a positive way that we could only dream of getting from other physicians.

We thanked him profusely for all instructions this charismatic orthopedist gave us. I decided to make us of his advice and book a visit with the female neurologist famous for her investigative approach to the ill.

The appointment with the orthopedist who to me was a Michael Rapaport's look-alike not only allowed me to regain my faith in doctors and a hope for a better tomorrow, but was also food for thought. By mentioning various possible illnesses during my visit, he activated in me a desire to search the Internet far and wide again, which I had somewhat neglected.

This tool, which I was using as the only and the simplest method for solving my problems, was often like a road to hell, albeit paved with good intentions. Though my mental clarity was deteriorating with every day, being a sentient creature, I could still tell if the advice shared by different people online was odd and not necessarily good. It wasn't easy. Many individuals suffering from various conditions were sharing their personal tragedies on different forums. There was always someone who was waiting for a prospective prey, like a predator hidden in the bushes, intending to steal the contents of the victim's wallet audaciously by promoting an unbelievably good supplement or a medication that would bring body and mind back to the original state from before the onset of a given disease. Not to mention individuals who were posting for some unknown reason bits of information that were utterly irrelevant, serving no legitimate purpose whatsoever. Although I didn't have the experience and my focus was not firing on all cylinders, my intuition still allowed me to walk past such traps, which on many occasions I found myself drawn to. I wanted to get free from my problems so bad, so fervently, begging the entire universe to help me.

The Internet was not the only source of 'good' advice; seeing my suffering and sharing it, my loved ones were doing their all to bring me relief even for a moment, too. They were offering me various literature intended to shift my way of thinking. Incredible techniques described by authors of such books were supposed to help me free my mind from pain. The principle was very simple. If I believed and imagined my dream goal while cleansing bad thoughts that were stopping my dreams from coming true potentially at the same time, everything that I wanted would suddenly become reality. The content of these works was highly promising and played more than just a minor part in maintaining hope that was keeping me alive.

If the content of each of these books is similar, there must be something in it, right? I must work, I wondered.

Unfortunately, no handbook that offers specific techniques yields results right away. Everything takes time. I felt like I had less and less of it, and whenever I imagined myself full of zest for life, free from all the problems I had, the more often I'd forget what that feels like. Perhaps the instructions contained there were changing in no time the attitude of those who had some blocks to obtaining success in business, winning over their beloved woman or quitting addictions. In my case, that still wasn't enough.

For this reason, I continued to seek knowledge in a bread sense that was concentrated in the virtual world.

Owing to the experience I had acquired as regards the course of medical appointments, I could save both money and time. I started thinking like a true doctor would, and predict next moves. I wondered what would the female neurologist mentioned by the orthopedist do, and what I hadn't done up to this point. I realized that until now, no expert had offered me an MRI scan of the neck, which was causing me so much discomfort, particularly after training, and which I had been flexing it in all directions relentlessly. Hence, I had a paid MRI scan of the neck done so that when I saw the neurologist again, the results would be ready.

Before I booked an appointment with her, staring at the computer screen, as usual, scrutinizing various websites and their content, I stumbled upon a term that had the word 'therapy' hidden within it in a sly way. Lately it was one of the most frequently looked up words in my web browser. This time, having entered a phrase, I saw the search engine suggested 'ayurveda'. Until that moment, I had no idea what that was.

When I delved deeper into the subject, I learned that ayurvedic therapy was the cradle of knowledge whose values were then adopted by conventional medicine and all other forms of alternative treatment. Having learned that ayurvedic therapy covers medical fields such internal medicine, psychiatry, or laryngology, which I had been familiar with for the previous several months, I concluded that I had to give it a try.

Therefore, I immediately started looking for someone who was practicing the oldest healthcare system according to WHO, that is, ayurvedic therapy, in my city. To my surprise, I didn't have search long, as I soon came across a website that persuaded me in a simple manner to enter a tab named "Contact us".

"We've been with you for over 5000 years." Math has never been my forte, but having counted swiftly on all my fingers and also my toes for assistance, I realized my city was founded as far back as in 1332, meaning that in 2014, they should've written, at best, "We've been with you for over 682 years."

That's just an error. 600 years is not bad anyway, they must have some massive knowledge. I'm going! I thought.

With my eyes closed, I was taking nearly everything that fate put on my way. My desire to get my health and normal life back obscured everything else, like my passion for weightlifting had in the past.

Although many times I had been returning from various facilities let down, disgusted and 'robbed' of hope, I was still hanging on to my faith that eventually, I'll get at a place where I will be saved.

As usual, my first encounter with a person practicing ayurvedic therapy was nothing like I expected it to me. My imagination was putting in front of my eyes various images of a therapist specializing in a different kind of medicine than the one I had been dealing with throughout these years.

As always, I taken by surprise, as upon my arrival I was greeted by a woman whose looks were to some extent bringing to my mind my mom. The elderly lady introduced me into the details of ayurveda.

"Ayurveda is a science about health written down over 5000 years ago in India. *Ayur* means 'life', whereas *veda* is 'knowledge'. The secret of our wellbeing and excellent health lies in balance, a state we can reach only by existing in agreement with the laws of nature. As you certainly know, our entire world is made of elements. Can you name elements?" she asked.

"Yeah, I guess, there's water, fire, earth, and air," I replied.

"Excellent! Very well! Elements are with us everywhere, they are within us and in everything that surrounds us. Elements aside, the entire nature that constitutes our world is also filled with things called *doshas*. These three energy powers of nature help us better understand the world around us and ourselves. *Vata, Pitta* and *Kapha*, for these are their names, are responsible for all our physiological functions. I think there's a *dosha* that's imbalanced in you, hence all the problems."

At that moment, it dawned on me that whoever developed the website for that lady surely made no mistake when it comes to numbers; however, I wondered why it didn't say that it would best if patients were well-versed in geography.

I didn't learn much on our first visit, which was more of a handshake, aside from completely abstract concepts that didn't fit in my head and which I found very similar to that the man practicing chakra therapy told me about. Nonetheless, I decided to give myself and the lady a chance and meet again to see what benefits our appointments could bring. The more often I was seeing her, the more I was convinced that I was wasting my time, yet again. Thought the woman's numerous elaborations made it feel like she very much in the right, for aside from definitions stemming from the realm of ayurveda, which oftentimes seemed to me totally out of touch with reality, she suggested that I change my lifestyle and diet, I knew I couldn't wait until my body, fed in a different way than up until now, catches on to the new rhythm and starts regenerating on its own merit. After several years of the fight, utterly exhausted, I still believed that in just a moment, in just a second, someone will appear from around the corner, who'd finally tell me what was wrong with me, retrieving from his pocket a cure-all for everything that had been eating me up from the inside. Back then, I didn't even think for a moment that changing what I eat could affect any of it. I was expecting a quick fix that would yield immediate results.

The elderly woman had such solutions to some of my ailments at her disposal, too. Learning more and more about me one visit after another, she told me what her diagnosis was.

"I think your *Vata* is highly disturbed; your *dosha* is not properly balanced, which in turn causes in you exhaustion, annoyance and anxiety that you talk about, but also muscle contractions and all atypical movements within your body."

The lady was referring not only to my ear-located tribulation, but also to fasciculations[15] visible to the naked eye. The entire 'gang' of the other symptoms that were ruining my life was joined by irregular tremor in specific muscles, which of all the weird sensations was least troublesome. Certainly everyone know the feeling when an eyelid suddenly starts moving a little uncontrollably and, oblivious to why that is, they take some magnesium to supplement its deficiency. The very same feeling began manifesting more intensely in various parts of my body, from the thighs up to the biceps, my mouth included.

"Your tiredness and fatigue are caused by *Vata* imbalance in your body. We need to unblock energy channels so that your life

---

[15] Fasciculation – muscle twitch.

energy gets back on the right track and starts flowing freely. To this end, we'll administer the cleansing massage *Abhyanga*, which will strengthen you, and your symptoms will soon alleviate."

I had no clue what that woman was talking to me about, but the optimism in her words was giving me no basis for suspecting it could be otherwise. And so, I subjected myself to this therapy, which involved pouring hot sesame oil on my head. Like any other massage, it was very enjoyable, but it also had a flaw, as it was very brief and I had quite a lot of oil left on my head, which was about enough to make some pancakes upon getting back home. I wasn't idle while waiting for the results of the new therapy. Even more than before, my state at the time wouldn't let me focus on one method only, especially given that I didn't fully believe that it works but I had to test it regardless.

There came just the right moment for seeing the female expert in neurology recommended by the orthopedist. Full of hope that just he claimed, the neurologist will not back down until she finds the reason behind my condition, I was on my way to meeting her feeling much better than I had during previous medical appointments. I was convinced that the female colleague of the charismatic orthopedist can prove someone much alike, yet specializing in a field that should in theory hold answers to my problems. As usual, I arrived with my security. Anna was also living in hope that this day was the day when, after all our fruitless visits and attempts, the person we were going to meet would end our search. Perhaps she would finally turn things around by overcoming the hegemony of the monster that was sucking everything best out of me. Sadly, once again, we got hoaxed. The colleague of the orthopedist who was eager to help and relatively committed to helping me was not at all like her fellow doctor described her, failing to live up to all his compliments. The neurologist's very common face didn't allow neither Anna nor myself to decipher even the smallest emotion. It was as if she wasn't even there and had no interest in anything that was going on at that moment. I didn't even want to try find who of all the human faces I knew she looked alike. Having listened to our entire story so far and, primarily, the description of my symptoms, there was not an ounce of compassion in her eyes, let alone a spark that would prove she had encountered a similar case in the past. Eventually, she uttered a sentence that showed that my previous move , like a significant factor, affected her emotions to some extent, clearly touching on an invisible sinusoid wave that pointed out to us that the grimace of the expert's face probably meant her dopamine just got boosted.

"I'm glad you had a neck MRI scan done. Without it, we'd have to meet one more time. I'd certainly ask you to have it done," she began examining the image on a CD.

"That's what I thought. I'm in a rush," I said.

I know it wasn't really true, though.

Had I come here unprepared, I'd probably have to book another visit, which would mean some extra earnings for the expert. She's either not one of those avaricious workaholics, or she's really being honest with me, I thought.

"I haven't seen a neck as pretty as yours the entire week; the line of your spine is just perfect; that's a really nice spine. Few patients have a spine like that one," she said. I didn't know what to say. Never before had I heard a compliment like that. If it was about my car or even my eyes, I'd know what to say back. This time, I had no clue how I should behave. Seeing that doctor can muster some human attitude, I asked her a question.

"If so, why all my ailments, doctor? Why all the prickly sensations that are like a knife drawn deep in my head? Why do I feel delicate tickling in the back of the head, preceded by that horrible sensation? Why do I keep tensing my neck like a bicep after a gym session? How is it even possible that I can contract muscles that keep my head up and why do I feel that awful discomfort like a stick that is blocking my every move? What causes that derealization and the sense of not being myself? For what reason I cannot do any physical effort anymore and keep suffering tremendously when doing ten knee pushups? I feel as if something was sucking my life out of me every single day! Are you capable of answering my question? Is any of you?"

"If all your other tests are fine, it seems to me, that you need to talk to a psychologist; in terms of neurology, you're healthy. No section of the spine can cause symptoms like that. That's all the advice I can give you."

Anna and I looked at each other. As thick as thieves, we could see in each other's eyes vast sadness and helplessness, but also hopelessness that had been our daily bread, which each of us interpreted in their own way. Regardless of how loving the people we have around us are, though they suffer with us, they could never identify with our subjective and real suffering. Everyone who had my back in my suffering could take a break for a while from the reality I was creating, be and live next to me, watch yet another TV series or attend to their daily chores. I, sadly, couldn't. My symptoms were not up for any vacation, they didn't intend to back down for a moment to hang out with their buddy Cancer or their girlfriend Asthma for a weekend. Although I still didn't know what was wrong with me or how to call that condition, I didn't give up and I didn't allow myself to get all emotional when hearing comments like that repeatedly from experts recommended to me. Paying two hundred *zlotys* for ten minutes, I was wondering if my presence was not making the neurologist inconvenient in any way. Meeting with her again was just not worth the hassle.

"Hold on, it'll be alright, you just need to talk to some psychotherapist!" these words would repeatedly come out of medical experts' mouths. Medical appointments started bringing to my mind the notion of a helpline that I heard of. The only difference between some doctors and the people on the line was that the commonplace lack of empathy and compassion, but most of all, a phone call like that was free of charge. Naturally, like many others did, I could avail myself of appointments covered by my health insurance plan, which wouldn't require me to pay extra money. But that would mean waiting several times longer in hope for my problems to be solved and to recover, and I wanted to do that while I was still young. For this reason, among others, I was turning not only to medical doctors for help. The desire to go through my youth healthy and strong was forcing me to seek further, including all possible alternatives.

After a few sessions and having my head all oiled up a couple of times, I couldn't tell any difference. On the contrary; I was feeling worse with every passing month, as usual. The tremors of specific parts of muscles that would seem my final symptom proved not to be the end of the story at all. The symptoms that developed over time became the new normal to me. Some of them were so annoying that they substantially affected my physical aptitude, while others were simply irritating due to their effect on my psyche. One of them was excessive, erratic sweating under my armpits – under just one on one occasion, and under the other one on another. This was particularly bothersome in winter, causing me to feel cold. I didn't have to wait long for yet another symptom like that to emerge. My body became a machine that was generating unpleasant sensations. For some inexplicable reason, my capillaries on the arms and the chest started being very reactive to changing temperature. This state aggravated to the point that each time I was taking a hot shower, I was getting horrible red patches on my torso whose irregular shapes were reminiscent of continents and islands. Over time, I noticed that these patches also appear after seeing doctors. I realized that the stress due to meeting with a healthcare professional (yes, stress; sadly, every subsequent appointment was making me embarrassed and terribly uneasy due to expecting a given medic to stare at me in disbelief, a reaction that usually ended in the same way it always had) was also raising my bodily temperature, causing the said patches to emerge. It dawned on me that if the orthopedist's colleague cast a glance at my red chest and neck, she might have assumed from the start that I was oversensitive and that my issue was solely psychological.

After several years of suffering and cyclically emerging new symptoms that were ruining my life, coupled with my ongoing search, my mental state was not the best. Everyone saw me only for a person struggling with headaches, completely disregarding the possibility that a mysterious devastating process could've been really happening inside a young male's body. It was still only I who knew that it had nothing to do with my approach to life and a compromised supply of happiness neurotransmitters. Not only repulsed, but also already accustomed for a long time to this turn of events, we were all calms and collected, knowing that we simply had to keep looking.

Hoping that the lady practicing Asian medicine would reregulate my *Vata* and at least some of my symptoms would improve, I kept seeing her. Administering massages and sesame oil on my head as she previously did, she also added to the therapy process her own herbs and tea intended to get me back on my feet and, most of all, help me stop the twitching and all other unwelcomed quavering that had been bothering me for ages. I strongly hoped that the applied hot oil had in it some power that would resolve the myoclonus that was murdering my ears every day. Waiting for the results of her treatment, I rolled with the punches and continued my marathon across healthcare facilities.

I often was lost in my thoughts, taking a good look at my life. *What would my life look like if I were someone else? Why do my loved ones have to suffer because of me?* I wondered. I could see that once a single individual is in pain, his entire household was in pain, too. Reflecting on myself only for most of the time, I had no clue what it was like when you look at someone close to your heart and you can see what he's struggling with, yet you're helpless. I could only guess what my family and those close to me felt like. My future was uncertain. I had no idea why all these things were happening to me. There were odd, selfish questions in my head that had been coming to the surface for some time now. To me, they didn't seem anything utterly inappropriate, but back then, they were surely something evil. Today, they make me feel embarrassed and give me the shivers. *Why me, and not one of my buddies, for instance?* I'd ask the universe. Considering incidence and other statistics pertaining to various diseases in Poland and around the globe, a very common thing is that there's one ill person in every five people. Although the boys and I have been always forming a pack of six, it didn't change my point of view in any way. Perhaps I was feeling great resentment towards them because of their lack of interest in me, or maybe there really was envy growing within me, because usually, I was the one who was getting his ass kicked. I was the one who had no luck with the ladies, I was the one who couldn't hold his liquor, I was the one who was ill most often, I was the one who often couldn't make it to the party, I was the one called "Shorty". I'll never forget our first summer-break trip abroad. For some it was their first unsupervised trip, for others, it was their first trip abroad. When I was fourteen, we were sent by our parents on a so-called 'team building trip' with other kids scattered across Polish cities. My buddies and I spent some memorable moments in magical Bulgaria. The scenes that we knew all too well, images taken, as usual, from adult movies, became real. We were all raised on movies such as *American Pie* and we wanted the same experience that protagonists of these coming-of-age comedies really bad. A warm beach, young people having sex in swimming pools, gallons of alcohol pouring in, drunk girls scampering along a bar table with sparkles scattered around, prostitutes offering their services regardless of our age, or drug dealers walking around the promenade in long coats filled with pills. That was just part of the dream world of every brainless teenager that we had at our fingertips for the first time in our lives. Yes, it all was available to us every evening. Though we could have availed ourselves of any of these 'goodies' during our dream summer break, trip, not all of them were within my reach, or affordable. One day, in the evening, I was walking with my three friends to a disco. We were approached by two young girls who offered us entry tickets with one free drink to a night club for a party that was about to take place. They handed the tickets over starting from one of my friends. Once they gave away all the three tickets to my buddies, who were head taller than the young hostesses and me, there came the moment when one of the girls extended her hand with a ticket towards me. Suddenly, for some reason unknown to me, she stopped halfway

"I can't give a ticket to you, you're too young," she said.

My buddies almost died laughing. I almost did, too.

"We're the same age! What's your problem?" I asked in English, back then quite poor, hoping that my petite dark gray mustaches would change anything.

"You're too small. I can't" she said and then turned her back and walked off with her girlfriend, leaving us behind.

The guys couldn't stop themselves laughing the entire evening. I found it funny, too, but some part of me and my ego got hurt. Because I looked significantly younger than I actually was, I couldn't have everything that was easily accessible to us there.

For a long time, I couldn't have what my friends did, that is, strength, good health and a normal life. For some reason, yet again, it was I who didn't get the 'entry ticket' to what life usually offers a man in his twenties. On that day in Bulgaria, I didn't get the ticket, but I still had my buddies who didn't take the chance to make the next step into adulthood only because they'd have to go there without me. I wondered why was their choice different now.

Every additional help and interest from any of my loved ones were just as precious as gold. Every suggestion and recommendation of an acquaintance who could help me or give some pointers were much welcomed. The fewer people were interested in what was going on with me, the fewer people were there around me, the more research had to be done and the more suspicions had to be made only by myself, and I was getting befuddled already. Given stories such as that from Bulgaria, my loved ones were still convinced that everything that was destroying my personality was because of unhealed complexes from my youth and, primarily, weightlifting, which they considered the reason behind most of my ailments. Considering the statements of all the experts in the field of conventional medicine so far, it was hardly possible to think otherwise.

I started getting somewhat fearful of receiving an answer to my questions from professionals practicing conventional medicine, as looking at me, all they could see was a person who had psychological issues. Pages in my biological calendar were turning as if it was an open book left on a windy day, making me older and older. Some of the medics I was seeing on an ongoing basis wouldn't even show that they regarded me as a twenty-something who was just stressed-up by life, while others didn't even bother and told me whatever came to their minds, right off the bat, oblivious to how profoundly they were hurting a young man, and how their clear incompetence can affect my life further down the line. Soon after, I could learn that firsthand.

Continuing my adventure with the lady practicing ayurveda, I hoped for even minor positive changes happening in my life. Sadly, the power of tea that I was getting and, predominantly, the gallons of oil that was poured on my head, proved not enough to improve my wellbeing even a little bit. There came a day when I decided to quit, not solely due to the noticeably low effectiveness of the treatments. Though we had already had a couple of sessions, they didn't abound in discussions. The woman who was massaging my head and ears with hot sesame oil wasn't most talkative. The last suggestion she made when finishing massaging my auricles made my imagination fire up way too strong. It is possible that the lack of common ground and the fact that the massage was administered to the rhythm of Indian relaxation music played an immense part in it.

"At the next session, if you want to, I'll show you how to make a son."

Sitting in a chair and gazing at the floor, I heightened all my senses, baffled at her proposition, wondering if I misheard her.

"Sure, why not, ma'am," I replied.

That was the last time I ever had contact with an ayurveda practitioner. It wasn't until after some time passed, when I was rummaging the Internet, that I stumbled again across the wisdom of Indian medicine that explores secrets passed on from one generation to another. These golden nuggets were describing a diet and various physical exercises that would trigger changes on cellular level inside the body, thus increasing the probability that a man would make the smaller and faster sperm cells with the chromosome Y. At that moment, I realized that the elderly lady didn't intend to do anything ignoble to me, but most likely all she wanted was to share that knowledge with me, which was highly significant back then and in my particular case.

Even if I dreamed of starting up a family with my Anna, back at that time, it wasn't possible.

How am I supposed to stand at the altar? I wondered.

I'm not talking about me manipulating my neck, which would surely suggest to the people and the priest that due to all the stress, the groom got quite wasted. It would be impossible because of my derealization and the sensation of being permanently locked inside a spacesuit coupled with the anxiety I had been fighting with a few years earlier, which slowly and noticeably started resurfacing.

Every man who's sitting next to his dream spouse in front of God would like that day to be exceptional for him. Though to me, God was a matter of marginal importance and I wasn't paying much attention to such events, it was important to me that Anna, my future wife, had one of the most beautiful weddings you can imagine.

I knew, however, that back at that time, I was unable to do it.

God, just don't let me get all anxious, don't let me run away. I knew from the get-go that thought like that would overtake my head. Anna knew that, too, and so she was waiting patiently.

The doctors whom I was seeing most often, aside from those specializing in neurology, were laryngologists, among others, whom I needed more than ever. My peritonsillar cyst took on its final form, making an impression that it wouldn't get any bigger. The spherical object in the form of a small pink transparent egg was clearly filled with something. Though I wasn't suffering in pain, feeling only slight discomfort when swallowing food, I was convinced that something had to be done about it.

Fearing that pain would show up, I kept seeking help among doctors specializing in such cases. Obviously, at every appointment, I yearned to finally hear one of them saying that he knew what was happening with my ears and that he'd definitely help me.

It wasn't easy for me; on the contrary, it was getting worse. Individual cases that were similar, which I encountered online, particularly on foreign websites, were gradually becoming my reality. The nightmare I started to experience only assured me that

I wasn't anywhere near the threshold of suffering that my body could still cause me.

Many times, I'd sit trying to recall the moments from previous years that I considered bad or even disastrous because I got an E on my test, got a stain on my brand new pants, had a fight with a friend, or got my phone scratched. Recalling everything that I used to see as the end of the world, I hoped that it would somehow make that which turned my life upside down look a bit better. Unfortunately, evoking the images of the worst moments of my life, I was unable to find any that would outdo my present negative experiences. Likewise, all attempts at positive thinking were not effective enough to help me. The world in which my loved ones started minding how carefully they should be putting their cutlery away or if they should put keys into their pockets was my world now.

Every insignificant noise that goes unnoticed every day by every normal, healthy man was bothering me. My ears were reacting more and more strongly to individual sounds from the world around me, but also were getting increasingly annoying after each word that got out of my mouth. Trying to save myself from unwanted scraping noises and prevent the muscles in my ears from supposedly moving around, I'd let a little bit of air inside by doing the Valsalva maneuver. It was the only thing that could calm my sensations down, to some extent. Sadly, this state would somewhat improve only until I swallowed saliva, as the air was disappearing along with it.

Another method that I came up with to get a relief even for just a moment was holding the index finger inside the ear canal. This way, some of the sounds that were causing the noise of a butterfly rubbing its wings on the walls of my inner ear rendered inaudible and I could take a breath. As you can guess, this wasn't a long-term solution. After only five minutes of holding my finger in my ear, my arm was going numb. I tried many things to remedy the inexplicable, disgusting 'madness' in my right ear that was showing me how much I had been in the wrong for thinking that so many things in life were irritating and that nothing worse could ever happen to me. All in vain. Still filled with rising pressure that was just an astound pain in the ass, my head was abused even more severely by constant, unstoppable movements of the muscles inside my ears. The constant unfair fight that I was fighting there by repeatedly contracting these smallest muscles in our body was giving me a feeling that my head was growing like a balloon.

The desperate war I was waging against my inner ears led me to develop a habit that resembled chewing. We all know what chewing a gum looks like or the sound we make with a mouthful of chips that we're chewing on. From then on, it seemed to me that my ears acquired some extra abilities unknown to humankind. Although using a finger like a stopper that was stuck into a hole was a temporary solution for one ear, nothing could make the noise of a broken speaker in the other one go away. The more often I was talking, the longer I was taking part in discussions, the more I felt that there was a swarm of angry mosquitoes and flies was about to fly right out of my right ear. Everything suggested that some force not only wanted to prevent me from participating in social life, but also deprive me of my voice. Yes, voice. Previously a person who wasn't usually the quiet one, I was gradually becoming more and more distant, not only locked away in my own room, trapped not only inside my own body, but also in subjective silence.

Silence, right after sleep for which I was waiting all days, became the one I most respected. In his poem *Na zdrowie,* Jan Kochanowski wrote that no one appreciates good health until it's gone. His words perfectly reflected my situation; I came to understand them as no one else, unaware that soon, I'd have to face yet another immensely powerful obstacle that twisted the knife in my wound, but also became my salvation.

Dear silence, no one appreciates you here, no one notices you. You're like oxygen, without which no one could be here. I lost you and sadly, I have to live on without you, I thought.

If someone told me that I'd spend the best years of my life on the road, I'd probably smile back and let my mind drift away, wondering what would that journey be like. Is there anything more beautiful than learning about different cultures and stunning places of this world? My twenties proved to be one big trip from one medic to another, both those trying to solve my problem and those pretending they give a damn about it. The only journey I embarked on was the one within myself.

All the new sensations that my body was causing me were like a test. *How much more can I take?* I kept asking myself. The more medical professionals I was meeting on my path, the more resentful and hateful towards them I was getting. *Hoaxers! Can any of you help me?!* I cried in my desperation. Before I met on my way a person who seemed solid, finally, I went on several trips across the country. Whenever I went, I heard the same thing.

"I don't see anything up there!"

"Your ears are clean and healthy."

"I can flush it."

"If I were you, I'd keep my hands off that cyst."

"It got there on its own, it'll pass on its own, too."

One day, I got at the office of a woman who was the first one of all the medics who had similar equipment to make use of it for a couple of minutes without hesitating and try identify my problem more from the inside, and not just superficially. To this end, she performed a fibroscopy.[16] By putting into my nose a long, thin tube with a camera on its end, the doctor was able to determine the condition of my Eustachian tubes and assess if they were clog-free. As one of the few, she was wondering if that was the reason. Having my previous test results at hand, she stated that she must assess physical condition using a camera, and not just figures provided by the tests such as a tympanogram. Seeing a doctor with such an approach and interest in my case, I felt a small rush of endorphins. The doctor put an anatomical ear model on her desk and used it to quickly explain the structure of the ear to me. Despite my exhaustion and the growing inability to concentrate, my

---

[16] Fibroscopy – a test that allows otherwise inaccessible parts of the respiratory tract to be inspected visually using a fiberscope.

head was working well enough to tell where the doctor was going with it. In my view, back at that moment, there were two possible scenarios. The first one suggested that having performed fibroscopy, the woman realized she had no clue what I was struggling with and wanted to save her face. She gave me a lecture on how the ear is built, shared her knowledge of otolaryngology with me.

Oh, so I'm about to learn that you're completely clueless as to what you're dealing with, I thought.

The other scenario was telling me that perhaps there's still hope that I was wrong, and the lecture was intended to guide me further into the topics of the diagnosis and the treatment to be done.

"These are the muscles you're talking about, but I don't think that's the reason," she said pointing at the plastic ear model.

To my astonishment, I didn't get sent off home empty-handed. I got a prescription for a sinus flush kit.

Sodium chloride in the solution I was to make was supposed to help me get rid of my problems. I knew that it might not be enough, but I gave it a try regardless. Two weeks of rinsing my sinuses didn't change anything, unfortunately. When seeing the doctor again when the sodium chlorine treatment was completed, I knew that the first scenario that formed in my head during the first appointment was closer to the truth. However, I'd never expect that the specialist's memory would prove worse than that in my head that had been getting foggy for some time now.

"Please remind me what issues you've been having," she said at our second appointment.

For a second, I was having yet another *déjà vu* moment. Is it really possible for an otolaryngologist who listened to me describing such a rare condition in detail to then forget it all after only fourteen days? Talk about breaking a record.

"Oh, oh right, I remember now. Well, then? Did it help? she asked me after I described my ailments to her again.

"Sadly, the rinsing didn't change anything."

"In this case, I don't know how I can help you. I really don't know what's wrong with your ears."

"How about the cyst?" I insisted.

"Please don't touch it, it should resolve on its own."

It downed on me that the equipment and the good impression that the expert wanted to make on me were not enough to help me. Although I already had the experience, I was still clinging to hope that one day things could be very different.

I didn't give up and trudged on following the trace left online, seeking experts who were the top of the top according to Internet users. My search led me to yet another city and yet another otolaryngologist, one of the few in my country that were handling cases of tinnitus. That condition, though better known in the field of laryngology, was just as difficult to diagnose and thus also to cure. My aunt on my dad's side was struggling with that awful issue many years. Persistent noise in the head that cannot be silenced can ruin life. My life was in shambles already, but taking into account tinnitus or other diseases in this world, I knew that others were going through worse than I was.

The next specialist I encountered on my seemingly endless road was known for providing assistance to people suffering from tinnitus. In turn, I was looking forward to her extensive knowledge of a condition as underdiagnosed as tinnitus is, hoping there was a chance that she'd confirm my suspicions and that we'd solve my unusual issue together.

The experienced doctor's features were reminiscent of a somewhat older version of Laura Dern, a young actress. The well-groomed woman with her blonde hair let loose, wearing high heels and big plastic safety glasses on her nose invited me in to her office.

We took our seats facing each other; smiling, she asked me the standard question of what brought me there. Having listened to my regular story, now updated and enriched with new sensations and symptoms, finally, she proved to be the first person in my country to know what I was probably struggling with.

"What you're describing sound like a myoclonus of the ear. I've already dealt with a case that was similar. There was a girl who suffered from a problem that was much alike yours. Sadly, nothing was helping. In the end, she had to have a surgery for middle ear muscle transection. I don't know how her story ended, unfortunately," she said.

I realized that my diagnosis, which I arrived at using foreign websites, could be accurate. Although I was very much hurt by how miserably poor the knowledge of the experts I had seen so far was, I was glad that finally, I found someone who could at least elaborate on the subject a little.

"Muscle transection?" I asked, wanting to explore this matter, which I had already did in my room.

I knew that the only effective solution for that defect of the stapedius and the tensor tympani is to have them cut; at least that was the information that was circulated by everyone struggling with that problem outside Poland.

"Yes. However, I have no idea where the girl's gone to have that surgery done. As far as I know, there's no one in our country who performs a surgery like that. Although there's one clinic that you can check if they're offering such treatment, but you'd have to wait long to get an appointment. But, there's still a chance."

"Of course. Thank you for the information. Lately, I've been practicing patience a lot. I'll definitely go there!" I replied upon hearing only positive remarks about the mysterious clinic that was handling ear-related conditions.

"This ailment afflicts one person in a hundred thousand. That's undoubtfully too few to allow laryngologist to get a glimpse of it, but maybe you'll get help at the clinic."

I didn't know if I should laugh or cry. I was glad though that finally, I managed to get to a laryngologist who had some knowledge on that topic. However, the information that I received was all the more depressing.

Lucky me! I guess I'm special, after all, I laughed sarcastically, in spite of everyone who still claimed it was all because of my complexes.

"Surgery is one thing. But, before you take measures like that, you have to try pharmaceuticals first," she added, offering to help me.

And so, hoping that the expert could alleviate my pain at least a little, I put my trust in her and followed the path she showed me. I started taking trimetazidine[17] to improve my circulation. I had no idea why would a drug like that be of any help for me. Yet, considering my other ailments that I mentioned, I was guessing that this was how Laura, as one of the few, was trying to solve some of my problems without having to send me off to a psychiatrist.

Additionally, I was taking tizanidine[18] to relax my muscles. According to the doctor, it was the only right treatment for a middle ear myoclonus before making the decision to take the ultimate measure.

It was a moment when for the first time in a long time I felt being handled by a competent healthcare professional who offered me a care of some sort and showed some interest in my case. The first attempt at non-psychiatric treatment of even a couple of symptoms from my long list made me feel relieved for a while.

That small euphoria didn't last long, though. One week into taking the medicinal drugs that were intended to help me, I had already experienced a nightmare that would case me the shivers every time I even thought about it later on. The torture that ruined and transformed the lives of many forever, including the life of my aunt, got me, too. The day when I heard for the first time in my life the characteristic sound that was not coming from the world around me but solely from inside my head was a nail in the coffin.

In my time free from delving deep into the wisdom on the Internet, I was giving in to my passion for boxing by watching punchers fight, often getting some ringing in their heads and ears, the difference being that whether they went off the ring with their hand up or not, the noise was gone, too. In my case, it was completely different, a hand raised in victory just my utopian dream.

---

[17] Trimetazidine – an organic chemical compound, a medicinal drug used for treating coronary artery disease, with cardioprotective properties (it protects the cells of the cardiac muscle).

[18] Tizanidine is a form of a hydrochloride used as a skeletal muscle relaxant.

That evening made the activities in my life that were the sole source of my pleasure started yielding one of the most persistent side effects of my new condition. Because of that, engaging in my last passion that didn't require any physical effort from me was never the same again.

On, God! I cried at the top of my lungs out of fear, panicking, as usual, not knowing what was happening to me. *No, no, no! Please! Everything but that!* I realized what was probably setting in.

I threw myself on the carpet, hands covering my ears, my forehead stuck to the floor, desperately listening to what was taking place inside. Although my eyes already got all watery in horror, I took a deep breath, relieved for a second. *Oh, my! I must be oversensitive,* I thought.

Having resumed watching the movie I had paused, I hoped that my imagination coupled with utter exhaustion were just playing tricks on me. Sadly, my alleged delusions proved more than just a hallucination caused by me being completely worn out, but the first stage of another symptom of my mysterious disease.

Watching the movie and experiencing the newly emerged problem in a more conscious way, paralyzed, I started crying like a baby. With every resounding special effect or a raised voice of a protagonist that the movie was feeding my ears with, the sudden jerking of the muscle aside, I started experiencing yet another anomaly that was reminiscent of the sound of a thousand tiny pins raining down from high above on a glass surface. The longer I was listening closely to this weird noise of imaginary needles coming through my head, the more I felt that the sound was getting clearer and clearer, and louder and louder. The fact was, the higher I set the sound of the movie, the more needles were falling down, twofold. It was as if you threw away hundreds of mental pins while standing on the stairs on the top floor of a high building, right into the abyss of the space between the staircase railing, waiting for it all to hit the smooth, shiny tiles on the first floor.

Assuming that it was just a consequence of my tiredness, I went to sleep, hoping I'd never hear anything like that again.

Thinking back again about the books I was reading, I was trying to send positive thoughts into the universe.

Please, make it go away! It's not there! Tomorrow, I'll wake up healthy ad well, with no noise in my head!

In the morning, I realized once again how ineffective my self-healing powers were.

The silence that had been filling my room up until that point, was replaced by a sound similar to the one we all enjoy on summer evenings spent in nature. Already awake, I had a feeling that in my room, there was a throng of crickets or grasshoppers that were running around, playing their tune like an orchestra of insects would on summer evenings. Though it was cold outside, and many would consider the sound enjoyable and give a lot to hear it in this time of the year, I wasn't that glad about it. On the contrary, I was terrified and even more depressed. My thought were permeated by fear and loneliness.

Although I was surrounded by people who loved me, I could feel the looming end of the world I was living in. Every ounce of hope I'd get sometimes somewhere on my way was immediately thwarted, my awareness getting slapped across the face so that I don't get too happy for too long.

It was as if some evil force wanted to make it known to me that it wasn't over and that everything I had experienced up to that point was just a beginning of my long road.

Whack! Right in the face. *Letting your mind drift away, pal? You think the doctor will help you? I've got something for you. There you go! One more problem in your collection. Don't thank me, you're welcome!*

God, why me? Why do I have to get torn down like that? More and more often, I'd ask questions addressed to the one I used to pray to in the evenings as a kid, but somewhere on my way to adulthood, I stopped feeling like doing it.

I can't recall exactly how and when I discontinued my relationship with God. That is, if 'relationship' is even the right term. I think it all started at the moment when I became old enough to taste the forbidden fruit more often than I could before. Being a young man raised in a Catholic household, I would occasionally go to church with my parents on Sundays. It's not a secret that I didn't see anything interesting in doing that, and spending nearly an hour at a mass every Sunday was like the ultimate punishment to me. That ritual seemed pointless to me.

Why would I need that? What's the point? Does anyone really believe in God anymore? After all, God was invented by someone to subjugate mankind, right?! I'd ask myself.

In truth, I was spending more time with my friends hanging out behind the church than inside, the sole pleasure that a holy mass was giving me being the chance to playing table tennis in the meantime. Yes! During a mass!

From the moment we were allowed to use a ping-pong table in the day room situated in the basement under the church, there was nothing else we could do but treat ourselves to it and occasionally enjoy a game on a proper table in the church underground instead of the brick table at the park in our neighborhood. After some time, the guys and I started playing ping-pong for money. While the priest was collecting mas stipend from his parishioners, we were passionately indulging in our juvenile, completely harmless form of gambling.

There were some of us though who, unlike me, first participated in the mass and only then did they come hang out with us behind the church. When it comes to me, in most cases, I'd go straight behind the building.

My parents were oftentimes unaware of the fact that instead of taking part in the mass, I was passing that time in a way that was different to what they expected, to how they raised me.

Knowing God only from the viewpoint of bricks and walls that I was looking at standing behind the church I wasn't aware that things could be otherwise. I had no clue that I could seek help and rescue also in a place where everyone except for me were heading to every Sunday. Soon, I learned that firsthand.

There was nothing else I could do but to immediately go out of the city again to see Laura. On my way to her, I was pondering on what could be the reason behind the recent situation. Perhaps it was the medications I got to boost my blood flow that contributed to the tinnitus?

"Tinnitus? How come? I was afraid it might happen."

"You knew?" I asked, perplexed.

"The myoclonus you have can be comorbid with various other conditions."

"Other conditions?" I asked. As if I didn't have enough of them.

"Yes. The ear is a very complex organ. I once had a patient who was fainted each time someone left a door open just a crack or opened a window. There was clearly something wrong with his bony labyrinth and inner pressure."

"Could the blood flow medication affect the tinnitus?"

"I don't think so. I assume it was just a coincidence."

I couldn't believe that the sudden cricket sounds that occurred interchangeably with the noise of falling pins was a mere coincidence. Though Laura was reluctant to talk about the cyst in my throat and she didn't have much clue how to remedy the myoclonus likely manifested in my ears, she was supposed to be one of the best tinnitus experts in Poland.

"You're lucky to have come to me. There's no one else more experienced than I am," she added.

"What should I do now?" I asked.

"You should continue taking the medication I gave to you, as it's administered to people suffering from tinnitus."

I didn't know if it was my derealization and brain fog that I had been struggling with for some time that made me unable too logically comprehend it, or if something was not quite right.

"Just a few days ago I didn't have any tinnitus, I started taking a medication for tinnitus and now for some reason, I'm getting the tinnitus. I don't understand," I said.

"That's what tinnitus is like, no one understands it and, in truth, it's hard for us to tell where they come from. The reasons can be plenty. From damaged hair cells within the inner ear through dietary deficits and injured cervical spine to massive stress," she explained.

Having read a lot about it earlier, I knew that one of the reasons could be the body's reaction to the drug. Still, the doctor ruled that option out from the get-go.

Though when I came to see the expert, my intent was completely different, fate had it that while seeing her, I had to start curing tinnitus, too.

One of the solutions was to continue my trimetazidine therapy.

"Is there some other method that you could suggest?" I asked.

"There is. Habituation.[19]

"Habi what?"

"You can learn to ignore the tinnitus, to live with it without paying attention to it. It's possible, but it takes time. This is achieved by using a sound generator, for instance. You can purchase one of those at my office. It works in the same principle a nightstand lamp does. There are several types of sounds already uploaded on the device. The thing is that you focus on a sound that does not come from your ear or head, on the specific noise generated by the device. This method consists in teaching your brain to receive noise consciously. Tinnitus starts being a problem when you put all your attention on it. The role of the sound that comes out of the device is to minimize the contrast between the tinnitus and the environment, so that you stop paying attention to it. This would be impossible to do in complete silence."

I realized that most likely, I was in a dead-end situation. Everything my aunt had been mentioning for years was like something taken out of a sci-fi movie that suddenly became a fact.

How am I supposed to not pay attention and not focus on everything that was going on with me? God! If only I could purchase a health generator that would drive my attention away from all my problems! I thought, addressing God more and more often.

---

[19] Habituation – the process of making oneself accustomed to a specific stimulus.

"Before you make the decision, I'll refer you for AMSA[20] inhalations. We'll try get your ears back on feet in this way. Though your test results don't show any impairment to the Eustachian tubes, we'll try to gently unclog them."

I was glad that despite all the evil, there was still some hope and an opportunity I could try that no one else had mentioned earlier. I thanked Laura and said goodbye.

As soon as I returned home, I rushed to google the inhalations the doctor gave me a referral for. To my surprise, no medical facility in my city had such equipment. Since inhalation therapy was supposed to take two weeks, I had no other option but to go somewhere where I could both get a break from my worries and undergo daily treatments. And so, despite my condition that wouldn't let me function normally and enjoy my life, Anna and I left for the seaside.

We both hoped that I'd manage to take a vacation from my problems, if nothing than just for a little while. Sadly, the monster that was still growing inside my body wouldn't back down even for a moment, striking more painful blows; this time, it sent me right to the boards like a powerful heavyweight puncher. With a couple inhalation sessions already checked, one morning, I experienced a nasty wakeup. There was a chirp of crickets that were waking up and going to sleep just when I did every day, drowned out only by the noise of a hairdryer throughout the day.

Initially, I thought that it was Anna or some neighbor vacuuming or drying heir next door. As soon as I realized that my fiancée was there lying next to me all the time, and my other senses recognized that few people take a vacation in the spring, I got up quicker than ever. Having jumped to my feet in a fit of panic, I stuck my index fingers in my ears to listen more closely to what had probably been developing inside throughout the night.

"Please! Anything else?"

---

[20] AMSA – a pneumatic inhaler that generates a vibroaerosol, that is, an aerosol whose energy is spiked by means of superimposition of an acoustic wave, administered under short-term hyperpressure.

With my hand on my head and my back against the wall, I slowly went down to the floor, weeping and crying for help to no end.

Hearing me in despair, my Anna leaped out of bed and tried to comfort me.

"Everything will be fine, you'll see. Don't cry."

It looked like Laura was right. I didn't have to buy the noise generator to silence the crickets that invaded my left ear. Like the siren of an ambulance, or perhaps more like a line of cars trapped in traffic, honking at one another on a busy street, a new sound appeared suddenly in my right ear, suppressing the seemingly unbearable tune of the insects with the horror and atrocity it evoked.

In spite of what was happening inside my ears, I continued the AMSA therapy while staying at a small seaside town. Some part of me was able to muster just enough strength to let me persevere. I had no other choice. Although the weather wasn't spoiling us, Anna and I were taking frequent walks on the beach to calm down a bit and enjoy as much iodine as possible before going back home. The sand on the beach, still damp after winter, reminded me more of the dark-gray surface of the Moon than one of Poland's golden beaches. Never before had I found myself so in tune with my surroundings, overwhelmed by my ailments like a cup filled to the brim. Fitting the color of the ground I was walking on well, I had a feeling that I came there on a NASA mission and not AMSA sessions. My uncomfortable spacesuit helmet was not only filled with extraterrestrial pressure, a storm that was striking me with thunders at random, and creatures of some alien civilization hidden inside my ears that were making fluttering noises in response to any sound; now, on top of all that, there were also invisible vehicles honking their horns at one another, surrounded by thousands of crickets.

The fog that was obscuring my reality make the water and sand around me seem unrealistic. It aggravated the sensation that my awareness did not belong to my body even more, making me feel as if I was playing the main role in a science fiction movie. The aching groin was reminding me that most likely, I'd never be able to kick an inflatable ball back to my son in the future, and the anxiety that was trying to break loose from its cage, as I still had the strength to stop it, was attempting to erase all my dreams about starting a family with Anna. Despite these burdensome ailments difficult put in words, I still didn't lose my own self.

On our way back from the beach, I noticed a young man retrieving a pizza box from a trash can; there was some sauce on the cardboard box, which he scraped off with his bare fingers. I knew that person was in great suffering and that he must've been starving. I couldn't watch it. I approached that young guy and gave him twenty *zlotys,* an amount that would buy him a fresh, hot pizza, my favorite dish. He looked at me.

"Oh, my! Thank you! I'll give it back as soon as I can," he said.

That made me very sad.

"No need! Get yourself something tasty," I replied.

Perhaps he was cold, perhaps he, too, was suffering from some illness. Though he was undoubtedly in a situation worse than I was, he still felt that he owed me. At that moment, in a sense, his suffering was no different than mine, and I was dreaming of any doctor to alleviate it even for a while. I'd be just as awfully grateful as that poor man was and my response would be similar, probably.

I'll pay you back! I could see myself saying to the doctor of my dreams.

Time passed mercilessly, as always, in the pace determined by the universe. Though I continued to take any and all attempts at saving that what was left, my ongoing battle was more like Sisyphus's work with no progress.

The AMSA inhalations and all other methods failed me. Trips from one healer or herbalist to another, whose treatments sometimes lasted months, yielded no desired results, likewise. My life took on a completely different meaning, bringing me into one of the worst states I could find myself in, and which I didn't want to experience at any price.

I lost all my hope, and the trap and the pain I found myself in owned me. Locked inside my own body like a prisoner, I was sitting on the window sill in my room, gazing at the sky, looking for Hope in a prison cell that entrapped me more than ever before. Looking through my imaginary lens, I was waiting for it to show up. It was a dream moment with the most perfect light that would seem impossible to capture to every photographer.

I left my tripod on the bed, my hands are shaky, but I'll try anyway. Focus, a proper frame and angle, I've got it all already. Will I do it? I'll take the risk! It's my only chance, and I won't let it go to waste! I did it, here it is, I managed to shoot it despite the bars in the window! Now I know what it looks like and I can show it to others! Look! There it is, that's what it looks like! Perfect and beautiful Hope!

Every time I cried, every time I begged, I couldn't do anything; no one was hearing me, while my dreams of hope that dies last were getting more and more out of reach, like an opportunity for ever being happy again. The more I tried to revive it in me and recall what it looks like, the more it was all futile, and the prison walls that I wanted to jump over every night were growing taller.

What's incomprehensible in all this tragedy is that every new symptom was turning into a cure for everything else. In all this torments and painful perfection whose only point was to test where the limit of my abilities was, some of my attention paid to the other issues would shift on the most recent one. Thus, in a way, it allowed some rest for that part of the brain that was otherwise constantly engaging in keeping my focus on previous symptoms. It wasn't an ideal solution that would work long-term, though, and I had to learn how to live in the new reality, regardless. Each day I was asking myself how to live. What was the point of waking up every morning to live another monotonous day in suffering? Someone might say, "Dude, come on, every moments there's something going on in your life." Maybe that's right; my life wasn't that monotonous at all. I was getting new symptoms every moment. That wouldn't let me get bored. Is that the dream life of a twenty-something?

Although more and more often, my head would get flooded with the worst thoughts, and the desire to take the most precious thing from myself – my own life, was not only something I saw in the evening news or repeatedly watched in the movies, I knew I couldn't be that selfish.

Gritting my teeth, I'd tell myself, *You can do it! You must! Not for yourself, but for others!*

I had too much love for Anna, my family and, most of all, for life, to cause them so much pain. And yet, I didn't tell them things had gone that bad. I knew that there was only one place my disease would drive me to, and we all know what that is. I was aware that if I get there, I'd have no more chance to get saved and the dreams of regaining Hope for a recovery would simply disappear, because I was still the only person who knew that I was ill.

Springtime in Poland can be wonderful and the climate we have there can often play tricks on us. Is there a place anywhere else in the world where in one year, April brings an African heatwave and winter on the next, so that we make snow bunnies in Easter instead of creating bunny-themed decorations? I love driving to my fiancée's in the spring, especially in the evenings, with warm wind flowing inside the car through a rolled down window. The state I found myself in took those brief moments, so insignificant for so many people. Moments that were something special to me.

This helmet invisible to others and my awful sensations that were rendering the reality I had known unreal, I lost what we refer to as "here and now".

I loved that feeling when a warm gust of wind got inside the car, gently caressing my head and making my hair all messy, cooling down my face that yearned for that favorite feeling.

Unfortunately, things weren't the same they used to be. I couldn't feel the pleasure it always gave me. It was as if everything became fake, and I, stuffed with nothing but bad sensations, had an invisible anti-pleasure shield. Though my emotions were still all over the place due to inexplicable, random fits of rage, for some time, I had a feeling that it was making room for an irrepressible desire to cry. Natural tears that I was previously able to shed when watching movies were replaced by tears of despair. Situations that I had no influence on, yet which I had always handled well, became unbearable. Although I was going to my Anna's less and less often, sometimes, spring and warm days would successfully convince me that the world wasn't over yet.

Still trying to make myself think of something different than just my conditions, I was going for anything that was at hand. Driving a car involved the risk of anxiety setting in. Unable to drive around numerous frogs that were crossing damp roads in their mating season (and often with no such possibility available), I had to take due account of them getting inevitably murdered under the wheels of my vehicle. Failing to hold back the tears, I'd drive on. I've always been a highly sensitive person, but never that sensitive. Undoubtedly, I've always stood out from my buddies not only due to my looks, but also the level of my sensitivity to the world around me.

One day, in my youth, one of my friends and I were occupying the ping-pong table at our meeting spot in the park. The ball that was served got carried away by a gust of wind and ended up right under a tall linden. When I was bending down to get the ball, I noticed three small nestlings. The young starling babies were covered in countless red ants that surely had no intention to help them.

"Look! We have to do something!" I shouted.

"Are you retarded? Leave them be!" my buddy said.

Despite my friend's odd response, I knew that I couldn't leave them like that. I quickly lifted the small birds off the ground and gently flicked the ants that were biting them off, and then put them inside a cardboard box after pizza that we had eaten a while earlier. Then, we took these tiny creatures to the Wildlife Rehabilitation Center, where we were told that if it wasn't for our help, the birds would've died in just a few hours from severe dehydration. Not to mention the ants.

With such everyday life situations in my memory, I felt like a small baby bird who fell out of the nest for some reason with no chance for survival. I couldn't comprehend why it is always me who has to be the weakest link.

Lying like a small vulnerable bird that cannot fly, I was mourning my fate behind closed doors of my room. Hearing me weeping, my mom, who was just walking down the hall, couldn't hold back her tears, too.

Time passed by and I had more and more reasons to cry. Because of the brain fog that was getting more and more intense, I was doing all I could to feel like a human again, even just for a while, often by coercing my fiancée into having sex (by insisting on it), and sometimes by simply self-abusing to online pornography. The world I had known, in which I used to live, became completely meaningless. I found myself helpless and alone. Though Tomek was trying to let me know remotely that I wasn't, I still felt resentment towards the others for not being around me anymore. Back then, I couldn't see what I already had. Anna and my family didn't even let me know for one second that I was right.

"How am I supposed to stand my ground when I'm outnumbered?" I'd ask uncle Andrzej. Of all my family members, he became the voice in my phone I was talking to most often while he was trying to uplift me. Because he went through a lot in his own life, he knew and he could feel that I needed it.

"Cheer up! We can make it!" he'd say again and again, making suggestions on what could the possible reason behind my issues be.

In moments of hopelessness, the closeness and interest of other people are highly important and it was exactly what I needed, too. Nonetheless, in the situation I was in, being my own doctor with no practice or experience, playing whom was proving ineffective time and time again, there was nothing else I could do but turn for help to someone whom I usually couldn't care less about.

Mom would always say, "When in fear, God is near!" In my case, these words turned out to be true like nothing else.

"Pray," my mom would say.

Crying desperately always brought an emotional cleansing that lasted a while, but it couldn't purge the destructive evil power from me that was going forward relentlessly, showing me its wide range of capabilities. New symptoms that I started experiencing were not only drawing even more tears of out of me, but also made me recall prayers that I had neglected over the years.

One of such symptoms that were causing me massive fear was an increasingly frequent sensation of walking into an invisible wall. For another person, it must've been peculiar to see the surprised look on my face. The moment when I was going forward and made a step, hitting with all my body into a 'wall' that wasn't there was something I couldn't put in words. I had a feeling that the number of ailments manifesting in my body was simply merciless and would keep tormenting me to no end. There were also symptoms that, all their awfulness aside, could make you smile, or maybe even a burst of unrestrained laugh. One of them was undoubtedly drying myself with a towel under shower with water still pouring down on me, which wasn't that often. No one could understand what I was struggling with.

If not for the periodical episodes of common cold and flu-like inflammations, I'd give up on seeing Dr. Armani, since despite the years gone by, the stance adopted by himself and his fellow doctors remained the same. There was nothing else I could do but turn on the survival mode inside myself, suck it up and hope for a miracle to happen.

I've always been a realist who didn't believe in miracles, considering phenomena described by people that cannot be rationally explained a figment of their imagination or a proof of lack thereof. Back in the past, people used to view a rainbow showing up in the sky as a miracle. To this day, I know several people who still believe that to be true. Not to mention a solar eclipse.

If anyone had told me at any point in time that God or another supernatural force intervenes in my life, I'd probably drop dead laughing or reply that it's either a coincidence. Perhaps this is why none of the healers I was seeing came up with a way to convince me their powers were real. It was difficult for me to try interpret things as divine interventions, particularly in the situation I was in. I heard time and time again that there was a 'plan' the Almighty prepared for each of us, implementing it slowly by means of what we call a coincidence.

"Everything happens for a reason," my mom would tell me repeatedly.

"If my wellbeing is some part of the divine plan, then God must really love me, mom," I'd tell her.

What would it be like if he didn't, though? I thought.

Back then, when each day was a fight for survival, sarcasm was pouring out of me in gallons, arising from my suffering. I wasn't aware though that soon, the world I knew, even the one on the big screen, would share with me something I had always considered impossible. Trapped in the subjective, egoistic prison of suffering, that was telling me every day that I was playing the lead in this drama, I realized that it wasn't true. I had become part of a script that many refer to as the 'plan' I had heard so often about.

"Why won't you just pray?" my mom asked me again one day, seeing that in all the pain, I started asking God for help.

If only it was that easy! I thought. I was doing my best to act like a man of honor in my life but it didn't always work out for me. I considered lying repulsive in others, yet I myself had lied on several occasions. Nonetheless, my biggest lie left a mark within me and a bitter aftertaste to this day.

The Our Father, the Hail Mary – that's virtually all I knew. Praying basically every evening in my childhood, if I wanted to, upon finishing every prayer, I added what my intentions were. I asked for the same thing practically every time, and nothing more. "God, I ask you for good health for my parents, my entire family, I ask you for rest for the deceased souls and, most of all, peace on earth," I prayed.

I was never self-interested. Even when reciting the Angel of God, I'd accentuate all the lines in plural, thinking about others, such as "our guardian dear", or "be at our side". And yet, there came a time when I made a small deal with God and eventually asked him for something special only for myself. Before my upcoming finals at the end of high school, I promised God that I'd come visit him for the holy mass every Sunday if only I pass the finals, back then, the most important exam of my life. I did pass, but I never honored my side of the our arrangement. Some bitter aftertaste about not being able to fulfil my promise stayed with me, and each attempt at an honest prayer was difficult for me. I felt ashamed and wondered how could God ever trust me again. This time, however, I didn't make any promise; I closed my eyes and begged for help.

In spite of me crying even more often and begging God for help as well as I could, nothing happened; absolutely nothing. More and more often I was trying to take a look at the Almighty from inside a church and not just by staring at its walls. Unfortunately, the anxiety I was still holding inside would activate as soon as I walked through the door to the temple. I couldn't stay there for more than a few minutes. I felt the same issue arising that I was afflicted by several years earlier. The days and months that followed passed by without any major changes in my life. The monster I was carrying inside was the only one who decided to not mislead me and never failed to show up with a new symptom, doing an excellent job. Aside from the ears, which were dysregulated to the point that touching my face or moving my head was enough to set the muscles in my left ear in motion without my consent, there came a time for a new symptom, one of the most unpleasant of all I had experienced.

Sudden mouth paralyses, each lasting for seconds, showed me that I shouldn't be underestimating the strength of my adversary anymore, not even a month longer. It was as if I was slowly losing my ability to speak. Fear and terror that started overwhelming me re-evoked within me a desire to penetrate the Internet even more intensely, as I could've overlooked something.

I mustered the remnants of my focus and reason that I had left. I sat in front of the computer and started analyzing what I could've missed.

The ears were trying to stop me by reacting to every hit on a key in the keyboard, but I knew that if I didn't help myself, no one would. In an attempt to mitigate the jerking in my left ear I put some music on, as it was the only way I could gently calm down the rebellious muscle inside my ear. Unfortunately, a cure for one problem turned out to be a trigger that set off yet another nightmare. A thousand pins were thrown yet again at me to the beat of the music that was supposed to help me unwind, their metallic sound most antagonizing.

That moment, though it wasn't different to my daily monotonous existence, made a light bulb suddenly go off in my head, turning my fate around.

My state of several years and its symptoms could be attributed to many diseases. Unfortunately, previously it was too hard for me to self-diagnose – up until that point, when the tinnitus that was adding to my overall torment probably revealed not only where it came from, but also the source from where all the symptoms were taking their destructive power from. That evening, I was closer to identifying the cause of my health problems than ever before.

Browsing one website after another, my PC got hot-red. Although I myself was very tired, I didn't give up and kept up the momentum. Eventually, ruling out one disease after another, as well as probable dietary deficiencies that I had been studying many times on my journey, I stumbled upon two suspects who could've contributed to my situation, namely, a compromised thyroid and Lyme disease.

Did I finally find the reason behind my issues? I wondered.

I went to bed, for the first time in ages considering that day a good one, regardless of everything I was struggling with incessantly.

It was definitely too soon for me to assume that my prayers had been delivered to the Almighty's office. Nothing big happened yet, and I was simply glad that after such a long time, I finally managed to come across a very plausible link that had gone undiscovered throughout all these years by Dr. Armani and his fellow doctors alike, claiming to be experts in their respective fields who help others.

My lost hope started waking me up from a coma and there was nothing else I could do but follow the newly designated path. On that path, there was a secret that had been previously kept hidden from me and from others, too; a secret that turned my fate around, but also had a profound impact on my Anna's life further down the line.

CHAPTER IV

How does it feel when you've been wrestling for five years with an unexplained situation that has been probably robbing you of the most beautiful moments of your life, and then you find yourself closer to the answer that unravels the greatest secret? I kept asking myself. To this day, I cannot answer it; to this day, I cannot recall that feeling. One thing is certain: shortly after, I regretted ever seeking the answer at all.

Back then, I didn't even realize what fate had in store for me. The reason of all my problems was a silent killer billions of years old that humanity still doesn't know much about. Although for several years I had been in a battle with myself and my symptoms that were emerging time and again in new forms that were depriving me of any strength to live on, I didn't know that I was stepping into the very middle of yet another war. I strongly hoped that my problem would be solved soon. Reality decided to toy with me even more than before by tossing me right in the center of a battlefield, between people upholding competing theories on my illness and treatment methods. I soon came to realize that my symptoms of five years were just the beginning of a road I had to take for some unknown reason.

Time was still ticking without warning; to us all, it had now a completely different meaning. After her graduation, Anna took up a job. Regardless of the fact that she chose life with a young 'hypochondriac', as many called me, she had to keep going forward and pursue her passions without paying attention to the fact I was sitting alone in my room crying all the time when praying. I totally get that. Many could see in me the several years of depression and the struggle it involved. Meanwhile, I was dreaming of going back to the gym, hanging out with my friends on a bench in the park – like in the old days, or simply socializing again like Anna was. Sadly, I couldn't. This was not because of my mental breakdown, but an entire range of ailments that were still unexplained. One day, Anna got back home from work with some great news.

"Honey, get dressed, we're going to see my client's sister!"
"Why?" I asked.
"The woman can diagnose people with some device."
"Some device?"
"Yes, some bio-resonance or something!" she said.
"Bio-what?"

With nothing to lose and a shorter distance to the finish line, I concluded that either way, I had to have my suspicions verified. And yet, I wouldn't be myself if I didn't take a quick peek into the source of knowledge that the Internet had become for me over the recent years.

I wanted to learn what bio-resonance is about before leaving with Anna. Sadly, the information I found online didn't encourage me to do so. Many articles that I came across were referring to this method, which can be used both for treatment and diagnostics, as satanic, lacking any scientific foundation, used by charlatans in their shady businesses. There were also studies whose authors were confirming that the device was highly effective.

In my situation, I didn't care anymore. Being a person of little faith, I didn't read much into these types of labels; on the contrary, I was completely indifferent, and epithets such as "diabolical machine", taken right out of some devotional websites didn't work on me at all.

And so we set off to pay the recommended lady a visit. We parked the car by an elementary school building and headed towards the main entrance.

"Where are you taking me?" I asked Anna.

"Don't worry. It's the right address," she replied.

Crossing the doorstep of the elementary school, I was getting more and more sure that at least part of the information I read online was not necessarily a lie, and that stories about shady bio-resonance businesses that people run are in fact real.

When we were descending to the underground story of the building, I recalled the misdeeds of my buddies and I by the church and started imagining that someone was definitely committing sins down there.

We saw a very short, stocky lady with some unusual features. Though I was never fond of women who were several times as bulky as I was, that one was undoubtedly incredibly charming. With her face reminding me of a bit bigger and better nourished version of Natalie Portman, the woman with white glasses and short-trimmed orange hair greeted us with a big white smile accentuated with some red lipstick.

Her smile wasn't the only big thing about her. She had some other attributes that were quite noticeably on display. Despite my growing disorientation, confusion and difficulty to think clearly, my manly radar was still working just fine. Natalie invited us to her office in the basement of the elementary school. On her desk, there was a very small device reminiscent of an old tiny radio or a modern cash register, with two cords plugged in.

The woman asked what brought us there. After a brief conversation, she requested me to fill out a sheet of paper with a list of questions. Some of theme gave me food for thought and I started believing even more that the things posted online were true. "What hurts you and where?", "Do you have any health conditions?", and the most delightful one, "What health conditions you suspect you might have?"

While completing the form, sitting awkwardly right next to my fiancée, I was taking hasty looks at the lady leaning on the desktop, putting more than just her bright smile on view. I realized that she must've been compensating in some way for those questions, which were all very telling for an intelligent patient.

"Now, please place your hand on the table!"

When she handed one of the cords ended in a copper rod over to me, I asked, "What's that for? Will it hurt? How does it work?"

"This device works based on electromagnetic vibrations at a specific frequency, which allows me to eliminate and also detect various pathogens, diseases or vitamin deficiencies in your body. You won't feel anything."

"How's that possible?" I asked.

"Every living being emits its own wave at a specific frequency, and each cell has its own dedicated electromagnetic frequency. All bacteria and viruses have their own specific frequency. It was determined long ago that all cells are constantly in motion, and so their membranes are vibrating all the time."

"But why do I have to be holing that?" I asked.

"The device is nothing else but an electromagnetic wave generator. It has programmed frequency for pathogen vibrations. The vibration range of all unwelcomed guests we have inside our bodies is very specific, and using vibration of well-adjusted frequencies I can detect a given pathogen in your body. This is the only way I can diagnose you."

I had absolutely no clue what she was talking about. Nonetheless, I subjected myself to the treatment without any second thoughts. She put in my hand (both were ice-cold for some time now) a copper rod that was plugged in to the bio-resonance device, an she grasped the other and began pinching it gently and painlessly using the end part of the other cable, which looked like a ballpoint pen. Three minutes into this acupressure, she said, "I see you have some issues with the thyroid, but probably Lyme disease, too."

How strange. That's exactly what I wrote down when I was honestly answering the questions on the form," I thought sarcastically.

"What now?" I asked.

"Now you need to go see a doctor to get a referral for testing and come here again with it."

We paid for the appointment, similar to what medical experts required for private visits. Since I was a wreck, I had no idea what to make of it all.

Is that what diagnosing and treating people using bio-resonance looks like? I kept asking myself. *If so, it means that Natalie got us hoaxed,* I thought.

One thing was certain: I had to go see Dr. Armani to show him the new trace that I had found, which after all was what he and his fellow doctors should've done, as it's the patient's doctor who should do all the investigation, and not the patient himself.

With every new trace and every subsequent appointment, I was feeling more and more like an idiot who, in doctors' eyes, has nothing to do and spends years convincing himself that he has diseases he really doesn't.

To my surprise, the now-older Dr. Armani had no objections and issued for me the referral for the necessary tests without any problems. Not engaging in any superfluous disputes with me, he still maintained his previous stance and considered all my suspicions yet another whim of a hypochondriac.

"You have no Lyme disease, but very well, here's your referral for the test. It's worth having your thyroid checked, but I doubt if that was the cause of your ailments," he wrapped it up.

To him and other staff at the facility he worked at, I was a legend and one of those patients they could probably laugh at behind the scenes.

When Anna and I were waiting to get the referral verified by a medical receptionist with the stamp of the clinic, one of the nurses who worked there recognized my fiancée.

"Anna! What are you doing here?" she shouted.

"Oh, my, good morning, I didn't recognize you!" Anna said to the woman who turned out to live in the same area.

"Why, darling, you've found yourself one ill guy!"

We all looked at one another, smiling. Thank God, despite all these conditions I was struggling with, life didn't take away my sense of humor. Though that joke was clearly inappropriate, the nurse hit just the right spot with it. *Good one!* I thought.

When we already got the referral we needed, there was nothing else for me to do but to go to a laboratory where I often had my blood tests done on very friendly terms after all these years.

Since an experienced employee of that facility noticed that the thyroid test the doctor ordered covered only checking the metabolic activity of hormones T3 and T4 responsible for the proper functioning of the human body, he also advised me to have some additional ones done, often done by people as part of the package. Therefore, I bought an extra test for antithyroglobulin antibodies called anti-TG and also thyroid peroxidase antibodies called anti-TPO, which are essential for diagnosing chronic inflammatory autoimmune thyroid disease – Hashimoto, which as it turned out, generates symptoms similar to those of Lyme disease.

"Thank you. It's a shame my doctor didn't sort that out," I said.

I received my results, yet I didn't understand them at all, given that my medical knowledge was based solely on online content and wouldn't let me comprehend what was written down; and so, after a couple of days, I rushed back to my local outpatient clinic.

Sadly, I didn't found Dr. Armani there, so I had to see his elderly fellow doctor with whom I had appointments just as often.

My every visit at Meggie Smith's office was very much like that at Dr. Armani's, the difference being that I was usually feeling even more embarrassed. It seemed to me that Meggie's age and experience are two things that were unquestionable.

What are you even doing here? Shouldn't you retire? I thought.

As usual, I got a 'warm' welcome, the forced smile on Meggie's face telling me one thing, *What have you come up with now, young man? What' brings you here, again?*

"I'm back with my test results. I think I've found the reason behind my health conditions of many years."

As usual, Meggie slid her glasses down to the tip of her nose and cast a glance at the results. Sliding the specs back up with her index finger, she leaned back in her chair, her face unnaturally serious.

"Tell me, young man, what's really bothering you?" she asked.
"I don't understand." I replied.
"Lie down on the bed, look at the ceiling and think about your life! Start living like a young person should instead of playing a detective. Looking for diseases is my job, not yours! Your results are very good. Get a life, young man!"

Although I wasn't as good looking anymore as five years earlier and my physique didn't look like that of an athlete, more like that of an ordinary guy who's often sitting at home watching TV, the doctor still considered me a picture of health.

In moments like that I dreamed of my hidden Mr. Hyde taking total control over me and offloading all the negative emotions and all the aggression that had been lurking within me. *For so many years, you haven't even lift a finger to help me, and now you're telling me that looking for diseases is your job?* I thought.

And yet, sadly, like Dr. Jekyll, I was humbly listening to Smith talking; my head held low, my eyes lifted no higher than at the level of her knees sticking out from behind the white desk didn't even evoke the slightest bit of empathy within her, no thought, "what if I'm wrong?", "what if that young man has really been in pain all these years?"

For years, when leaving each doctor's office, I was imagining myself walking out upon leaving his phone number on their desks like a police lieutenant in a movie, saying, "If you happen to recall anything, call me, please." Unfortunately, roles in this script were completely reversed, and as the victim, I couldn't play the good detective. It was a total paradox in my entire situation of several years. In just a moment it turned out that I wasn't that bad in that role, after all.

After seeing Dr. Smith for the last time, I had no idea where I should go next. My body was in shambles, my life was hanging by the thread, and my results, as the doctor mentioned, were very good. Though I weren't that sure about the bio-resonance business Natalie was running, in truth, there was nowhere else I could go. I decided to go back and see what her opinion about my test results would be.

"It looks like I don't have Lyme disease, and my other results are excellent," I said right at the start.

"Michal, I cannot help you. You need to go see an endocrinologist."

"I thought you can examine me using that device?"

"Yes, I can, but in order to implement suitable treatment, I need to hear a medical doctor's opinion.

If so, I had absolutely no idea what her job was. Nonetheless, I was glad that at least, I got some good pointers, something I hadn't gotten from a primary care physician for a long time, and maybe I've never had.

"One more thing. As I've mentioned before, the compromised thyroid aside, I suspect you may have Lyme disease," she added. "Please ask your doctor for a referral for Western blot[21]; the test you had administered is ELISA[22], which is one of the oldest methods for diagnosing Lyme disease, but also the least effective. In that method, blood serum is tested for the presence of Borrelia antibodies. Research shows this test to not be as reliable as we would like it to be, though."

"How come?" I asked.

"ELISA was administered to many people, including a group of individuals suffering from a certain type of Lyme disease, as evidenced by the so-called erythema migrans, with usually a negative test result in 40% of those tested."

"But that means I could've just as well toss a coin, right?" I asked.

"Unfortunately, it does," the woman replied.

"Erythema?" I added, intrigued.

I had heard of Lyme disease on several occasions in my life; having learned that term from a coursebook back at school, I didn't have a clue how vast and mysterious a subject it pertains to, though.

---

[21] Western blot – a method used in molecular biology for detecting specific proteins.

[22] ELISA (enzyme-linked immunosorbent assay) – an enzyme-linked immunosorbent assay, one of the most common tests in biochemistry assay, both for scientific and diagnostic purposes.

Also, I didn't have a clue how destructive the disease I was probably struggling with was, and, on top of that, if it really was that particular disease at all.

"Yes. Did you ever happen to have a suspicious red area on your skin?"

"No, I didn't"

"Exactly! Erythema migrans often manifests as circular red rings at the site of a tick bite. However, in many cases, it can take the form of red rash with irregular borders, commonly misdiagnosed as some other skin disease. Sadly, erythema migrans shows up in only few lucky patients. Studies show that only a quarter of tick bites cause it."

"Lucky patients?" I asked.

"Yes, the lucky ones. Erythema migrans serves as unquestionable proof that the body got infected. The sooner an action is taken, the more there is a chance to avoid the suffering that you've experienced, for instance. If you are infected at all, and I suspect you are."

"You've mentioned ticks, right?"

"I have. Have you ever been bitten by a tick?"

"No, never."

"You could've never noticed."

"How come?"

"Suffice that you fell prey to a transitional form of the tick called the nymph. In order to transition into the adult form we usually hear of, the nymph has to fill itself with blood. Due to its small size about that of a poppy seed, it is sometimes a greater threat than the adult form. But enough about that. You should get additional Western blot testing done. Like ELISA, Western blot detects in the blood antibodies produced as a response to the infection. Both these test determine the presence of IgM antibodies, which evidence there's an active infection, and IgG antibodies, which show if there's already been contact with the bacteria. Your ELISA result is negative. In this case, doctors see no point to continue diagnostics. If you got a result that was borderline or positive, they'd most certainly order additional

Western blot testing, which very often serves as phase two in the diagnostic process."

Although the lady's knowledge seemed to surpass that of many doctors I had been seeing in the past, I still couldn't get it what her job really was all about. It looked more like consulting an enthusiast of healthy living than charlatan wangling hard-earned money from the ill. After my second appointment with her, I still didn't know where I stood and what I should do next. I had to continue going down the path I had chosen for myself based on online research, though.

Therefore, I went to see an endocrinologist, albeit it sounds odd. I hoped that my issue lied in compromised thyroid, which for a layman sounded better than Lyme disease, as the latter didn't seem any easier to tackle given Natalie's descriptions.

As usual, to save myself the pain, which I had already experienced in excess, as well as not to wait several months in line, I chose a path that was less difficult, albeit more expensive, and booked a private appointment with a female endocrinologist who had quite a few positive reviews. At the visit, it turned out that my thyroid test results were very good, just as Dr. Armani's elderly colleague pointed out to me. Additionally, I had an ultrasound done, which confirmed nothing bad was going on with my hormone-producing gland. As usual, it came with some good advice.

"I suggest you find a really good psychiatrist," said yet another expert on my path, having listened to the story of my journey of almost five years and the theories that came to my mind lately.

Since of all my conditions, anxiety seizures were the one that continued to reoccur even more intense, the physician decided to help me by means of prescribing propranolol, which has anxiety-reducing properties.

Because the situation was getting worse and worse, I decided to resort to the medicine to help myself. Unfortunately, as previously, the drug had no effect on me.

Hearing yet another person claiming I was whining instead of enjoying life, I started self-reflecting. My brain started a war of thoughts with me, but owing to my conversations with God that I had implemented sometime earlier, I wasn't talking only to myself. *What should I do, God? Am I really mentally ill? Is everything that's happening to me just my mental creation? If the ELISA test was negative, perhaps there's nothing I should be looking for?* I wondered.

Regardless of how many times I cried, there was no answer. I could feel, though, that it wasn't the right time to give up, and that I had to keep going. I knew I couldn't go back to Dr. Smith and ask her for a referral for Western blot, as she'd probably never give it to me, and confronting her unquestionable diagnosis yet again was not something I needed. Seeing Dr. Armani again wasn't the best idea either, but I had to take the risk; after all, there was nowhere else I could go.

"Welcome! What do you need this time?"

"I'd like to ask for a referral for Western blot for Lyme disease."

"But you've already had a Lyme disease test."

"Yes, but I'd like to do a different one called Western blot. I've heard it's more reliable."

He sighed.

"I don't consider that necessary. ELISA is a really good test. It's not only quick, but also highly sensitive and specific. If you had a bacterial infection that causes Lyme disease, we'd certainly be aware of that. The result was negative, so I see no need for you to had any extra testing done."

I had a feeling that I won't get the referral for the additional testing, not even from Dr. Armani. For this reason, I had no other option but to have the testing done again, at my own expense.

I don't recall the feeling that overwhelmed me in the moment I got in my hands the result of the test that would determine the road to my healing further down the line. I certainly asked myself, *Why so late? Why not five years ago?*

Just as in the case of ELISA, the result for the IgM class that indicated of the was an active infection with Lyme disease bacteria was negative. However, the IgG result was quite different, which informed me that I had contact with the bacteria. The total score that antibodies are given within the reference interval that determines the result showed that it was a borderline result. Despite the results still being uncertain, there was no smile on my face; I could feel though that finally, I had a small answer. That tiny yet very significant bit of information forced me to put even more mental effort and commitment into rebuilding everything I lost. For a while, I felt a fresh breeze of optimism, which after all the previous years made me believe that I could recover.

If the tests confirmed past infection, why wouldn't there still be some bacteria inside me? What if I still have it? What if they are the reason behind all my health conditions? I wondered.

Although I still had no answer to the questions that were bothering me the most, I was much closer now than further to getting it. I wasn't aware yet that in my struggle with the mischievous pathogen that had been possibly ruining my life I'd be on my own, and I'd have to fight my way through to recovery.

I couldn't wait to see how the doctors at my outpatient clinic would react to the results and what they would tell me. Though I could never act boastful, glowing with pride, over someone who should've admitted I was right in any situation that required it; despite my terrible condition, some part of me didn't want to take them all down a peg or two.

"I've found something, after all!"

Maybe we should swap places? I suggested in my mind, watching Dr. Armani checking my results several times.

"Indeed, there's no doubt you could have had contact with the bacteria," he remarked, nodding. "However, a borderline result doesn't determine whether you have Lyme disease or not; you have had contact with the bacteria, that's for sure. I can't tell you if you're suffering from Lyme disease. You need to go see an infectiologist. I'll give you a referral to a clinic."

Couldn't that be done straightaway? Did I really have to go through it all so that one stupid piece of paper dictated who should come up with further diagnoses? I pondered.

I didn't see any trace of remorse on Dr. Armani's face or any other gesture that would evidence he was feeling stupid, or one that would tell me, *Forgive me. You were right.* I was satisfied though that I got my way and that most likely, I solved the mystery that proved too difficult for him and his coworkers to handle.

Leaving the outpatient clinic, I ran into Meggie Smith who was walking in, and greeted her by nodding my head. Though I felt like a walking dead man, I mustered an unusual wide smile that I sent her way, my eyes showing grief I had towards that lady. It was the last time I met that woman.

I think that each one of us experienced at least once that wonderful feeling, a kind of a reward for the time and effort vested in some task or idea. My peers or friends, as continued to call them, were executing their plans or projects of many years, or simply graduated, experiencing an inflow of all the positive emotions linked to being committed for years to something that finally gets finished or implemented in the way they desired; I was trying to generate that excitement within myself, too. Unfortunately, I couldn't, I was unable to enjoy my small success. Is that even the right term? Success? The greatest success I had managed to attain up until that point was probably self-diagnosing.

Well done! I thought sarcastically.

"What are you talking about? Look how long it's been tormenting you!"

"We're glad. Now, all it takes is to find the right doctor who'll help you!" my relatives said.

Even if I was capable of re-evoking the feeling of excitement, which I used to know very well in the past, it wouldn't last long. The small flame within me that some part of me was trying to turn into an inferno of joy, with all my loved ones were tossing matches in, would soon get put out. The right doctor that would eventually save my life that was falling into pieces proved no different than the others.

"Welcome. What brings you here?" she asked me at an infectious diseases clinic.

"I come to you with a huge problem," I relied in a worn-out voice that was emphasizing the state I was in most excellently. "I suspect I have Lyme disease."

"Have you been bitten by a tick over the last several months?" she asked.

"I've never had any contact with a tick."

"Then why the suspicion?"

"I had a Western blot test done. Please, take a look at the results."

"You had that test done out of boredom?"

"No, I've been suffering from a series of symptoms that have been ruining my life for almost five years now."

"Five years?" she asked, her eyes showing she was somewhat surprised.

"Yes,"

"And have you ever noticed on your body a red circular mark?" she asked.

"I've never had any marks like that," I replied, my voice trembling.

"And do you get joint pains?"

"Joint pains?" I was flabbergasted, losing my grip due to all the stress.

"Yes, joint pains. If you had Lyme disease, your knees, wrists and elbows would hurt. There's this thing about Lyme disease, it attacks primarily the osteoarticular system."

"No, ma'am, I have no joint pains, but I do have lots of other symptoms that won't let me live."

"And yet, you're alive and talking to me, are you?" she replied with a hint of sarcasm.

I went silent for a moment.

"Very well, tell me what's bothering you."

As usual, I was overtaken by extreme emotions. I hated telling them about all the things that had been happening to me. After all that time, it felt like stripping down, revealing all the intimate secrets to the amusement of for the public healthcare professional sitting in front of me. That moment when you feel you're just another number in the waiting line, and you can see in the doctors' eyes that they're wondering what to cook for dinner, was still making me unbearably uncomfortable even after all these years.

"Sir, your Western blot proves nothing. If you had active Lyme disease, your joints would've been in pain, and you would've tested positive for the IgM. Your result shows that your body have produced antibodies to fight the bacteria, but that just as well could've happened back in your childhood. Owing to the immunological memory of plasma cells, antibodies can remain in the blood for decades. What I'm trying to tell you is that you definitely don't have Lyme disease, and your immunological system overcame it long time ago, that is, if it had any contact with it at all, as your test result is borderline."

"So what do you suggest, doctor?"

"Young man, if you had Lyme disease, I'd put you on an antibiotics for a month. However, in this case, I don't find it necessary. If you really have had contact with Lyme disease bacteria at some point, and today, you're experiencing any related symptoms, we could be dealing with the so-called post-Lyme syndrome[23], assuming that your body got rid of the bacteria and healed on its own."

"Post-Lyme disease?" I asked, surprised.

"Yes. It's a condition that persists in many people who either went through Lyme disease or cured it in one way or another. This means that the reason behind your ailments lies elsewhere."

"Where 'elsewhere'? What do you mean?"

"I suggest that the symptoms you're talking about be treated at an outpatient clinic specializing in neurology or psychiatry, but when it comes to me, I can't help you. One thing's certain, though: you don't have Lyme disease."

The doctor's opinion closed a chapter in my life in which I could decide my fate for myself, and my intuition, which was usually telling me healthcare staff was not always right, remained silent this time. Both me and my loved ones were highly confused by that situation, which had been taking a toll on us all. Each of

---

[23] Post-Lyme disease, also called post-Lyme syndrome (PLS) or post-Lyme disease syndrome (PLDS) is a group of symptoms typical of Lyme disease that remain persistent after the end of the treatment.

us had already lost track of that incomprehensible drama that I was most afflicted by. Although I could still go see Natalie again, I found that option pointless.

After all, if I go see her again with the opinion of the infectiologist, I'll only spend money unnecessarily, just to hear her say that she's unable to help me or that her bio-resonance therapy results were wrong, I thought.

Although the woman seemed to have some expertise backed by the online reviews, I still couldn't understand why did she ask me to write down on a piece of paper names of diseases I suspected myself of; that wasn't something I'd expect of bio-resonance therapy. That highly odd situation made me give a serious and careful thought to it, rendering the physician's words the sole reliable source of information, yet again, and the only accurate direction further down the line. In turn, I decided that the lady who was using an electromagnetic wave generator for diagnostic purposes was just ridiculous. I fell into a spiral of monotony that after many years of guessing and struggling, I got spit out back on the road deprived of any hope.

"What shall we do then?" my loved ones kept on asking me.

"I have no idea," I'd reply.

"You must take a decision! You can't continue living like that, you can't go on suffering like that!" they said.

I knew that my family and Anna had only one solution in their minds.

We were all aware that no neurologist would help me, for most of those I had seen just pointed at their fellows specializing in psychiatry.

I had no other option. The constant fear I felt when watching my hands that were making me even more anxious than before, to the point that I was unable to drive or socialize, the incredible uneasiness in my neck, or the powerful sensations of having my head squashed that was making me unable to do any physical effort – it all was just a small fraction of all the atrocities I was carrying around within myself, which forced me to dial the number of the medical expert who was Tom Selleck's look-alike.

When the year 2015 started, I still had no clue what was causing my nightmare. I felt like the last piece of dominoes, standing on the verge of a precipice, the only thing that was allowing me to not fall into the abyss being that the piece behind me, which had been pushing me towards it over the five years of this destructive cycle, hadn't been completely knocked down yet. That was not what I imagined my life would be like.

It's not what anyone's life should be like, I thought watching my yet another friend starting a family. Being twenty-eight already, my main thought that was filling the hopelessness of my daily existence was, *Will I make it to my thirties?* My heavy spacesuit, which couldn't be taken off me even for a while, was making it feel even hotter, and I felt weaker and weaker. I was as if I stepped into some unknown land on an alien planet where gravity is even more powerful and temperature is much higher. Though I had already wrestled with an occasional sensation of my face all burning in the evenings, it became even stronger and more annoying. The sensation of cold hands that I had on a daily basis would momentarily turn into an unpleasant wave of heat; it was just as if my hormonal system completely lost it. I had no other choice; taking note of the prospect of falling down into the dark abyss, I didn't wait any longer. The amount of negative feelings forcing themselves on my helpless body caused me to start choking and panicking when I was alone, and realize that I couldn't do that any longer. Dead while still alive, I got dressed and, with all my test results that I had done up until that point under my arm, I went to see Selleck again after a break.

Walking through his door again, I could see myself from five years ago, my hand on the doorknob of the first psychiatrist as if it was yesterday and it wasn't five years later at all.

"Help me, I beg you! I can't take it anymore! Please, do some quick therapy! I beg you!" I cried holding a tissue, tears rolling down as if I were a kid, asking the man to bring me some relief.

Trying to make the doctor recall my entire story and to describe to him what I had been struggling with additionally, I realized I just couldn't. Each day was only worse and worse. It was as if my command and control center was gradually getting broken, while the aggravated brain fog was preventing me from mapping out my present situation to anyone, slowly gagging me like a hostage.

There was a reason why I was impressed by how my first appointment with that psychiatrist went. Though I expected it to be completely different, his professional approach and dedication to his job put him in an even better light.

"I'm not convinced if any therapy would help you," he remarked, having studied a sheet of paper with the list of my symptoms on and all my test results, primarily the borderline result for the Western blot. "If you really do have Lyme disease, and the symptoms you're talking about can suggest that, I'm very sorry for you, because I know you still have a long, arduous journey ahead. I could begin a therapy with you but I'm afraid it might not be of any help to you, and if you do have a bacterial infection, its time-consuming nature could only compromise our therapy, preventing you from starting proper treatment."

"What are you talking about? Man, have a heart! Everyone's thinking I have some neurosis. Please, at least give me some meds, if nothing more! I can't take it anymore!" I continued to beg him.

On that day, I couldn't comprehend that things could've really been different than what everyone was saying. My growing inability to focus coupled with brain fog made me forget my suspicions of these several years, and most of all, my counterarguments that were based on my intuition. It was as if I forgot that it wasn't a matter of what was happening inside my head but an intervention of some monster that only I believed in throughout this time. Suddenly, the script for my journey of several years changed dramatically, and the psychiatrist that everyone were sending me off to, was now sharing my conviction, causing all the more confusion in my head.

"What do you suggest then? Can you give me something that would help me, even just a little?" I asked thinking of pharmaceuticals, my voice trembling.

"As I've just mentioned, if you do have Lyme disease, I see no point in putting you on meds that will not eliminate the underlying cause of your issues. You must not stop and go get yourself properly diagnosed somewhere. If the test result was borderline, perhaps it's worth doing it again?"

"Please, give me anything, only for some time!" I insisted in my suffering, completely disregarding my previous beliefs, not fully understanding Tom's opinion.

"Very well, if you want it that bad, I'll prescribe one of the latest drugs. It's a very expensive one, but with my prescription and seal, you'll get it at a little less. It's called Valdoxan."

At that moment, I could think about nothing else but taking anything that could help me and bring me relief for a moment. However, I didn't expect that the long list of my symptoms would now also include one of the main side effects of that drug, reported in a fraction of patients, which was the biggest nail in the coffin I could've get for myself.

Sleep was still the only thing I could find solace in after having wrestled with my existence days on end; to me, existing became a challenge of sort that I had to take up every day. For most of us, sleep is merely part of our lives that we don't pay attention to. Closing eyes, we wonder what the next day would bring when we open them again. Going to bed on every Thursday, somewhat excited, we're thinking about Friday, followed by a wonderful weekend that offers numerous possibilities that we just can't wait for. In my case, it was nothing like that. To me, sleep was the only way to escape from my awareness available to me, right into a different reality where nothing was bothering me; a reality that was my unfulfilled weekend. Though I didn't always dream of being a better, healthier version of myself, I hoped that the state of repair and reconstruction that resting for several hours a night entailed would turn my fate around on the very next day. The day when I embarked on the deck of Valdoxan undoubtedly changed the days that followed, sending me off to an even more distant planet of incredibly severe symptoms and experiences where I had to face ruthless insomnia.

Jesus Christ! Everything but that! Mentally devastated, I was asking God out of my subjective helplessness, *Why? Why do I have to suffer so much? What did I do to you?*

I had to take up another fight. I knew that if I leave the ship of the latest medication, which would probably bring me some relief later on, there would be no change for improvement. Sadly, I couldn't win that battle. After fourteen days of sleep deprivation, I felt like I was disappearing, as if my spacesuit was being consumed by some alien wetland previously unknown to me. I felt as if I were a pencil drawing that someone starts slowly erasing for some reason. Insomnia combined with a whole gang of enemies that were taking my life away was like the ultimate weapon that had only one purpose. I got trapped and there was no way to escape. The lack of sleep caused my head to reflect on the purpose of my worthless existence more and more often, making me type at nights on my keyboard, "How to kill oneself?" I was like that little black cat that years ago, like a suicide, simply got run over. I, too, hoped to get 'saved' like that. My day was now twelve hours longer, making me feel everything twice as intensely, while my brain was unable to hold back a roaring army of various thoughts. One of them was my mom's words that she'd tell me repeatedly, which apparently got stuck in the dense thicket of my thoughts. "Everything happens for a reason, son."

Repeating this line in my mind like a mantra, I could feel that it calmed me down a bit, allowing me to focus a little more on my prayer to God.

Lord! Help me, please! I'd cry inside my head more and more often.

During these nights, with my laptop on my belly, staring at the screen, I was surfing the Internet trying to drown my thoughts in the abundance of information. On the night that turned my fate around, moonlight was making its way through the slats of my blinds, making the entire room bright, as if it wanted to tell me that one day, I'd get out of my darkness.

Despite the vast amount of resources available on the Internet in 2015, there were few websites dedicated to Lyme disease. Finding any online forum that had some specific information was little short of miraculous. I'd force my brain to penetrate pages in language different than my native tongue, but it would rebel against me more and more, causing me to feel more and more sore. After making some intellectual effort for just a while to understand a foreign language, I was feeling massive exhaustion. It was as if I trained for an hour only one body part, such as my bicep, to then find myself unable to move my arm. At one point, miraculously, I stumbled upon a website of the Polish Lyme Disease Patient Association. *"We are people suffering from tick-borne diseases, as well as the loved ones and friends of such people. We live in every part of Poland. In our search for help for ourselves and our loved ones, we set up an association that represents us in contact with medical, political and social circles, as well as public media. We undertake to help everyone who feels lost and alone in their illness. We advise on what to begin you fight for the good health of either you or your loved one. We don't seek to replace doctors, but we are happy to share our own experience. We collaborate with medical professionals across Poland and strive to establish cooperation with new ones who are ready to undertake the enormous challenge of battling Lyme disease and other tick-borne diseases."*[24]

Perhaps it was Valdoxan speaking, perhaps it was my yet another prayer to God, but something led me to that website. Back then, I didn't know the answer to that question. However, back at that moment, for the first time in ages, I felt that I wasn't all by myself, and the moonlight not only did illuminate my room, but my soul, too.

First thing in the morning, I went online and contacted the association. *"My Dear Ones, help! I suspect that I might have Lyme disease. Blood test results show I probably had some contact with the bacteria. Sadly, the infectiologist thinks otherwise,"* I wrote in the e-mail. I got the following reply, *"Hello, Michal, it is crucial that you contact an ILADS doctor! If you are suffering from Lyme disease, there are usually two paths to choose from. There are two methods known in the world for approaching this condition. One of them was developed by IDSA – the Infectious*

---

[24] https://www.borelioza.org/onas.htm

Diseases Society of America. It is a standard method used by healthcare professionals dealing with conventional medicine, including infectiologists, one of whom you've already seen, most likely as a result of getting a referral from your primary care practitioner." I wrote them back, "*I have. The infectiologist has already expressed her position as regards my health condition.*" The reply read, "*In this case, there is nothing else for you to do but to contact one of the doctors of ILADS. It is the International Lyme and Associated Diseases Society, that is, a group that associates people using the ILADS treatment method, who question the standard IDSA method.*" Immediately, I wrote back, asking, "*They question it?*" The member of the society replied, "*They refer to a number of scientific studies that confirm that Lyme disease is very difficult to diagnose and requires intensive treatment. IDSA has a completely different standpoint. I will provide you with a list of doctors you can visit. You won't find help beyond that.*"

I'd never guessed that identifying any disease is that hard for physicians these days. Hearing of limb, heart or kidney transplants, or even distant plans to transplant faces or human heads, which was on TV, I didn't realize that there are still medical issues that we as mankind cannot handle.

I was all the more unable to comprehend how you could even split into some groups, arguing who's right, at the expense of other people suffering, left to their own devices. Then, I remembered though the problems of this world that I had heard of since forever, yet they were never discussed as often as the successes in the medical field and plans for the future that would seem impossible to implement. I always wondered why people want to go looking for water on distant planets if they're unable to deliver it to places where it's most needed, given that there's not that much of it on earth. After all, lack of access to drinking water kills several thousand children every year. Why every year one-third of the global food production ends up in the trash, while every several seconds kids around the globe are starving to death? Reflecting on such global issues, I recalled the deadly malaria, which I heard of last time back in college, and which was taking fifty children every hour to the other side in the very same time when I probably found the reason behind my problems.

According to UNICEF statistics, in 2013, nearly two hundred million cases of malaria were reported, of which over five hundred and eighty-four thousand people died. That awful disease is caused by parasites that belong to the genus Plasmodium, transmitted from one human onto another by the world's most efficient and ruthless killer – the mosquito. That tiny but horribly annoying insect is believed to kill two million people around the globe every year. Back at that moment, I didn't even think of the fact that the mosquitos that I had been brushing away every year at summer barbeque events with my family or friends back in those better days could've caused many years of anguish, let alone, after having heard repeatedly of the possible cause of my problems being the tick. As it turned out, that was very likely, and, what's worse, it was not only malaria, transmitted by the vampire we all know, that could bring death.

Therefore, I put the contact details I received from the association to use. It could seem that its members knew much better than healthcare professionals did where I should seek help and rescue. Anna and I went to a mysterious doctor affiliated with ILADS which, according to the Internet, was called by most healthcare professionals a "charlatanism".

Nice! Does everything that opposes mainstream medicine have to be linked to black magic? I thought. Soon after, we realized though why that is.

Despite the fact that time was passing mercilessly, one thing was certain and constant: still, to see a doctor, even at a private visit, you had to arm yourself with patience. Life so far taught me a lot. One of the skills I acquired, which didn't use to be as well-developed as it is today, was patience. Eventually, it was our turn and with hopes for an end to this journey, which was very painful to me, I opened the door to an office of a female neurologist who was on the short list people who could help me. I didn't realize, though, that it would be one of the worst appointments up to that point and that the meaning of my journey would completely change for us all. Behind the door, we were greeted by a very petite, elderly woman. Although my focus and memory had been failing me for some time, and my brain fog wouldn't even let me compare people's faces to those well-known to me from the big screen, I could still identify that one. The neurologist, who brought to my fogged mind a Polish version of the English actress Helen McCrory offered us seats by her desk.

"What brings you two young people here?" she asked.

Already on the verge of physical and mental exhaustion, and sleepy most of all, I was trying to keep invisible matches in my eyes so that I wouldn't nod off in the lady's presence. Knowing that I could have some problem telling everything to the only person who could help us, Anna didn't wait long and decided to begin the conversation for me.

"We suspect that Michal has Lyme disease. We're asking you for help. We got your number from the Polish Lyme Disease Patient Association.

"You suspect? Have you done some diagnostic testing for that disease, yet?" she asked.

"We have. A Western blot, with came up borderline. We've also been at the Infectious Diseases Clinic, but according to the doctor, Michal is healthy," Anna replied.

"I know it's not a test that says if I have bacteria inside of me, but I really don't know what could be the cause of my problems. Help me, please," I chipped in, my voice tired, my elbow resting on my knee, my face hidden behind my palms so that I wouldn't let my head drop due to all the fatigue.

"The Western blot shows that your immunological system has produced antibodies to fight spirochetes that cause Lyme disease, and that tells us a lot already. Please tell me what's bothering you. In detail."

For some time, there wasn't even any need for me to tell doctors what was bothering me. I used a sheet of paper on which I would note down all my symptoms, from 2010 to the present. As soon as something new came up, I modified the list of symptoms.

"Please take a look; this is all that Michal has been struggling with for the past five years. No one can help us. Everyone's sending us off to a psychiatrist, every time," Anna said.

The doctor looked at us and nodding her head, smirked at us, as if it was not the first time she saw a case like mine.

"Sir, I'm convinced that you do have Lyme disease, and not only Lyme disease."

Astonished, wondering if one of us misheard Dr. McCrory, Anna and I looked at each other, and then once again at the doctor.

"What are you saying, doctor?!" we asked.

"A young man who, instead of enjoying with his girlfriend all the sweet essence of his youth (she cast a glance at Anna) spends his time wandering from one doctor to another for five years, has some mental disorder, indeed; he must've fallen ill with something or he's simply carrying at least one or several pathogens."

"Assuming you're right and that's really how things are, why didn't the infectiologist help us and why didn't he recommend any testing?" Anna asked.

"The answer is very simple. The Polish Association of Epidemiologists and Infectiologists forms all recommendations and regulations on the treatment of Lyme disease in accordance with the guidelines of IDSA and its European counterparts. For IDSA experts, Lyme disease is very simple to diagnose and cure, whereas a diagnosis that is easy to make, often based on the patient's convictions or sometimes only based on a single questionable test result is dismissed by a medical professional who uses the guidelines for 'proper diagnostics and treatment'. That is the system for treating Lyme disease that we have in this country, but not only here. To this day, many European countries have no idea what Lyme disease is. It could be said that you were lucky after all to be in Poland. And there's no reason to be surprised why primary care practitioners do what they do; they simply don't know much about it," she said.

"You're a neurologist, so why the other doctors specializing in the same field whom we visited didn't help him? And why opinions about you are so different?"

"For many doctors, a young person who looks good but feels bad is abnormal, so they were trying to send you off to a psychiatrist. I'm a neurologist but I am a member of a group that is considered charlatans who poison their patients with too much antibiotics over too long periods of time in line with a theory that we are said to have invented. But there are other diseases of affluence treated by the IDSA doctors by putting their patients on just as many pharmaceuticals and then it's okay. So why then there's a problem? When does it work?! In our view, treatment with antibiotics should be implemented after every contact with a tick, which others consider unjustified, too. When I say 'to contact', I mean 'to get bitten'. Erythema migrans, as you know, is like roulette, whereas a tick, though it isn't the only carrier of spirochetes, can play the role of a carrier of pathogens that get inside the body of its victim with its saliva, causing slow destruction, as in your case. Sadly, few people commence treatment right after being bitten or right after erythema migrans appears. In one month after the inflection, the disease becomes increasingly difficult to eliminate."

"After every contact? You've also mentioned 'spirochetes' a couple of times. So it's not only ticks?" I asked in disbelief.

"When it comes to medicine based on 'evidence', most recommendations do not allow for our methods to be used. What's recommended is that the treatment should be administered only if the patient shows specific symptoms of the disease confirmed in the 'right' way, and usually that doesn't go anywhere beyond thirty days of administering antibiotics. If you were in yet another 'lucky' group, and your ELISA or Western blot results were positive, you'd probably get put on doxycyclin[25]; it cannot pull anyone out of chronic spirochete-caused Lyme disease though, and not only Lyme disease, for that matter, in just a month. Yes! Spirochetes - most likely, the reason behind your nightmare; one of the oldest bacteria on planet Earth. Until this year, as many as fifteen

---

[25] Doxycycline – an organic chemical compound, and a semi-synthetic tetracycline-class antibiotic.

genera of that bacteria were identified, made up of hundreds of species. Four of them wreak havoc in a man's life. One of the best-known is *Treponema pallidum,* which causes syphilis, a disease you've probably heard of. Many researchers in the world suspect that spirochetes are the underlying cause of many conditions that are commonly known, such as Alzheimer's disease and some forms of cancer. What we are interested in though is *Borrelia,* as it causes Lyme disease, primarily the species called *Borrelia burgdorferi.* We don't know much about these bacteria, but one thing is certain: they're not carried only by ticks. Most people believe that the main reservoir of these bacteria are wild animals, such as the mouse or the red deer. Unfortunately, that's not true. We can get infected with that spirochete also by drinking cow's milk, whereas the infection can be also spread by other arthropods that bite, such as mosquitos, mites or even flies. A tick bite seems the main way in which it spreads, though. This is why it's so important to act immediately after being bitten by that insect."

"You've mentioned a 'lucky' group. Is there some other 'lucky' group aside from the people who get erythema migrans?" I asked.

"In your case, the result was borderline; some other people get results that are completely negative and yet they do have the bacteria and they feel awful, just like you do. The lucky ones with a positive result, who can also be denied treatment, for there are such cases, end up in hospital for three, four weeks of antibiotic therapy, and after the treatment, which is considered the only right methods, they are discharged and go home, often with aggravated symptoms, with a letter specifying they now have what's called the post-Lyme syndrome. There's no such thing as post-Lyme syndrome. What you probably have is chronic neurologic Lyme disease of many years."

"Chronic neurologic Lyme disease?" Anna asked.

"Yes, if you've been in pain for so long, it is safe to assume that you have a chronic disease that has caused numerous inflammations and dysfunctions across different systems in your body over the years. It is very common to assume that Lyme disease attacks primarily human joints, which you've seen for yourself while seeing the infectiologist. Sadly, the truth is that many people are affected by what happened to you, that is, possibly, an infection of the central nervous system and other organs. Many struggle with various neurological disorders caused by *Borrelia*. People suffer various forms of paresis, have paralyzed limbs, rheumatoid arthritis; many suffer from depressive disorders. There are some cases in which people are kept alive only owing to a respirator that breathes for them, and there are even cases of death. In the early stages, people infected with *Borrelia* know something's wrong. You knew that, too, five years ago. Unfortunately, it is very uncommon for them to get an accurate diagnosis. After some time, neurological issues are obvious, whereas the ability to think and function in general get severely impaired. Oftentimes, Spirochetes also eagerly visit the brain, where they then wreak havoc, often misleading healthcare professionals. In medicine, there a condition called demyelinating disease, which involves decomposition of the protective cover of nerve fibers, also known as the myelin sheath. The best-known demyelinating disease, which is most likely known to you, too, is multiple sclerosis. In the recent years, MS has become the most common misdiagnosis of Lyme disease. As you can guess, a patient who receives the wrong treatment has no chance to recover, and the wrong treatment leaves the field clear for *Borrelia*. All that because of the bacteria that still live inside us."

"You've mentioned that you're convinced that Lyme disease is not the only thing Michal has?" Anna chipped in.

"Sadly, that's where the problem lies. *Borrelia* is not the only pathogen that wreaks havoc."

"What do you mean?" I asked, terrified.

"I meant the so-called co-infections that make diagnosing and treating Lyme disease even more complicated. Usually, carriers of bacteria of the genus *Borrelia* also have inside several other organisms, just as unpleasant, that cause co-infections, which they probably got at the same time when bitten by an insect.

"Why didn't the infectiologist mention that?" I asked, perplexed.

"That's a question for that doctor, not me. If according to a medical professional from the Infectious Diseases Clinic you're not infected with *Borrelia*, do you really think she'd be excited about elaborating on other pathogens that are possibly ruining your life?"

"What are these organisms?" Anna asked.

"The most common co-infections include *Chlamydia, Mycoplasma, Bartonella, Ehrlichia, Babesia, Anaplasma, Rikettsia,* and *Yersinia*. All these bacteria are occupants that most likely contributed to your current condition along with *Borrelia*," the doctor replied, listing the pathogens one after another, their names as if taken out of this world, as if from other planets. "If we confirm Lyme disease and the co-infection, your treatment will take more time than recommended by European scientific societies or most neurologists and infectiologists, unfortunately. You must know that such treatment is considered unjustified by the vast majority of health professionals."

"What do you mean exactly?" Anna asked.

"You'll have to undergo a long-term antibiotic therapy."

"So where's the problem? I've been on antibiotics many times," I asked, confused, referring to my previous experiences with the antibiotics prescribed by Dr. Armani for my flu-like inflammations, among others.

"Unfortunately, treating Lyme disease is a bit different than you might imagine. You'll be put on several different antibiotics that will be replaced with others from time to time. The antibiotics will be administered in the form of pills, but also intravenously," Helen said.

"What do you mean by 'long-term antibiotic therapy'?" Anna chipped in.

"For mainstream medicine, the reasons behind your condition remain unknown. The infectiologist presupposed that if you really suffer from something, it could be post-Lyme disease syndrome, suspecting that your symptoms can be a result of permanent, spirochete-induced tissue damage or an immunological reaction against *Borrelia*. Today, no one has conclusive evidence that would allow your symptoms to be linked to an active infection. However, we do see patients' condition improve after extended antibiotic therapy. Some of them regain good health after undergoing the therapy for several months, while others need to be taking antibiotics for a couple of years, or even remain in therapy for their entire lives."

"A couple of years?" we asked simultaneously.

"All microorganisms that get inside a man's body encounter a unique ecosystem that is very different for every person. Hence, the course of Lyme disease is a bit different in each case. This means that antibiotics, but also herbs that work for one person can prove ineffective for another, or act on her in a different way. There is no one universal treatment method. The treatment you're getting is the so-called symptomatic treatment."

"Does it mean it only alleviates the symptoms?" Anna asked.

"Unfortunately. There's no guarantee that you'll fully recover. Our goal is to get you back to a state that allows you to function."

"Does it mean I might have to live with Lyme disease my entire life?" I asked.

"It does, sadly," Helen replied.

Hearing the answer I didn't expect, I could feel myself falling to pieces. I was unable to imagine going through all that hell and torment for the rest of my life.

I won't be able to live like that, it can't be true! I wondered, looking the doctor in the eye.

"Well, antibiotics disrupt intestinal flora, which can compromise immunity, right?" Anna chipped in, trying to figure it out.

"You have to consider if you want to save your immunity, that you don't have already possibly as a result of bacterial infections, using antibiotics, or whether you want to leave it as it is, hoping for a miracle to happen, and that you'll suddenly feel better. You can see for yourself that no one can help you. You can't spend your time wondering if a large number of antibiotics would make you lose your immunity. It's worth reflecting though why you didn't have any up to this point. It's all understandable, though, and the decision about taking up such treatment lies solely with you. What is the status between you two?"

"What do you mean?"

"What's your relationship status?"

"We're engaged."

"If so, you have to do some testing, too," she said to Anna, making us both snap out of a reverie.

"What? What do you mean?" Anna asked.

"Sadly, spirochetes *Borreli* are very often transmitted from one person to another. The bacteria of the genus *Borrelia* very quickly colonize the bladder in all animals, humans included. This is how they get excreted from the body in urine. This mechanism allows them to survive, but also to get transmitted onto other carriers. Sexual intercourse is yet another way a person can very easily get infected. Plus, scientists have determined that the DNA of *Borrelia* is also present in the sperm. If you have sexual relations and you two do have Lyme disease, most likely you've been infecting each other," she added.

At that moment, we both looked at each other, our eyes a bit watery, surprised and, primarily, terrified by the woman's theory; I froze and my mind drifted away.

One hour before the test, one of the people waiting in line had to leave for some reason. Then, out of nowhere, the vacant place of the fifteenth test-taker was taken by the most beautiful girl I've ever seen. I got infatuated with and hypnotized by her face. Her height, dark hair, blue eyes, and white smile... In our all-male company, the impression she made while standing in line couldn't have gone unnoticed. I imagined every guy in that moment saying to her in his mind, Look at me! Look how cool I am! From the moment she joined the line, time started flowing even faster and even more pleasantly. The girl retrieved some chocolate and started sharing it with all the fifteen of us with a smile. Perfect, I thought. Obviously, I didn't mean the taste of the chocolate, but that modest girl whose looks were nothing short of incredible, smiling to every person standing in line, winning them over instantaneously, I recalled the moment I met Anna for the first time.

"To sum up all the things you've said, does it mean I could've get Anna infected?"

"Yes, if you were really the first one to carry the bacteria, that's what could've happened," she said.

Recalling times with my fiancée back before the onset of my disease, I could never forgive myself that I might have infected her with anything. I couldn't live with the thought that the woman I loved more than anything would have to go through the same hell I have.

The dialogue that Anna resumed with the neurologist became inaudible and my mind drifted away; still operating, it got flooded with desperate thoughts at the recollection of the second time I met my sweetheart.

I could only watch the bus driver close the door behind her. Raising our hands up, we both waved to each other goodbye through the window.

Lost in thoughts, I regretted that I hadn't let it go back when our buses departed in opposite directions; maybe I could've prevented our lives from being ruined.

"Please. We'll deal with if when we get to it. Now, we need to have you both additionally tested."

"If given Michal's clinical diagnosis you're almost sure, then why any additional testing?" Anna asked.

"As you know already, serological tests that Michal has done do not identify the source of infection directly. Therefore, by looking at the test results alone, I cannot determine whether Michal has live *Borrelia* inside or not. However, the test results show his body was protecting itself against spirochetes. The immunological system recognizes chemical structures called antigens of all bacteria unknown to it that break into its 'territory', and starts producing antibodies. To produce antibodies that are capable of fighting, the immunological system must be healthy and efficient enough. If Michal's immunological system was not, there's high probability that he still carries it inside. What's more, spirochetes are the most intelligent bacteria in the world that can hide and camouflage themselves."

"Camouflage? Like soldiers?" I asked.

"Yes, like super-intelligent soldiers equipped with cutting-edge technology. They can connect themselves to human antibodies in a way that makes them undetectable to traditional tests like ELISA and Western blot. These bacteria hide from the immunological system in smart ways by situating themselves only in the brain or joints, for instance. Therefore, additional testing is required. And, besides, we have to get you tested, too, ma'am, for the good of both of you."

"How can you know all this? Why are you interested in that subject, while other neurologists have no interest in it?" I asked.

"I myself have Lyme disease, too. Many doctors do. And, sadly, more and more people are going to have it. Humanity is oblivious to the fact that it carries these bacteria, passing it on by means of donating blood, for example. At least in our country, blood donation centers perform no control tests and thus, by taking blood from the donor, they contribute to infecting others," Dr. McCrory said.

I knew that the vast majority who were sending me off to a psychiatrist should head there themselves, but back at that moment, Helen's words triggered more profound thought in my mind. After the first conversation with the neurologist, I knew that there was no point continuing Valdoxan treatment, as I had to get some sleep. My last five years were like a nightmare! For half a decade, I was bouncing back and forth like a ping-pong ball. The participants of that game (which could seem comical to others, but not to me) that most often resembled mixed doubles, were medical experts considered one of the best in their respective fields. Bouncing from one side to the other, I was not only trying to comprehend what was going on with me, but I was also experiencing firsthand that healthcare in broad sense was not working as it should. While I was wondering how I could escape the already five-year-long nightmare that my reality had become, physicians were sending me off to the other side of the net to be taken over by a psychiatrist, usually within the five minutes their patients were granted during appointments. Although some of them were most certainly exceptional at their job, none of them had any idea about Lyme disease.

Or, maybe they simply preferred to not know? I wondered.

After what I heard from Helen, Natalie or even the infectiologist, I wanted to turn back time myself, and not know about it. I hoped that my several-year-long journey through pain and suffering would end beautifully; in turn, yet another, exceptionally painful issue was added to my life, already overflowing with problems. I couldn't handle the thought that I possibly infected my fiancée. Almost certain what the cause of my issues was, I knew that there was no point going back to Tom Selleck, but for the first time in my life, I felt that this was where I started needing him. And then, with tears in her eyes, Anna asked a question that changed our way of thinking.

"But what if I got infected first? What if you're suffering because of me?" she asked, recalling the words of lady cat-eye from years before, who described her as very ill. "What if Ewa was right?" she added, all in tears.

This turn of events didn't evoke the same emotions in me. Prior to meeting Anna, my life had no meaning, and she changed it for the better. I knew that even if that was true, and if I could turn back time and take a different path, I wouldn't hesitate to go stand in line with Tomek again, waiting for the number fifteen to arrive, as it has become all my life. For, as my mom used to say, "Everything happens for a reason."

I was walking around my room the entire night, still experiencing the side effects of Valdoxan. In my mind, I could hear Helen saying, "Immunity disorders, or even chronic stress that everyone has been telling you about, can boost the growth of bacteria inside us that we may not know of even for most of our lives. The bacteria of the genus *Borrelia* can survive many years inside the human body without causing the immunological system to react whatsoever, until there comes the right moment for them, and then a man ends up in a wheelchair."

Back at that moment, there was nothing I wanted more than to get free from the pain I had been living with for so many years. I was overwhelmed by an even bigger fear of the suffering these organisms could cause my Anna. We were looking forward to getting tested, which I was more afraid of than ever before, but given that probably a greater evil could happen to us, we both knew there was no other way. And so, we had a series of tests recommended by Helen done, and quite soon, we went for our second appointment with the ILADS doctor to learn what her diagnosis was and start treatment; as she remarked herself, no one else had any idea how to help us, let alone the willingness to do so.

Unquestionably, the last several years gave me a hard time; I became a completely different man. Sometimes, one moment in life, one gesture, one sentence can affect how other people perceive us, how they will feel in our presence, what they will expect us to be like. Although I realized that in many situations it wasn't me who was controlling my body but a bunch of alien organisms that were terrorizing me, operating the rudder of the wreck that I was turning into, I was aware that everything that I experienced, and what my loved ones experienced because of me, will forever remain in our memory. Recalling the words of one of the psychiatrists, "soon we'll both laugh at it all," I was wondering how many people, not including myself, are just about to embark on the same journey or are already at that specific point, hearing the same things from their doctors. Recalling situations where I was breaking plates in front of my parents, punching walls in a fit of rage, or got slapped across the face by my sister, who was terrified, trying to protect herself from my uncontrollable aggression, it was but a small fraction of the mental suffering that I was about to face. American movies that were still the sole source of my amusement and contact with the world, titles such as *Virus*, *Pandemic*, or all those with the motif of evil forces of nature taking control over humans, took on a completely different meaning in my eyes.

Most guys who watch romantic movies with their sweethearts doze off for half the screening time, and throughout the other half, they closely watch their women reacting to the moment they have been waiting for since they saw the poster of the upcoming premiere. Before we even know that the main lead is played by one of the handsome Ryans – meaning only either Gosling or Raynolds, obviously – we're standing with popcorn in one hand, already half of it gone, handing two tickets over to the clerk who sizes us up and says ironically, "Enjoy the movie!" Obviously, that moment is the one when the two protagonists, who are meant to fall for each other soon, come very close for the first time to enjoy a passionate kiss. Since neither Anna nor I ever got bitten by a tick, we were convinced that our first passionate kiss ruined our lives. We did know, however, that we couldn't continue living like this, poisoning ourselves with thoughts like, "What if?", "What would've happened if?", even with due account of the words of healers we were seeing. And yet, we were oblivious to the fact that these visits could've had an influence on the ramifications that affected us in the near future.

"If we made it through it all, we'll make it through everything, together!" Anna would say.

We entered yet another period of time that was very difficult to both of us. It proved not as optimistic as my fiancée was; the words that our second appointment at Helen's office started with definitely transformed our life as a couple, never to be the same again.

"Well, now we know everything, dear ones! You both carry not only *Borrelia*, but also *Chlamydia pneumoniae* and *Yersinia*," McCrory said, looking at additional serological tests determining IgG-class antibodies, which were informing us all of the mere fact that we had been in contact with these organisms.

Nodding, yet again in her life she was looking at results that were not conclusive, and at two young people who were in pain, wondering where it all came from. She knew that though there was no perfect test that would dispel our doubts, there was only one reason, and the treatment had to be commenced without waiting any longer.

Aside from the trace of the co-infections usually comorbid with *Borrelia* that was left in our bodies, ensuring her that her diagnosis was accurate, she also based her conclusion on a quantitative CD57+ lymphocyte assay, which is an auxiliary test used in Lyme disease diagnostics.

"Your low lymphocyte count possibly also shows that you're struggling with a chronic infection. Now, all you have to do is reconsider everything that has been said and decide whether to start the therapy or not."

"I guess we have no choice," I remarked, wanting to cease my pain as soon as possible.

"Yes, we probably don't," Anna said.

"You should know, though, that it's not an easy, pleasant way."

Helen was not lying. Although our life got turned upside down long ago and wasn't spoiling us, it decided to toy with us a little more and go from the 'difficult' mode up to 'advanced'. In all that suffering, which was not only experienced by myself alone, Anna was incredibly patient and loving. Though she wasn't feeling as awful as I was, she knew that she had to undergo the therapy that was involving the risk of upsetting all the bacteria that she had in her body, now asleep. I knew that Helen's words didn't affect her at all and that she wasn't afraid that one day, her occupants would blow up like an unexploded bomb waiting for an external stimulus. I knew that she was doing it all just for me. Like most women, she dreamed of having a beautiful wedding with her prince charming. Although I wasn't even close to being that, and all signs were telling us that our dream wedding was not about to happen anytime soon, I felt that despite the deficiencies caused by the disease, that was exactly who I was in my fiancée's eyes. Amidst all that Lyme-themed tragedy that happened to us both, people who seems to be able to help us forgot to mention one more 'lucky' group that Anna and I turned out to be part of: we could afford to start the therapy. The various antibiotics prescribed to us in massive amounts coupled with herbs, supplements and probiotics were not reimbursed by the National Health Fund; meaning that every month, we had to allocate enormous funds for treating that disease. Combined, our prescriptions for whole bags of medications that we were leaving the drug store with every month were worth several thousand *zloty*. If not for the business my parents were running that allowed them to pay for my therapy, I wouldn't have been able to afford proper treatment. Anna's situation was completely different; regular daily struggles aside, she wasn't particularly suffering from any torments. Although both her parents and mine wanted to help her out, in her stubbornness, she was setting her earnings aside for her treatment. From then on, Anna had to spend all her life savings on medications, and the dreams she had been saving money for had to wait. Unlike her, I had no such option. Although I really wanted to get back to the world of the living and earn for my therapy at my parents' company, I simply couldn't. Neither could I commence the therapy on my own. "What's difficult about that?" you might ask. "All it takes is to swallow the pills and *voila*! It's not rocket science!" Sadly, our treatment turned out to be quite unusual, and due to my inability to focus coupled with general derealization I was unable to memorize all the steps that had to be followed as part of the antibiotic therapy.

It didn't matter how hard I tried, I couldn't remember when, what, and at what time I was supposed to put into my body. Several antibiotics, often of different types, taken in the course of a single day alternately with various herbs and supplements, were causing a total chaos in my head. Day by day, Anna and I were swallowing tens of pills like it was M&Ms. Sadly, they weren't as sweet and tasty as we'd like them to be.

While we are on the topic of sugars and tasty food, it weren't only us that took a serious beating, but also our stomachs. Our diets changed drastically. Not only was it necessary for us to take the bacteria-killing antibiotics, but we also had to be put on antifungal drugs and pharmaceuticals that support liver regeneration.

"You'll have to give up not only all sweets, coffee, black tea, but also fast foods," Helen said during our second appointment.

"Give up chocolate?" Anna asked, regretfully.

"Yes, primarily chocolate. All you'll be allowed is dark chocolate and maybe xylitol, which can substitute the taste of sugar. Antibiotics involve the risk of developing fungal diseases, and excess sugar would only facilitate that."

It was very rare for Anna to share chocolate with strangers while waiting in line, but it was still a delicacy that she couldn't image her life without. Unlike her, I couldn't imagine movie nights without a double cheese Margherita, a frequent guest at my home. The lack of training and poor nutrition made me gain a few extra pounds, which then disappeared into thin air over several months that followed. From the moment we began our ILADS therapy, my weight was going down at a head-spinning pace day after day, and I was getting smaller and smaller. Over six months into this new lifestyle that we both found extreme, my weight was similar to my fiancée's – I lost almost forty founds. Given her petite physique, Anna didn't have much weight to lose. In her case, what could be considered a loss was her wellbeing, which changed drastically in the course of the antibiotic therapy.

The previously unexplained pain in the legs, particularly in the knees, that she was suffering in her teenage years, returned twofold.

"Now you know where the sudden knee join deformity came from," Helen told her at a subsequent visit.

"But why now, why does it hurt so bad?" Anna asked.

"It is a normal reaction of the body triggered by microorganisms that are dying on a mass scale during the treatment. Your symptoms might become more severe, but not necessarily. Not everyone treated for Lyme disease and co-infections experiences the Jarisch-Herxheimer-Łukasiewicz reaction."

"Herxheimer?"

"Yes. Commonly referred to as 'herxes'. When cells of pathogens become fragmented, they release toxins that contribute to a temporary aggravation of symptoms. These toxins are expelled from the body by means of the liver or kidneys. When these organs fail to discharge the massive amounts of toxins as fast as it should, this is how the body lets you know that this is taking place. Not everyone feels worse in treatment, though, but it's better if you can tell a difference – that way we know that the therapy is working."

"What if that reaction is too strong?" I asked.

"Please. Let's cross that bridge when we come to it. If any overly severe reactions occur, we will use adequate measures," the neurologists calmed us down. "What's important is that you drink lots of water, go on walks, or even use sauna to sweat as much toxins out of the body as possible, because the liver might not be able to handle the large amount," she added.

The pain in the legs aside, which resurfaces after years, Anna noticed that she had a rush that was growing month by month, now covering the cleavage, the shoulders and the back, causing her more and more mental discomfort, but also oppressive headache and overall fatigue.

In turn, when it came to me, aside from unquestionably smaller purulent cyst inside my throat, substantial weight loss and even more aggravated exhaustion, I didn't feel any more significant changes that the ILADS therapy was supposed to bring into my life. However, my liver had a different opinion, its functioning and the enzymes it produces monitored every month.

With every month, in contrast to the positive and normal liver values of my fiancée, mine were getting worse. Although we were following the diet most devoutly and our meals were easily digestible, so it would seem my liver wasn't overly burdened with an excessive amount of redundant metabolic waste products, apparently too much of antibiotics was doing a bad job, which soon forced me to take certain steps and decisions.

Meanwhile, Helen was trying to reassure me by saying that many people get much worse results than mine when in the ILADS treatment, and that I had no reason to worry more than I already did. She was concerned about one thing though, or rather lack thereof.

"One thing bothers me," she confessed at one of our appointments, several months into the therapy. "Considering all your symptoms, I believe that you two carry also *Bartonella,* which is usually the reason behind the symptoms that are reminiscent of anxiety and depressive states. It is often the case that results of serological tests don't change until a 'provocation' is used, thus changing the result to positive. I strongly believe that both of you have *Bartonella,* one of the most common co-infections. Together with *Borrelia, Bartonella* forms a destructive duo. Both these bacteria are the hardest to eliminate. Sometimes, *Bartonella* can spread more destruction than *Borrelia* alone does."

Borrelia, Bartonella, Chlamydia, and all these other weird names of monsters sitting inside my body were irrelevant to me; I didn't feel like asking where they come from, their characteristic or anything else that was related to these bacteria. I had enough of it. I couldn't even memorize how to spell them correctly. Once I found the reason behind my issues, I couldn't care about anything else than to get these evil occupiers out of our bodies.

"Well then, what do you suggest?" I asked.

"You need to do the test again, so that we can determine the right antibiotic therapy for you further down the line."

More testing and more antibiotics meant less and less money for our pockets, but also worse results for my liver. It weren't only the drug prices but also the monthly monitoring of the toxin-eliminating gland that were draining our wallets. Yet another examination for verifying liver condition was ultrasonography, which was essential. As it turned out at one of such examinations, the expert performing it, who additional took a quick look at my gallbladder, encountered two quarter-inch polyps, which according to her had to be monitored every six months from then on.

"The liver looks good, but you need to keep an eye on these polyps. If they get much bigger, a surgery will be necessary," she said.

Anna and I were doing all our check-ups and liver function tests at places that were closest to each of us. Though I was awfully resentful towards Dr. Armani and the healthcare professionals at the same facility, as for all these years they were unable to identify the reason behind my ailments, I was going there every month. I cannot hide that Helen's words helped me change my attitude to this situation, "there's no reason to be surprised why primary care practitioners do what they do; they simply don't know much about it." This made me adopt a more understanding outlook on certain things. Therefore, I took the opportunity and immediately after having my first ultrasound done, which didn't bring any good news, I decided to consult it with Dr. Armani, whose door to the office was half-open.

"You do know that long-term antibiotic treatment ruins bacterial flora, which has a protective role, and triggers the formation of antibiotic-resistant strains," he said straightforwardly upon hearing what kind of therapy I was getting.

"What do you mean?" I asked.

"When the bacteria situated in the intestine share the environment with an antibiotic during many months of therapy, what takes place is a natural selection of strains capable of surviving in that environment. You're completely oblivious to the fact that you're becoming a carrier of bacteria that are not harmful to you, but possibly deadly to others."

"What does it mean exactly?" I urged Armani to answer, knowing all too well where he was going with it.

"Undergoing antibiotic treatment for preventive purposes or simply undergoing long-term antibiotic therapies has no rational foundation and, most of all, is plain harmful to you."

Now you're playing the medical doctor? I thought.

"But I don't have any other option! Unless you have an idea," I replied.

As you can guess, he didn't have any. He had none for five years and he couldn't have one now. Shortly after, he showed me that he was still capable of shocking me and doing things that changed my mind about that man forever. They put him and the entire healthcare service in the worst light I could ever imagine.

Despite being six month in the ILADS treatment, I didn't stop looking for possible ways that could lead me, and now also Anna, to recovery – except for the one path that appeared to be the one. I was an exhausted man slightly heavier than one hundred and ten pounds, who was still having all the symptoms despite the six-month-long antibiotic therapy. I could feel that I was running out of steam to persevere in spite of the entire package of symptoms, carrying that burden on as if it was a spacesuit. I spent the previous six months rummaging the Internet.

Maybe I will find a cure-all for Lyme disease? I thought.

Sharing views with many individuals online, I found that apparently, aside from the ILADS and the people who offer bio-resonance therapy, there was no one who could help me.

Bio-resonance? Oh yes, I do know your diagnosis, I recalled the appointment with Natalie.

There were moments when all my terrible experiences intensified by the ILADS therapy would simply knock me down. Helpless, I'd let gravity control my body, unable to beat it, often lying still here and there, without any strength to move.

There came a day though, when I stumbled upon the website with the ranking of all the best-known healers in my country. Despite the previous odd incidents involving such people (such as meeting Ewa), I decided to take the risk and once again, look for an individual bestowed with supernatural powers who could heal me. My mom, still intrigued by what lady cat-eye had said, wasn't that sure if that was a good idea. Both she and my dad would give everything to make me healthy again. "Don't worry, if we have to, we'll sell everything to make you recover," they'd say. Watching my woman toiling at her job to spend all the money she was making on her therapy, driven by the thought that we'd both overcome that nasty disease and live a good, happy life, just like most of our peers, I had to change something despite the massive crisis that I had been in for years.

I was watching my parents, who were getting older; my dad could just as well retire, but he kept working, thinking that soon I'd take his place. I couldn't come to terms with my fate and everything that was happening to me. In hindsight, I don't know to this day how I did it, but I found some strength within me that many times allowed me to get back on my feet and, wiping tears of despair off, muster what was left of my ability to focus, buried somewhere deep. Instead of wasting time for following the ups and downs of fictional characters on the big screen, I started watching my dad's endeavors, gradually, step by step, like years ago, but this time, with a stronger will to act despite the disease. Each time I tried to help him even a little, the outcome was not the best, or none at all.

Terrified by the fact that my antibiotic therapy still didn't yield any expected results, I couldn't sit idly any longer. I grabbed my phone and booked an appointment for both Anna and I with a healer who got the best reviews and accolades for helping many ill people in my country. The words I heard on the speakerphone not only made my mom intrigued again, but us all, too.

"Please come at 3 a.m.," a female voice on the other side said.

"You mean 3 p.m.?" I asked, assuming that I misheard her.

"No, the gentlemen are seeing patients only at night and early morning hours."

That's really strange, I thought. Never before had I had anything to do with anyone who for some reason was seeing his patients or clients at night, when everyone's still asleep.

Without delay, we set off for a nigh-time trip into the unknown.

Anna and I weren't the only ones who were struggling with health issues; my mom was bothered by pain in her spine and intestines, for instance. We also invited my aunt to come with us to meet the healer. Suffering from insomnia and gout, she was convinced that her issues weren't caused by Lyme disease, but solely disturbed acid-base balance in her body, which led to excessive accumulation of uric acid in her joints, causing inflammation. In my mind, I could see myself traveling back in time, standing by my aunt like a spirit from the future, watching the moment when tiny, almost unnoticeable nymphs go down a floral wreath she was wearing on her head, and penetrate her body, while adult ticks, unnoticed, go into the wide legs of pants worn by her friends', with whom she was relaxing on the grass, listening to songs by Janis Joplin. Having all the information I had gathered, from time to time, I'd try provide some guidance to various individuals and convince them to have their health conditions re-diagnosed, thinking about the concealed *Borrelia* that was likely responsible for many human problems. But in cases such as my aunt's, the answer I used to get was different.

"Michal, even if that's true, I'm too old to go on a search and undergo a treatment like that."

As anyone else, despite having her own mind, my aunt hoped that any of the doctors who would see us at small hours could alleviate her pain. We all hoped for that. Having left the last town that we had to drive through behind, we found ourselves on a quiet asphalt road cutting through a gloomy forest. The farther we went into the darkness, the more remote the last source of light got, cast by the streetlamps of the town we left behind, getting more and more distant.

"Where are we going?" my mom asked.

"Don't worry. We're almost there," I replied, taking a peek at the navigation app.

Although the healer was seeing his patients at atypical hours and outside of my city, we managed to arrive at our destination on time, and even five minutes before the appointment scheduled at 3 a.m. When we got to a dimly lit parking lot by an old, single-story building of a color that was impossible to tell, which reminded me of a typical elementary school or junior high, we noticed that there were quite a few cars parked already. When we got out the car, we saw an exceptionally long line of people, their dark silhouettes poorly illuminated by a barely glowing single old streetlamp that was doing its best. The long line was formed by tens of people, both young and old, some of them supporting themselves on crutches.

What's going on? How good that healer must be? Each of us thought.

I was afraid that we'd have to stand in line like that forever. Curious about what was happening inside, we couldn't see much through a single window with lights on and a door through which the ill were going in and out quite fast.

Then, we realized that the line of people was pushing forward as such a fast pace, because apparently, the healer didn't need much time per one ill person.

At the moment when we went through the door, time started flowing even faster, until there were only several women before us. Driven by curiosity, I leaned forward and peeked to see why he was so fast. I realized that I thought that I misheard not only the time of our appointment, but also the number of healers, since the words of the lady on the phone, "The gentlemen are seeing" proved to have nothing in common with a slip of a tongue.

Now I know why people go in and out so fast, like those who were waiting in line waiting to get a sausage at a state-owned store back in the times of the People's Republic of Poland, I thought.

All the ladies I had come there with entered the office with two hustling men in only for a minute, like everyone who waited in line did. It was my turn.

In a tiny room decorated with a splash of color in the form of a red carpet and red curtains, there were two men, one elderly, the other not much older than me. They both reminded me of the agents from the super-secret FBI unit known from the movie *Men in Black* because of smart black suits they were wearing. The protagonists of the Hollywood production, which I knew very well, were chasing immigrant terrorists from the outer space who had some sinister plans. Undoubtedly, the intentions of all the bacteria listed by Helen that decided to take us for their target were just as evil. The well-dressed gentlemen, though their physical appearance was reminiscent of only some movie characters, didn't have much in common with them.

"What's bothering you?" the older one asked, the only one of the two to engage in a conversation.

Aware of how fast that visit was about to go, I couldn't tell too much. In a much condensed recap, I described my most exhausting symptoms along with where they were located, without mentioning the bacteria I was carrying. It was a time when my ears were acting out more than ever. Therefore, I asked them to focus particularly on my ears, hoping that the gentlemen would put on sunglasses, retrieve a memory-erasing device from their pockets and turn it on, like the fictional FBI agents who were treating in this way the trauma of those who experienced an unpleasant encounter with an alien form of life. Perhaps under the influence of the antibiotics and the emotions that my hope was evoking in me, my imagination was getting out of hand. However, seeing the crowds of people lining up like for no appointment ever before, I really hoped that the two men could help us. Having listened to my swift description, the men proceeded to act by placing their hands on my body. Suddenly, I felt somewhat uneasy, but not because some kind of healing power was flowing through their hands, but because I had never been touched by two tall men before. It sounds weird, but it could look even weirder from an outside perspective. The older bioenergy therapist placed his palms on my belly, while the younger one on my loins. They both began administering a massage of some sort, making their hands vibrate.

"You have an issue with your spine," the more experienced healer said, and then put his palms on my head. "Drink Saint John's wort and take vitamin D supplements," he added, and then expressed their appreciation for my visit.

"How much do I pay?" I asked, looking at a small bowl filled with coins and several banknotes.

"You don't pay us anything!" the older man looked at me and, having grabbed me by the arm, walked me to the door, smiling, and then asked the next person in.

"Thank you!" I replied, surprised.

When we were leaving the building, we were passing by the crowds of people who were still lining in for an unusual, brief visit. Driving off the dimly lit parking lot, we went past cars that were coming in, one by one, shining their lights on the unlit street on a night that was just as dark.

On our way home, we all started sharing our views and experiences that each of us had in the presence of the two men.

"Boy! I didn't leave them anything, not even a single coin!" I recalled, shamefully.

"Don't worry, I paid for us," my mom said. Before leaving the office, she filled the tiny bowl with a bill of decent denomination.

Nonetheless, we all had the picture of the bowl filled with coins in our heads coupled with the enormous line of people seeking help.

As soon as I learned from the girls that the men didn't correctly diagnose any of them, and labeled each of us as having issues with the spine, I knew that something was definitely not as we expected. Saint John's wort or vitamin D are commonly known methods for problems related to neuroses or depression.

How simple! Everything's on the Internet now. Maybe that's why the bowl was filled only with some coins? I thought.

On the way back home, none of us considered it reasonable to go back to the mysterious duo of bioenergy therapists, as we could see all the ill people lining up in our minds. What happened for both of us in the hours that followed the sleepless night spent in our beds, changed our minds completely and made us want to go back for another appointment.

Anna and my mom didn't have any unusual experiences after receiving the energy of the two healing FBI agents, unlike my aunt and I, as we both had a completely different feeling about that. Already in bed, at the moment when I closed my eyes, I noticed a black void that each of us certainly has, which was filled by a revolving green spiral. It made me feel somewhat stressed and fearful of yet another anomaly unknown to me that seemed completely insignificant and thus safe. Watching it spin clockwise, I simply fell asleep. In the morning, when we were sharing our views again, I got a call.

"I slept like a baby!" my aunt said, very content because, her gout aside, she had been also suffering from insomnia for a long time.

Aware of what it feels like, I was very happy that at least in her case, the received help proved effective in a sense. The green spiral phenomenon had never occurred again, while the power of the energy that we allegedly received, if any, had no positive impact on our health condition. However, we were convinced that we wanted to set our alarm clocks again and see these mysterious therapists at least once more, and were very eager to do so.

Knowing from experience that you can't get everything right away, I accepted that I had to give myself some time, and perhaps give the healers one more chance. Everything had its meaning and was a distinct, time-consuming process, primarily the ILADS treatment. The very fact that *Bartonella* was identified, hiding from Helen and us like an assassin until it eventually showed to us in the serological tests proved that everything takes time. Our antibiotic therapy was expanded to include those of fundamental importance in treating tuberculosis, also tasked with bombarding *Bartonella*. As you can imagine, my lover, unlike Anna's which continued to give us no suspicious symptoms of intolerance, was not happy about it. Sadly, the next step and, consequently, the next level of treatment that we had to begin as part of the IL-ADS method, forced me to make one of the hardest decisions of my life. It also triggered a breakthrough in my nearly six-year-long journey through pain and suffering, since for the first time in ages, I could take my astronaut helmet off to take a breath of fresh air.

"To protect human health and life, to mitigate suffering, guard dignity and not tarnish it in any way." These are the words that Dr. Armani said before taking his position. I'll never forget the day when the Hippocratic Oath took on a brand new, different meaning to me. It all started on a day when Helen made us realize that it was the time of the least enjoyable part of the treatment method recommended by the society that she was a member of.

"It's time when we need to include ceftriaxonum[26] in your treatment," Helen said.

Accustomed to taking large doses of antibiotics with several days off in-between, we didn't consider that to be anything unusual.

Issuing the first prescription for that drug, she asked, "Do you prefer intramuscular injections or intravenous infusions?"

I've never goggled that bad in my entire life. I was unaware that there would come a time when I'd have to undergo any treatment that required sticking a needle into my body. Taking blood samples alone, which we both had to do every month, was not the most pleasant moment. Like most men, I was not a fan of needles.

"Is that necessary?" I asked.

---

[26] Ceftriaxonum – an organic chemical compound, an antibiotic which is a third-generation cephalosporin that has antibacterial properties.

"Unfortunately, it is. Taking this antibiotics in the form of pills would significantly prolong the treatment, and if time is important to you, it's the only way," Dr. McCrory explained.

Obviously, time was important to us; everyone who's suffering for some reason wants to get that reason off his back as soon as possible. With our backs against the wall, with no other way out, we had to make that choice.

"Now, you only have to decide which form of administering ceftriaxonum you prefer."

As you may guess, they both seemed terrifying to me.

Anna, who of the two of us was the tougher one, albeit whose memories of taking intramuscular injections were not good either, swiftly decided to go for time-consuming drips. Unlike her, despite having more patience to everything, a skill I lately acquired, I chose the other method, which was much faster. I hoped that the injections would be quick and painful. As it came out in the wash, I soon learned to take all decisions by analyzing them twice, mostly those I wanted to take to save much time.

"I'll go for the intramuscular injections," I said.

It was one of the worst decisions I've ever made.

Also, we were oblivious to the fact that Helen was not the one who'd be giving us the shots or the IVs.

"Now, you need to find as soon as possible someone who can safely give you the antibiotic."

"What do you mean?" Anna said.

"I mean a qualified nurse who'd administer the IV drips or the injections. You have to do that under professional medical supervision. You can't give the drug to each other with no experience. When it comes to intramuscular injections, you have to know how and where to inject the needle so that you don't cause the patient any harm. Same with introducing a venous catheter."

"Where do we find one?" I asked.

"Ask in outpatient clinics, the hospital, private medical centers. Surely it will be possible to find one somewhere," the neurologist replied.

Completely flabbergasted by that entire situation that we suddenly found ourselves in, we had no idea what to do. We started looking for a nurse who could dedicate a few quarters of her time to us and administer ceftriaxonum daily for an unspecified period of time. Though Anna's younger sister began her journey as a nurse and already had some practice, it was not enough to help us. Helen's words were echoing in our heads, warning that anything could happen. As it soon turned out, she wasn't wrong.

There came a day when Dr. Armani turned from a primary care practitioner into primary abuse practitioner in my eyes in just one moment, making me lose all my desire to ever contact that man again.

"Doctor, my fiancée and I are looking for a facility where we could have ceftriaxonum infusions or shots done," I asked for help, all agitated, knowing Armani's attitude towards my therapy.

"We don't do such things here. I won't order any of the nurses who work here to do that, sorry," he replied.

Not knowing where I should turn for help next, I hung my head in helplessness.

Perhaps Dr. Armani felt some human emotions, after all, as he said, "However, you can ask one of the nurses at our facility. If any of them agrees to do that in private, I won't be standing in your way. But you must come with your own antibiotic."

Glad to hear that, I got up and rushed off to the hall, looking for a nurse.

Though things between me and the women working there were not always rosy, most of them were very likeable. When I asked for help and explained myself, I wasn't turned down; on the contrary, two ladies expressed their willingness to help me with a smile on their faces.

"Sure, Michal, no problem. Please come to the office. We can give you the first shot right away," one of the nurses said, surprising me with her optimism and eagerness to act.

Why not? I thought, since I had taken 0.07 ounce of ceftriaxonum with me to show it to Armani. *At least that would be one less to go.*

So I sat down and started talking with the nurse, who gladly listened to my most recent experiences with the ILADS therapy and shared her own short story with me, too.

"Do you really know how to do that?" I asked, stressed up a bit.

"You know, after working at a hospital for twenty-five years, it's a little like riding a bicycle – you don't forget how to do it. Obviously, each day I thank God that throughout all these years, I've never caused any harm to anyone," she replied.

"That's quite reassuring. Will it hurt?" I asked.

"Intramuscular injections are definitely not the most pleasant ones, but at least you'll have one less to go."

I got up and lowered my pants, waiting for the first buttock injection in my life.

"I'll give you 0.07 ounce; half of that is a really small dose, and the sooner we get it over with, the better for you."

Obviously, I didn't care one bit if there was any way to make my treatment end any sooner, I was always a 'yes' man.

Unfortunately, neither I nor the nurse with her twenty-five years of experience had been informed that 0.035 ounce of ceftriaxonum, right next to vitamin B12 in the form of cocarboxylasum is one of the most painful shots. The injection of the needle was no big deal for me. However, what started happening a while after the shot not only earned me the label of the local legend at that outpatient clinic, but also made me unwelcomed there.

"Oh, God! What's happening?!"

Slightly confused in the beginning, I was overwhelmed by a sudden fit of pain in my thigh, initially quite bearable.

"Easy, Michal, the injection's already working, that's why you're feeling some discomfort, it's soon be gone," the woman said.

It's not going anywhere! It's getting stronger! I started panicking a bit, feeling that the pain was getting worse and worse.

With the powerful pain radiating across my right leg, I could see the nurse, who didn't seem as calm as she had been, and I started panicking even more, while the pain kept growing stronger. I felt as if someone put a grenade into my leg, the explosion of which was ripping tissue layers apart inside my thigh.

Never before had I experienced a pain so bad. I was unable to determine whether my current, almost anorectic condition and general physical exhaustion additionally made that feeling even more intense. One thing I was certain of, though. I thought that my leg would explode in just a moment. I jumped up off the couch and started running left and right, shouting and crying in pain.

"God, it hurts so much! I can't take it! Do something about it!"

Suddenly, another nurse ran into the room, the one who also had had no objections to administering the shot.

"What have you done?" she asked her colleague.

"What do you mean? I've given him an intramuscular injection," she replied, agitated. "I really don't know what could've gone wrong."

"Are you sure you've injected the needle the right way?" the other one asked.

Listening to them talk, I didn't know what to make of it. The pain was unbearable, while their conversation was making me even more confused and panicky.

"God! Help me, people! I'm going to pass out," I yelled.

Then, a young female doctor appeared in the room, whom I had been seeing, too, from time to time.

Seeing me very pale and in great suffering, she chipped in.

"Well, what do we do, girls? Call an ambulance?"

"Let's wait a little longer, he'll surely get over it in just a minute. Look how thin he is, that's why it's hurting him so bad," one of the nurses said.

Then, one of the nurses came up with an idea to call Dr. Armani for help and ask him to decide how to help me and if an ambulance should be called or not.

I was close to jumping on the wall like Spider-Man due to the immense pain I was in; I regretted that I had decided to get the shot, but I regretted even more that I chose my outpatient clinic as the venue. The words I was about to hear Dr. Armani say made me hate not only him, but the entire healthcare service, even more than before.

Stepping into the room that my moans where coming from, Armani took a good look around it to assess the drama that was taking place. Then he spoke.

"I didn't recommend that!"

He turned his back and slammed the door on his way, leaving me in pain, accompanied by his flabbergasted, helpless colleagues.

After dying for about a quarter, I started feeling the pain in my leg subsiding. Terrified, the nurse started apologizing to me for the entire situation.

"I really don't know what went wrong."

I have no clue whether years later, she realized that 0.07 ounce was too big a dose, as Helen remarked later on. Despite this blunder, I felt no resentment towards that lady. All my negative emotions were targeted on a person who in my opinion shouldn't even call himself a doctor.

On that day, Armani crossed the red line. It also showed me that the life I had known so far, especially that on the big screen, was nothing like I imagined it would be. Armani made me realize that the fact he hadn't diagnosed my condition in any way was not only due to his lack of knowledge, but also because of the faulty system that allowed him to take a false oath. Although many times I wanted really bad to go see that doctor again only to shout what I really thought of him right to his face, I never did. Later, I regretted that profusely, for coming a few years back in my memory, I could recall the dark, rainy night, the exact moment when I didn't stop right away to check on the elderly man who was lying still. Seeing in my memory the line of cars, none of which stopped by the soaked man either, I could imagine Armani in one of them, on his way from work, passing the man by, saying, "I didn't recommend that!"

The grief and anger towards doctors that I was experiencing were growing stronger. Armani's misconduct, who outdid himself, was not only one of the instances that affected it, while Helen's words that I was trying to recall had no power of making me feel any human understanding of the other person anymore.

I was filled with immense suffering, but also with anger that was boiling within me, which I soon vented on a young female laryngologist at a mysterious clinic that was addressing ear-related conditions only, whom Laura mentioned to me one year ago.

To some, waiting a year from the moment they book an appointment would seem extremely long, but there were people who waited even up to two years. When I got there, my attention got caught by numbers that were handed out to patients upon their arrival, so that they could watch them appear on screens hanging on the walls by the entrance to each office to tell when it was their turn. One year, over sixty miles and nearly a hundred minutes of staring at the screen, only to hear, "I'm not sure what you're talking about. Also, I don't know how to help you. I've never heard of cutting muscles inside the ear and I'm afraid no one in our country does a surgery like that. There's one thing I can do for you, and that's to get you an appointment with our psychiatrist who deals with ear-related problems," a very young-looking female doctor said

The words I heard elevated my blood pressure like nothing else.

"A psychiatrist specializing in ears? Why didn't I come up with that myself? Why didn't my sister go see a psychiatrist specializing in the spine, when she was suffering from hernia? Maybe I should recommend my aunt to see one, she has gout! And my dad, who suffers from eyelash mites, maybe go see one, too! If no one can help me, what are you even doing here? Isn't it true that you help people recover from hear loss, that you can insert an implant? You guys were on TV. Is there really no one who could help me?" Irritated, overflowing with negative emotions, I put my cards on the table, backing my words with the information that I managed to find out about that facility.

"I really don't know any other way I could help you," she said.

Perhaps it I was because of my bad luck, yet again, that I got an appointment with a newly minted otolaryngologist; at least she seemed newly minted. It could seem that even at the top expert clinic in Poland, there was nothing for me. Nearly six years had passed from the time when I heard the words "I don't know" for the first time from a doctor who was sending me off to a psychiatrist, and nearly ten months since Anna and I started our therapy under Helen's watchful eye. As you can guess, after my incident with the intramuscular injection, I forewent that quicker yet more painful way of taking the antibiotic. Anna and I managed to find a nurse who offered care in the home at competitive prices, who was kind-hearted enough to charge us both as if we were one person. It was a great idea, because neither Anna nor I had to go anywhere and, despite the unpleasant process of administering IVs, we were passing that time in a cozy atmosphere. Despite our arms being all bruised after the IVs, and although my veins were gradually refusing to cooperate, and that downtown, people were looking at us every step of our way like we were patients who escaped from a hospital, I would do it again without hesitating.

Up until now, I haven't been able to tell what exactly contributed to the first more significant improvement that I noticed, and though I don't know if it was owing to one of the antibiotic or the drastic diet alone. One thig is certain, though: the time when I started feeling like a human again was one of the most beautiful periods of my life. I cannot tell exactly the day or the hour when I felt lightness inside my head. It was more of a process that made me realize one day that my severe brain fog, extremely high pressure, inability to focus and, most of all, derealization, which had been slowly making the world around me seem completely alien and blurry – all these symptoms were gradually improving, releasing their grip.

It was as if I could finally take off some of the burdens I had been wrestling with off my back. Holding under my arm a helmet filled with the ailments I had been suffering from for so many years, watching the sun setting behind birches on a green meadow in the hills, the landscape of my fiancée's family village, I was enjoying that beautiful moment, wanting to hold onto it. For the first time in ages, I could feel my connection with nature, as I had in the past. After such a long time, I could finally take a breath of fresh air into my lungs and exhale it without wondering if the visible vapor was mine or not, or whether the sun on the horizon was real. With tears in my eyes, I realized that it was a beginning of something good, at last. Sadly, as always, nothing good lasts forever.

"That's great! I told you everything would be fine!" Tomek shouted once he came back to Poland again. "Talking about your problem and Lyme disease, I'll show you something," he bent down and pulled one of the legs of his pants up. "Look! Something bit me and now it looks funny. See?"

Showing me what was definitely a site bitten by an insect, I gasped in disbelief. There was a huge mark that definitely looked nothing like a typical erythema migrans accompanied by redness that was almost purple here and there, evidencing that something very bad happened or was still happening with Tomek's leg.

"Bro, we have to do something about it!" I got concerned, seeing the size of the bite, the shape of which was reminiscent of a several-inches-long spot.

"Come on, I'm fine. It doesn't hurt, it's not itchy. I only wanted to show you this because it's interesting."

"I'm not having this discussion! You have to go show it to a doctor, an infectiologist, on top of that," I was not backing down as I knew the consequences a bite like that could have.

"Leave me alone, I'm not going anywhere," Tomek protested.

I happened to feel much better on that day, so despite the anxiety seizures that were still attacking me out of nowhere, I decided to drive the car. With another person by my side, I felt more confident behind the wheel and I knew that if something happened, he could drive instead. That day, Tomek didn't have to do that, the only thing I expected of him being to act reasonably and agree to my firm request.

"We're going to the ER!" I told Tomek while parking the car by the hospital of infectious diseases.

His disgust and discontent were saying it all. He knew, though, that he had no other choice. He was aware of the fact that the keys to the car were in my pocket, but he was also keeping track of my history. In my head, I could still hear Natalie informing me of irregular marks of a tick bite, but also Helen's elaborate on other insects that could've left a whole bunch of ill-willing monsters inside Tomek's body.

"Okay, fine. I'm doing this only for you!"

On that day, Tomek was oblivious to how bad I wanted someone to take me somewhere nearly six years ago, to anyone who could stop all these pathogens I had inside of me from growing. He couldn't have known that, as he couldn't even imagine what I felt like. No one could.

We were lucky and quite soon, Tomek was admitted into the hospital. We didn't have to wait long for the doctor, who took him to her office. I was not allowed to go in, so I went back to the car. My friend's visit in the doctor's office didn't take long.

"Go!" he said.

I started the engine and set off back to our homes.

"Well? Tell me!"

"The doctor said I just caught some allergy."

"Allergy? That's it? Is that what an allergy looks like? I asked in disbelief, recalling the huge, irregular, purple discoloration with what clearly was a bite mark left by an insect in the middle.

"Yes! It's only an allergy, and I got an ointment for it."

"Well, did you mention the ticks, Lyme disease, me?"

"I did!"

"And? Did she at least order some tests to be done? Serological ones? Anything?"

"No, she said a tick bite doesn't look like that and that it's only ticks that carry Lyme disease. She also added that she was busy and that next time, I shouldn't bother her with some bullshit like that."

Since I knew him well, I knew that the doctor likely didn't use these exact words, but I also knew that he wasn't lying. I wanted to make a U-turn and shout my history to that woman's face; what if every 'lucky' person that Helen and Natalie mentioned was treated in this way, too?

Although Tomek saw tears in my eyes more than just once, he didn't even have paid serological testing done. We were both adult men and I wasn't persuasive enough to talk him into doing it. I had no right to be angry with him. I don't know if he had a chance to convince me, back when I was healthy, if our roles were reversed. I knew that in order to understand this nightmare, you have to experience it firsthand, in your own body or at least in my case, also in my liver, which caused me to make one of the more significant decisions I ever had to take.

For some reason, my organ tasked with detoxification, metabolism or simply filtering of all the filth wouldn't stop informing me every month that its condition was getting worse and worse. When I was having my liver function tests done for the last time, the liver texted my always-dependable intuition, saying, "You're the only one who decides what happens to me next."

Concerned that my organ could get damaged and, most of all, that it would lose its regenerative abilities, I had to reconsider whether to continue the ceftriaxonum infusion therapy under the supervision of the ILADS expert, or to discontinue it. It wasn't the easiest decision of my life. Helen didn't see my results as tragic, as she kept on suggesting that such scores in people who continue the therapy get even worse, trying to discourage me from the idea of discontinuing our sessions. She was assuring me that nothing regenerates as fast as a liver does. I had to make a strong decision immediately. Although I didn't want to have anything to do with Dr. Armani, I could still hear him warning me that my treatment could end bad for me. Aside from my concern for the fate of my liver, I found making this decision hard, among others, because of my feeling that except for the ILADS method, there probably was no other solution or people whom I could contact to get help, but most of all, because of my awareness of the fact that I wasn't alone it in all; my sweetheart, who was carrying around a ticking bomb inside of her, too. She could easily continue to walk this path. I knew that if I give up, Anna would do the same. I felt responsible for both of us, not only because I was still tormented by negative thoughts that we could've hurt each other, but because knowing my fiancée, I was convinced that she'd follow suit.

I really wanted to continue walking that path. After all, I failed to find anyone else who would be capable of diagnosing me and helping me out. Owing to Helen and her method, considered by many a charlatanic doctor role-play, it was possible to obtain the first positive results in several years. Although throughout the extraordinary long period of drug-taking that she recommended I didn't manage to fully recover, I knew what I got back and what I'd never be able to fix.

Therefore, I decided to part ways with Helen, at least for some time. She wasn't happy about it.

"If that's your decision and you know what you're doing, I won't be holding you back."

Obviously, we had no clue what we were doing. We had no idea. We didn't know that realm as well as she did. Not surprisingly, Anna forewent the therapy, too.

"I go where you go, and I do what you do!" she'd say.

I had no idea what to do. I didn't know whether I should talk my woman into continuing a therapy consisting in taking vast amounts of antibiotics, or whether I should wait for the right moment when she'd have to decide for herself whether to follow Helen (who was suffering from Lyme disease, likewise) or not. One thing was certain: my fears exceeded all my expectations, and this extremely difficult decision was taken with the assistance of a specialist I went to see to have my liver diagnosed. I had no desire for running into Dr. Armani, so I chose a completely different facility in the area Anna was from. The man who performed the ultrasound testing of my liver not only confirmed Dr. Armani's words, stressing that I could make things even worse for myself, but also told me about liver problems that I didn't want to face in the future.

"You don't have two polyps on your gallbladder. You have four," he remarked, adding to my issues, as if I didn't have enough of them.

"Is it possible that they grew over the course of one month? I asked, surprised, thinking about the previous check-up at the facility Armani was working at, where I had been testing myself every month up until that moment."

"That's rather unlikely. The other diagnostician simply must have overlooked them."

"Could my antibiotic therapy result polyp formation?"

"Everything's possible but you won't be able to verify that now. Maybe that's just the way you are," he concluded.

I didn't know what to make of it all. Despite my supportive loved ones, whom I never saw for whom I should've always seen them for, and who were trying to guide me somehow, I still wasn't sure if I was doing the right thing. I had enough of all these misdiagnoses, erroneous opinions, slip-ups that I had experienced in my contact with healthcare professionals. I was afraid that Helen could've been wrong, too. I didn't see any errors, though, in the last resort available to me, which to me was the duo of mysterious, elegant bioenergy therapists whom we saw a few month earlier. I think they were one of the reasons why I made that decision. Although it was only my aunt and I who experienced something unusual on that night, Anna and my mom both hoped that next time, the healers' hands would make them experience something that could be considered a healing power, too. Unfortunately, there was a bitter aftertaste we all experienced after our second appointment, which triggered in us some concerns; not only did they make us part ways with Helen, but also everyone who went with me again at night, tired and sleepy, didn't want to have anything to do with bioenergy therapy ever again.

On our way for the second appointment, we didn't need to use the navigation app because my Anna was with us, and she has an innate sense of direction. It's amazing, really. Wherever she was once, her brain, like a computer, memorized the route and the area of a given town or city where she had been before even just once. The first time I noticed my fiancée had that highly useful ability, I was scratching my head, wondering how that's even possible. This time, she led us straight to our destination, too. A line of cars that suddenly appeared out of the dark on the gloomy road, lighting the darkness in front of us and scattering mist that was flowing right above the paved surface, telling us that we reached our destination. This time, the number of cars with plates from all around Poland was several times higher than the last time, while the line of people who were suffering, each in his or her own way, seemed even longer than the last time, too. Anna wasn't the only one who had exceptional memory. The way each person standing in line was welcomed was surely impressive.

"Well? How do you feel after our last time?" the older man asked. He was still the only one who talked.

"Same," I replied, surprised that the bioenergy therapist remembered me. I couldn't get it how was it possible that among hundreds of people these two men were seeing from time to time, of all these tens of faces that were hoping for a miracle on that night, it was my face that he recalled best.

"Give me those ears!" he added, causing thoughts in my brain to race even more.

That's impossible! How does he do that? I thought.

"Are you drinking Saint John's wort?"

He killed me with that question.

This time, well-prepared, I put a banknote on the bowl, which didn't contain much, as usual. When I went out to the hall, the older healer followed me out of the room and took me by the ears.

"Give me those ears for one more second! Here, some more of my energy," he said.

Though many people had been attended to before me, I never noticed the two men to act like that. It was quite nice of him.

Waiting for my companions, who this time entered the room right after me, I was looking around for cameras hidden in the building, as I didn't notice any at the office. I was certain that they had to be there somewhere.

I couldn't believe that my face is so memorable that they could recall who I am and everything we talked about at my first visit. After all, I was accustomed to healthcare professionals who showed me repeatedly that even a young guy with an ailment as uncommon as my ear-related condition can be forgotten within two weeks.

"Well? How was it?" I asked Anna.

"Weird!"

"Meaning...?"

"He recalled me perfectly and basically, that's that."

We waited for my mom and aunt who entered the office right after Anna.

"How do you feel about it?" we asked them.

"Nothing unusual, aside from the fact that the gentlemen perfectly recalled my case," my aunt replied.

"As for me, my experience wasn't what you'd consider a good one," my mom said.

"How come? What happened?" I asked.

"I'll tell you on our way home," my mom was not content with it.

On our way back, once again, we all started sharing our experiences. This time, no one went through anything extraordinary in the healers' presence, aside from their astonishing ability to identify human faces and recall their cases, which each of us found intriguing.

"How about you, mom?" I asked.

"This time around, I felt an odd sensation. The older gentleman, holding me by my head, made his hand tremble and asked me if I felt his energy. 'No,' I replied. Then, he grabbed me again, this time using a bit more force, and said blatantly, 'Feel it! You feel it now?' I saw discontent and anger in his eyes, and the way he was talking to me was inappropriate, too. It wasn't pleasant; frankly, it was very unpleasant," my mom said, somewhat frightened.

On that morning, I could see in her eyes the very same look that she had on the day I took her to Ewa. Although I didn't always agree with my parents, I could tell that their misgivings about some situations were accurate. Anna and my aunt had no opinion about that; I started feeling some negative emotions, too, but once I returned home, the green spiral that was haunting me last time never showed up again. Although my aunt was the only one was satisfied, as her insomnia issues got resolved, we had to make one more difficult decision.

I knew that I won't heal my fiancée with Saint John's wort alone, but it wouldn't help me tackle my bacteria, either. The way the healer recognized us was unquestionably astonishing, just as the number of the ill coming to see the duo from all around the country was.

Maybe the bowl filled with coins was not at all so that we could pay for the visit, and the duo had a different way to have their mysterious debt paid back? I thought.

Nighttime visits only, crowds of people coming in and waiting in line to be touched, the green spiral, my aunt's cured insomnia and, most of all, my mom's symptoms started moving our imagination to the point that we all began seeing these appointments as a certain form of idolatry. We were not the most devout Catholics, but there are some images that everyone had to do with in their life, and they came upon us for some reason, putting each of us in a meditative place; a place that torments the conscience.

CHAPTER V

Undoubtedly, the mental clarity I regained in the course of the ILADS treatment was a factor that affected my most recent decisions. If not for that substantial improvement, which allowed me to look at the world through clean glasses again, probably, I would've kept wading through the antibiotic treatment without paying much attention to what happens to us further down the line. I recall neither the day nor the hour when, taking yet another look at my hands, I didn't feel the overwhelming anxiety and derealization anymore. When my mind went back to the state that made me capable of spending more time in the world around me and enjoy the good things, particularly the little things that I had never noticed before, my aching body and soul stopped shedding so many tears. In sickness, Anna and I got to know each other even better and learned to appreciate our closeness, and the closeness of those who were supporting us became even more valuable to us. We were more and more convinced that my mom's words, which she would repeat time and time again, meant much more than we thought. *Maybe everything did happen for a reason?* We pondered. My 'sick' love and passion for training, which used to be my whole world and was now discontinued, simply disappeared. Naturally, I still missed being active and exercising, but I was no longer enslaved by the oppressive thinking that whatever happens, I need to go to the gym. Despite the other symptoms that were still there, ruining my life and annoying me every day, the will to survive that was within me and my hope allowed me to focus more often on the important things. Unquestionably, one of them was my job and the family business. Although the date of our yet another appointment with the two mysterious bioenergy therapists was near, we all decided this path, albeit highly intriguing to us all, should not be pursued anymore. Secretly hoping for my body to quickly recover after the antibiotic therapy, I wished to see Helen just as soon, as she seemed the only lifeline we had. I took her claim to heart, believing that most likely, we wouldn't recover from chronic Lyme disease and the co-infection as long as we were alive. I knew there was nothing else I could do but continue seeing her occasionally, giving my liver and myself some time to regenerate.

Our lives, which had been turned upside down over the course of the previous years, were still one big unknown. *What's next?* We were all asking ourselves the same question that no one could answer. Everything in our lives was changing, and time was passing at the same pace. More and more of our peers were getting married before God. Their enamored eyes were shining with the great joy and happiness at the thought of sharing their future and the process of building a loving family. Leaning on a church pillar for support, I was exhausted, still fighting my anxiety. Imagining that one day it could be us, I was watching Anna scratching her itchy places where a catheter and an IV drip were in just a moment earlier.

God, if you're really there, I beg you, make my Anna happy, I asked the Lord, seeing my fiancée of many years, who forewent a better life to be with me, fall into a reverie, her eyes showing tiredness. Unexpectedly, a miracle happened, which I still failed to link to my prayers to God and assumed it was a coincidence. We began the year 2016 with more hope for a recovery than ever before.

"Michal, have you heard of antibacterial lamps?" one of my clients asked me, who sometimes, seeing me, could sense the power of the bacteria that were devastating my body.

"Lamps?" I was puzzled.

"The daughter of the guy who installed a staircase at my house suffers from Lyme disease, too. They say the girl went blind, and today, she goes to work as if nothing happened. As far as I know, she cured herself with some kind of a lamp. I can ask the carpenter for his daughter's phone number, if you want."

The words I just heard came to me dazzling like a bolt from the blue. Having parted ways with Helen, I was convinced that there was no other solution that could help us in any way whatsoever. I had no clue what the client was talking to me about, and the method he mentioned seemed a completely abstract idea.

I hope they won't put me on a tanning bed! I thought.

"Of course. I'd be much obliged for that person's number," I replied.

As soon as I got the phone number of the girl who allegedly got her vision back, I didn't waste a second of time, and called her immediately. As it turned out, it all really happened, and the girl, like me, had been wrestling chronic neurologic Lyme disease for several years. Up until that point, I considered Helen's words just a theory that I heard of, but talking with a person who went through a nightmare similar to mine, or perhaps even worse, made me all the more afraid of my occupants. The advanced stage of her disease, which partly resembled mine, caused her to lose her vision in one eye. The raging bacteria attacked her optic nerves, as a result of which she woke up one day to one of the biggest nightmares you can imagine. Unlike us, she identified the cause of her condition sooner but, as she claimed, no relatively easily-accessible treatment method helped her.

Just like we did, she underwent long-term antibiotic therapy that proved ineffective and lasted much longer in her case. For two years, she was also in bio-resonance therapy, as diagnostic purposes aside, bio-resonance is often applied for eliminating pathogens. All in vain. When she was about to lose hope for a recovery, she stumbled upon a plasma lamp called Rife's machine, which made her miraculously regain vision only two weeks into therapy. With Helen's words echoing in my mind, claiming that there is no one specific method for treating Lyme disease, I was very skeptical about what that young woman was telling me on the phone; but, at the same time, I found it all fascinating. Most things she told me about were consistent with our previous experience with *Borrelia*. However, at some point, my attitude became even more skeptical.

"As far as I understand, when you regain your vision, you were convinced that the machine works, but how did you learn that it over?" I asked her.

"A bio-resonance diagnosis," she replied.

At that moment, there was one thing on my mind: massive uncertainty. My most recent experience with bio-resonance didn't yield any desired results, and the diagnosis Natalie offered me was quite comical. I decided to share my experience with the girl on the other side of the phone.

"I don't know where you've been, what device you've been diagnosed with, or who carried out the test, but one thing's certain: it had nothing in common with what I'm talking about. The true test doesn't take a couple of minutes, it can take up to an hour. Contrary to what you've heard, the diagnostician has to be really focused and pay much attention to diagnose pathogens correctly. I'll recommend the facility I was diagnosed at to you and give you the number to the people who have Rife's machine."

"What about the lamp? What is it exactly?" I asked.

"I wouldn't know; you'll certainly learn all about it when you get there. I know that this device generates various radio waves that kill the bacteria. I know that nothing helped me as much as that machine did, I know it."

Talking with her made me feel ecstatic and all fired up about a better tomorrow for the first time in ages. I believed her words and wanted the same outcome for myself. Then, I recalled that doctors can be very different, and so why would unconventional therapist be any different? I knew there nothing else I could do but to make an appointment with the people who diagnosed that girl and, primarily, to go see those who had the mysterious plasma lamp.

Being a man of little faith, despite listening to the young woman's account of her recovery, I continued to seek some reassurance. This was not solely because of my belief that most likely, there was no machine that could destroy the bacteria, but also because of my experience of six years that left a mark on me.

That happens only in movies! I thought, and I had seen many.

I also took Helen into account, who was suffering from Lyme disease longer than we did, and whose experience and knowledge certainly wouldn't have let her ignore an invention like that. Therefore, I got back online, seeking any information about the said machine relentlessly. Sadly, back then, there were few of them out there. Eventually, though, I found it.

On one of the online forums where people would leave various questions and someone interested in a given discussion would post a reply, one of the users who initiated such a dispute on Rife's machine decided to leave his e-mail address for those who'd like to learn something more about it. I didn't hesitate and contacted him right away. Soon after, we started conversing, also via phone. The boy was the second person I met who experienced the great power of the machine right after undergoing the ILADS treatment, which was ineffective in his case.

"Antibiotics helped me a lot, especially for my tinnitus. Unfortunately, like many others who suffer from *Borrelia* and *Bartonella*, it seemed too resistant to antibiotics. Even one year and six months into the antibiotic treatment, I couldn't eliminate *Borrelia* or *Bartonella*, which were causing me horrible anxiety."

"You had anxiety, too?" I asked.

"I did! Terrible one, I'm telling you! I have a pilot's license, I can fly planes. Sadly, I had to leave that passion behind. Having uncontrollable anxiety when you're behind the wheel is awful, but on the day I got an anxiety seizure at the controls of an airplane, I realized that I wouldn't be able to just park it all of a sudden. It was then that I started seeking the cause of my problems. Anxiety in Lyme disease and co-infections is one of the most common symptoms. I know a story of a guy who loved mountaineering, but not in the sense of taking a longer hike in a beautiful mountain scenery. The dude was climbing summits with protection gear.

He's been doing that since he was a kid. One day, attached to the wall of a mountain summit, he looked down and felt something he had never experienced before in his life, which was a very strong fear of heights. He couldn't understand why he got it all of a sudden. It was all due to Lyme disease that he later managed to identify. When I learned about Rife's machine, I had to give it a try. I was in therapy for nearly two months, several times a week, several hours a session. It was worth it! *Borrelia, Bartonella*, and most of all, my anxiety, were all gone, and I resumed flying. It didn't improve overnight, though, it took some time."

As you may guess, in my mind, I was almost home. I didn't need any more accounts to embark on a new journey on the road to our full recovery. However, before we entered the world we had never even known of, since undoubtedly, the machine aside, there were a few surprises that were still waiting for us, Anna and I decided to tell Helen about it all, since we had been through a lot with her over the last year, and she herself was still looking for a cure against the bacteria that were tormenting us all, too. Sadly, despite our sincere desire, surprisingly, our best intentions were misinterpreted.

"I have no idea what you're talking about, and there's not much I know about the bio-resonance method, either. I do not question the physical foundations of the way it is applied, but to me, a medical professional, the way such results are interpreted, or rather misinterpreted, which I come across quite often, is simply unacceptable. If the device you're talking about really exists, maybe I should quit antibiotics and ILADS, listen to you two, and then start sending my patients off for treatment with bio-resonance and a plasma machine?" she said with a hint of sarcasm, somewhat disappointed with our approach and the decisions we made.

We didn't understand her attitude. We wanted to share these accounts with her, because she might wanted to give it a try. Soon, we realized that the war between infectious disease specialists and ILADS doctors could easily involve also other methods of unconventional treatment. As fate would have it, for some reason, we had to make our way though that battlefield. But then again, was it fate, really?

As Alfred Hitchcock used to say, "A film should start with an earthquake, and then the tension is to keep on rising incessantly." I think that my brutal journey through Lyme disease unraveled in the exact same way, starting from 2010. However, if I could take a camera in my hand and record everything that was happening inside my head, I'd start with that specific moment.

F***! F***!" I was standing and gazing at the miraculous painting of Our Lady of Czestochowa at the Jasna Gora monastery, and my thoughts were being overtaken by an inexplicable flood of profanities I couldn't hold back. A paralysis; my legs all trembling; inner confusion; massive shame, and, most of all, my impulsive, profound apology, and my eyes cast down in embarrassment, making me unable to maintain eye contact with the sacred icon – it was all just a fraction of what I was experiencing back then. That moment of terror lasted only for a couple of minutes, for I couldn't hold for any longer, having entered the Sanctuary of Our Lady of Czestochowa where Anna and I would come ask for help every weekend from the time we started our new treatment.

"What's wrong?" Anna asked, seeing me jerking my head left and right, as if I wanted to get bangs off my face.

"Same thing again, we have to leave!" I replied, admitting to my anxiety. At the same time I lacked the courage to tell her what I experienced a moment earlier, and what then turned into my another problem.

The one-eyed girl, as I called her when talking about her with others, didn't lie, that's unquestionable; she was also right about bio-resonance therapy and Rife's machine. My previous diagnostic testing performed by Natalie had nothing to do with the test that was done later, and the people to whom we turned for help, recommended by the young girl with the past, made a great impression on us. They were very well-versed in the subjects of health and health-promoting lifestyle in general, which in our case was necessary for our recovery, and in the case of healthy people, essential to keep them this way. This approach to life was exactly like that of Asian cultures, where right from the beginning, you're taught how to not get sick, in contrast to the western approach in medicine, which teaches you how to cure a disease. The former was definitely much more to my liking. The abundance of information these people had and the form in which they conveyed it all undoubtedly hit a chord with us, like an arrow hitting its target. Never before had I seen expertise that unrivalled in any of Hippocrates' heirs. This was probably due to the fact that usually, doctors had no time to chat, even those who took enormous sums of money for private appointments, some of which lasted only a couple of minutes; or, many the system each of them was part of, Armani included, didn't allow them for some reason to give health-promoting guidance that could help me.

Maybe it's only me who was so unlucky, and the other healthcare professionals are the right people for the job? I thought.

With my brain fog gradually cleared up, because of my awareness of everything that had happened, my imagination and the images my mind was generating, my hatred for the healthcare professionals grew even more. All the people who couldn't afford treatment were often on my mind. I could see mothers, giving the last money they earned to medical experts to get their children saved, and the doctors who would then reply without batting an eyelid, 'I don't know' or 'Please go see a psychiatrist,' to then take the money like the punks who were stealing flowers from the elderly man by a busy street, and simply leave. My unexplainable irritability and fits of anger that I had been experiencing for several years transformed into contempt and resentment that I started feeling towards healthcare professionals.

I would have never thought that despite all the tragedy and suffering, the body is capable of adapting to a given situation so swiftly. You're in pain, you wake up like that day after day, and you have no way out, there's nothing you can do about it. Your problem is not going anywhere and, sometime later, it becomes an inherent part of your life like an annoying shadow. My life took on the same format that the main character in the romantic comedy *Groundhog Day* directed by Harold Ramis had to put up with; for some unknown reasons, his fate played an unpleasant trick on him. Each day the protagonist was exactly the same, to no end, making him re-live everything yet again, from the very beginning; in order to break the cycle, he had to understand a lot of things and change many things about him, too. The feelings I was experiencing were not a comedy, though the doctors I had been seeing at the expense of my health made me laugh on many occasions. Before I, too, came to understand why my life had taken that particular course and not another, which happened quite soon after, I heard the following words.

"My dear patients, I'm sorry to inform you that you both carry many pathogens specific for diseases of affluence, including the so-called tick-borne diseases, which you need to address before they cause you massive harm," the diagnostician said, unaware that we perfectly knew we were infected, and the harm he mentioned had been already taking its toll for some time now.

Thistime, however, putting words of the people who recommended I take this path to the test, I decided not to share my story at the bio-resonance session right away with the enthusiasts of alternative medicine who were diagnosing us. I wanted to hear them saying that diagnosis without giving them any reason to think that Anna and I could have any bacteria or any diseases whatsoever. Although Anna and I hoped that after nearly one year in ILADS therapy, referred to by many as pseudoscientific, the diagnostic test wouldn't detect anything, to our surprise, the test results were perfectly consistent with our former serological results. What is more, they showed that aside from the pathogens we'd been fighting up until that point, we were also carrying *Rickettsia* and *Mycoplasma* that Helen had mentioned, which were not identified in our previous blood tests. Before we ventured off to try Rife's machine, despite the accounts of people just as sick as I was, I was still skeptical about bio-resonance.

Everyone must be getting the same results! I thought sarcastically.

Without waiting too long, Anna and I sent several relatives at the same facility to verify our suspicions. As it turned out, results were not the same. Some of them got excellent scores, their bodies not encumbered with *Borrelia* and Co., while others learned from the test that they had the same ticking bomb inside them, ready to go off anytime and turn their lives upside down.

I didn't need any extra evidence to open the door to yet another method of our treatment. However, I wasn't aware that once Anna and I pass through that door, we'd step into the world we had never been in before and which we had never experienced before, and which undoubtedly had been wide open and ready for any of us from the first days of our lives. For me, that first step into the unknown proved extremely painful.

The people who confirmed that Rife's machine worked weren't lying. With my very first encounter with that device, which to me was reminiscent of a prop from a spaceship taken right out of a movie back from the 1990s, I could feel it was working. Funny looking gauges showing many different values, several knobs or a miniature screen displaying frequencies that were changing nonstop are only several features of a quote large, silver box. Above all, there was a plasma lamp filled with argon (a noble gas), emitting a very warm, orange glow, the essential part of that device whose healing effects were mentioned by my client. Lying with Anna in the same relaxation chair, we were undergoing treatment that involved Rife's machine every weekend; by means of electromagnetic energy transformed into a plasmatic wave of just the right frequency, the device was penetrating our bodies to target the adversarial occupants that were inside.

"Is that all we have to do? Just sit there?" I asked at the first session.

"Yes! Exactly!" a very likeable boy replied, who together with his wife was running an alternative medicine office offering diagnostic testing based on bio-resonance and elimination of tick-borne bacteria using Rife's machine.

"Are we going to feel anything during the therapy?" Anna asked, concerned about her condition, as her rash and the pain in her legs, which tormented her during the antibiotic treatment, and which were getting more and more intense with every month.

"The plasmatic wave of a specific frequency affects various cell structures in pathogens by resonating with them. At the moment when a cell gets affected by a wave that is powerful enough, has just the right frequency and duration, a phenomenon called polarization takes place, which cases irreversible pores to form in the outer cell wall. This way, Rife's machine can cause deformity in the cell and make it disintegrate, as a result of which a large amount of toxins gets released into the body. This can make you feel aggravated symptoms or experience discomfort."

"You mean the so-called 'herx'?" Anna asked.

"Exactly!"

"Cell disintegration?" I asked out of curiosity.

"Indeed! A properly selected frequency destroys cells of all microbes, causing the bacteria of the *Borrelia* genus and other pathogens to disintegrate. Every living organism has its own unique frequency at which it vibrates, and that frequency makes its all cells, tissues, organs and systems healthy and efficient. For many years, Royal Raymond Rife was trying to find the reversed value of that frequency, until he finally did it. He built a machine that annihilates pathogens. Let me give you a better picture; an example often used by Rife himself to visualize how his invention works. Imagine an opera singer who uses high vibrations of her powerful voice to break a crystal glass into pieces. All it takes is for her to find the specific sound vibration and keep it for a specific period of time, and she can make the atomic arrangement of the glass weaken and disintegrate. Bacteria break down in the exact same way.

"That's fascinating! Why haven't we heard of that man?" I asked.

"Maybe it'd just you who think you haven't. Royal Raymond Rife was born in 1888. Only forty years later, he went down in history. His life calling was to see what a human eye cannot see. He was convinced that if he succeeded to see bacteria and viruses, mankind would be able of inventing a cure for any disease. Rife was one of the greatest inventors of the early 20th century. Before he turned forty, he already had received fourteen state awards for scientific accomplishments. Owing to him, for the first time in history, humankind could see a living virus under an optical microscope that he built. Once he did that, he made some observations, and identified the virus, which in his view was responsible for causing cancer. Pursuing his own studies, not only did he invent a machine that allowed him to annihilate viruses, but also found the right frequency that was killing cancer cells and he also determined those that were eliminating other conditions. His discoveries could've cured all humankind," the boy said with excitement, making that mysterious scientists better known to us.

"Cancer cells?" Anna asked.

"Yes! Sadly, as it was usually the case in the history of humankind, some matters couldn't just be let out in the open. The technology that Rife constructed concerned the pharmaceutical lobby, who could lose millions of dollars because of him. For this reason, he was proclaimed a mad scientists who tried to sell people bull. Please, believe me, this is not bull, and it's not a joke, either. The machine works and you will be able to tell that for yourself."

Perhaps Armani and Co. only continue that sick system that oppressed Rife, I thought.

"How can we be sure that this device will help us?" I asked.

"The plasmatic discharge it generates affects the entire body, reaching to all tissues and annihilating not only bacteria that wander the circulatory system, but also those that hid from antibodies or antibiotics in the nervous system. Certainly, you'll feel the Herxheimer reaction firsthand, just like I have. Typically, this reaction manifests as two or three weeks of painfully aggravated symptoms caused by vast amounts of toxins released from microorganisms into the body," he replied.

"Do you mean you had Lyme disease, too?" Anna asked.

"Most of people who start to delve deep into this subject by offering some kind of treatment, either suffer or have suffered from this condition. Although the top-tier doctor provides a person suffering from Lyme disease and its co-infections with massive amounts of support, relationships like that are very hard to find, unfortunately. Most patients never come across such a person, and for many others it is nearly impossible. I, too, had some issues with that, and the antibiotic therapy, particularly the drastic diet, was slowly wearing me down. Up until then, humanity had learned a lot but we all still know very little about these bacteria, especially about how to successfully eliminate them. My wife and I stumbled upon Rife's machine in my worst moment; shortly after, it helped me get back on track and regain balance. To this day, I've no idea how it was possible. There are many people of there who are just like me or you, like you, they take matters in their hands and come to us seeking help, but often it's already too late."

To me, everything said by that young man, whose face reminded me of actor Breckin Mayer, was like a release of a new science fiction movie, but about ten minutes after the machine was first started, Anna and I felt as if we were having a 4D movie theater experience. Staring at the orange light of the plasma lamp that was tuning itself to the frequencies changing on the screen, embracing each other, we were listening closely to the sound made by Rife's machine, trying to relax. Looking at Anna, who was simply dozing off like a baby, all of a sudden, I felt the power of the device. In an area inside my head that was already well-known to me, there was an odd tingling sensation cutting across with its characteristic force, which always manifested right before every instance of a painful prickly sensation in my head, evoked unexpectedly, with immense intensity I had not known before. No bioenergy therapist, healer, or antibiotic had ever caused a sensation like that inside me. It was just as if the frequencies immediately started beating down the resisting bacteria that were really located in a place inaccessible to the antibiotic. Owing to the ILADS therapy, my perception, including my compulsive habit of comparing people to actors, were back on track, while my other problems were still looking to be resolved by the recently discovered, mysterious method of treatment that, like many others before, seemed to us to be our last resort.

The sensation of having the area of my head intensely penetrated, which I experienced at the very first session that lasted several hours, was a prelude to Herxheimer reactions that Mayer mentioned, which continued for three weeks. Every session with the machine ended for me in my body responding in a very strong way. Each time we were leaving the building where we were treated I felt as if I was walking out of a club after being there for several hours straight, mostly at the bar. Then, I recalled Helen saying, "Not everyone feels worse in treatment, though, but it's better if you can tell a difference – that way we know that the therapy is working." I felt uplifted. Though back then, she was talking about antibiotics, which work differently on every person, as she mentioned, I knew that in this case, it must be like that, too. I firmly believed that at that moment, for the first time, I learned what it feels like when bacteria die, and all my cumbersome ailments related to the neck and the head that I kept flexing and turning in all directions additionally turned into an unpleasant, dull pain and recurring episodes of moderate haze. Such symptoms would then persist for two, sometimes three weeks, just as all experts in Lyme disease mentioned. Already extremely exhausted, after all those experiences, and with the symptoms that were continuing to harass me, I didn't know whether to cry or laugh. "That's a good sign!" they said time and time again. However, the therapy using Rife's machine had a completely different impact on my Anna. Most sessions were making here sleepy, the sole Herxheimer reactions that she noticed being an aggravated rash across her entire neck and cleavage, and osteoarticular pains in the legs.

From time to time after several-weeks-long therapies, Mayer's wife was making a very specific diagnosis based on bio-resonance. To this end, she was using a device different than the one applied by Natalie or the people recommended to me by the carpenter's one-eyed daughter. This difference aside, the device showed the exact same set of bacteria that Helen identified in us and those whose presence was detected by the diagnostician recommended by the carpenter's daughter. My lack of faith and doubt in whether these devices are effective gradually turned into certainty that the 'charlatanic' technology works and provides reliable results.

With every passing weekend that Anna and I were spending on a trip to Czestochowa, I imagined Rife's optical microscope and the cellular structure of the bacteria that were disintegrating into pieces to the sound of frequencies affecting our bodies like a distinct voice of an opera singer, leaving no trace behind.

Shortly afterwards, I was affected by the same feeling. I spent the previous two years opposing the ruthless, microscopic monsters that had been destroying me both physically and mentally. There came a time when I started feeling that the remains of that which is referred to as 'being human' was falling apart. I wasn't perfect; I made a few mistakes in my life and I was nowhere near being a 'noble man' who could become someone else's authority figure. Though I had no textbook relationship with God, I considered myself worthy of the label of a true Catholic, as I wasn't breaking the Christian rules that my parents instilled in me in my childhood, until my subjective spirituality got knocked out harder than I could ever imagine. The several previous years were like twelve rounds of a fierce, unequal boxing fight with my opponent, who was physically one-upping me in every possible aspect. And yet, it was only now that I started begging for someone to drop a towel on the floor, thus saving me from what we had to face aside from everything else.

The history of the world shows that every living being seeks God and expresses a need for prayer to someone whose existence he or she is aware of, someone who is above all forces, above all evil. It is undoubtedly a common denominator that we all share. We all have a sense of morality, shame, or conscience that help us tell the difference between good and evil since childhood, and when facing a threat, we all start calling God for help. As Winston Churchill used to remark, atheists are nowhere to be found in a lifeboat.[27] Like my mom, who would repeat time and time

---

[27] R. Carswell, *Pytanie o Wiare*, 2012, e-book, p. 6. A Polish-language version based on R. Carswell's *Grill a Christian: Answers to tough questions about Christianity, God and the Bible*.

again, "When in fear, God is near," Mr. Churchill was not wrong. I wasn't an atheist, more like an agnostic. Despite my very little faith and questions that were still bothering me, like, "Why me?", "Why us?", there was some massive force that was pulling me to the painting of Our Lady at the sanctuary in the spiritual capital of Poland. In contrast to our peers, who were spending each and every weekend accompanied by family or partying with their friends, unwinding and recharging my batteries for the days to come, we continued our treatment, sitting and staring for hours at the orange light of the plasma lamp, hoping for a better tomorrow. At first, Anna and I were driving eighty miles only to have one therapy session with Rife's machine crossed off and then, often at night, we would go back home. However, one day, Mayer and his wife suggested that we should have sessions on weekends, too, and book some place for a night. And so we did; we found this solution definitely more convenient for us, as it allowed us to undergo treatment using the machine on daily basis without having to spend a couple of hours on the road every single day. Contrary to what you might expect, in a town that was not the most attractive to tourists, finding a place to stay overnight was difficult. In the end, we managed to come across very nice people who were offering rooms for people on a pilgrimage to the Sanctuary of Our Lady of Czestochowa. It so 'happened' that every weekend, we were falling asleep several hundred yards away from the location of the miraculous painting famous for its hundreds if not thousands of cases of people healed from various types of conditions. Naturally, the force behind it all was not the old painting but Jesus Christ, who was requested by the Mother of God herself to heal the sick, as people were convinced. I've never believed such stories to be true; hearing of someone who was allegedly healed, I'd say, "And so what?" and proceed to live my everyday life completely disinterested. However, there came a time I'd give everything for becoming a protagonist of such a story.

Despite not feeling well, Anna and I would spend every weekend away from our families. We were free to use the time in-between therapy sessions any way we wanted, that is, to entertain ourselves, as young people do. But for some reason, my heart and brain were telling me we should go pray before the holy painting.

Anna had no objections; taking me by the hand with much enthusiasm, she navigated our way to the sanctuary, though her sad face was saying it all. She was well aware of my reactions in public spaces, where I'd most often get all anxious for no good reason, unable to overcome it on my own. On that day, it wasn't only anxiety that got in my way, but also something much stronger that I was unable to comprehend or explain in any rational way.

Already at our destination, I felt that I'd have a meltdown soon. I only wanted to approach the sacred icon, look at the Mother of God's face and ask her to relieve us both of all our ailments. Nonetheless, the thing that happened to me there was awfully painful. In one moment, when I was fighting my anxiety with every passing second while expressing my intentions to Mary at the same time, inexplicably, some curse words started popping up in my thoughts. It was as if there was someone hell-bent on feeding some unexpected lines to an actor reciting his part on the stage. I could feel my mind getting filled with filthy epithets insulting the Mother of God and I couldn't do anything about it. Unable to admit to Anna what was happening to me, I ran outside the temple doors to get some fresh air. Then, I got overwhelmed by massive fear and a feeling I can't put in words. Yet again, arising in my head, there was the question whether I chose the right path.

Maybe Armani and his colleagues were right, after all? Maybe I really am mental? I wondered by the shrine. And yet, some part of me knew that I just had to end up there. Despite the shame that flooded me, I knew that the Mother of God knew all too well that those words were not mine.

I was aware of the fact that I couldn't give up at that point and just run away from the altar like a coward. Every time I was experiencing something highly unpleasant, my mom's words were like a weapon I used to fight back. "Everything happens for a reason!" I'd say time and time again.

Much time passed before Anna and I realized that all the signs that had been appearing on my way were not merely a coincidence. I felt that I should've folded my hands, knelt down and lost myself in a prayer long time ago, since whatever the thing that decided to torment me in front of the Mother of God was, it wasn't about to give up easily. Meanwhile, I told Anna about it all, and we both knew that we had to dedicate every moment not spent in therapy to praying in front of the sacred icon. And so we did.

Every weekend, after every session when the bacteria were 'bombarded' with plasmatic waves, Anna and I would go to Jasna Gora to make requests and apologize for what was going on inside my head. I recalled movies such as *The Omen* starring Gregory Peck, where a little antichrist would get a full-blown attack of hysterical panic in front of church doors.

God, do I have the same thing? But it's just a movie, I thought.

With every passing weekend I felt that I could endure a couple of minutes more praying. It was just as if my completely unjustified anxiety that would show up whenever it pleased started to ease up week after week. The same thing with 'my' inexplicable thoughts that were tormenting me in front of Mary. The more often Anna and I came to see the icon, the more it receded. I didn't understand what was going on with me and how was it even possible. One time, the man whose place we were staying at (with whom we found some common ground and shared our story with) mentioned that near Jasna Gora, in the direction to our city, there was a Dominican monastic church in a village called Gidle. He said, "Jasna Gora is famous predominantly for conversions, while Gidle is known for physical healing." He added, that the healing of the body is the work of a wooden figurine of the Mother of God shrouded in myth. After what we had experienced in Jasna Gora, we didn't take much time to deliberate and on our way from yet another weekend session with Mayer and Rife, we'd make a detour each time and head to Gidle only to kneel for a while in front of the wooden statue depicting the Mother of God with baby Jesus. Just like water is essential for fish, the vast silence of the monastery was much needed for my tinnitus, which was trying to disturb me when I was making requests. Every time I appeared before the figurine or the holy icon in Jasna Gora, I could feel that it was only in the spiritual capital of Poland that something was forcing into my head words that weren't mine; nonetheless, in both these places I could hold for a longer time that I had before. Visiting each of these sacred locations, Anna and I would look at the votive offering brought over the years by the healed. I wondered if one day we would make such a gift, too. Back then, I didn't feel any need to do so, as I didn't feel healed. Even when taking a look at my watch, which was informing me I managed to endure less than an hour without anxiety and curse words in my head, it didn't make me think much. Despite what had affected me and subsided for some reason, I didn't feel any divine intervention; what's worse, shortly after, I forgot about it. I wanted to be physically healed so bad that I wasn't interested in anything else, particularly in what I didn't understand. After several weeks in Rife's therapy with Anna, we got the first news from Mayer's wife, which was extremely positive.

"Dear ones, say goodbye to *Mycoplasma* and *Chlamydia pneumoniae*! I sense neither of them anymore!" she said during our check-up.

Maybe this is why my anxiety and horrible inner dialogue disappeared, too? I thought, wondering if it was owing to Rife's machine or the small pilgrimage tours that we were going on every time we came for a therapy session.

The words of Mayer's wife were not merely a theory the young woman deducted from the bio-resonance results. Anna and I could still feel the effects of the wave generator on our own skin. After the lengthy herxes that I experienced following therapies, there was an inflow of positive sensations. The longer we were in Rife's therapy, the more I could notice a substantial improvement. The unpleasant prickly sensations inside my head significantly eased up, while speech problems and instances of mouth paralysis that were up to several seconds long started subsiding. The enormous red spots on my torso, visible to the naked eye, the shape of some was reminiscent of continents, which manifested, for instance, when I was taking a hot shower, started simply disappearing from one therapy session to another. I felt that finally, I was getting some good moments in my life. Taking note of the clearly visible improvement and the subsidence of some symptoms, I decided to exercise tests every month to see how much I could handle. I would get into a plank to do pushups that used to be an inseparable part of my athletic lifestyle to test myself. I would watch the reaction of my head and neck, which after every effort were causing me sensations that were hard to describe and bad enough to even make me feel not present. Unfortunately, it wasn't the right moment yet. With the words of the carpenter's daughter still echoing in my head, I realized that every form of treatment against Lyme disease and its coinfections will always have a different impact on every individual, and the results will not always occur at the same time.

The wave of news that was quite positive for us seemed to have no end. I received a call from my sister, who had been living in Germany for a couple of years, and heard some good news.

"I booked an appointment with a terrific laryngologist who saved ears on many occasions, mostly those of professional divers. The guy is said to have cut muscles many times; you said they could be the reason behind your troubles. Pack your bags!"

Having no luck with doctors specializing in ear-related conditions in Poland, I felt that I had no other choice but to go on a brief expedition abroad to talk to the expert who had dealt with a similar issue. Fortunately, my derealization and brain fog, that left me when I took off my subjective helmet during the ILADS treatment, allowed me to focus on English to talk freely with the doctor, my only hope for getting rid of the maddening mess that was going on inside my ears, without resorting to the help of a translator, that is, my sister.

When I was already there, the green light that all the good news had on its way suddenly turned to red.

"It seems to me that you've diagnosed your problem very accurately, and that without question, all your terrible sensations are caused by the muscles. I'm surprised by your great knowledge on the subject, which indeed can sometimes surpass that of some doctors. Still, you should know that if I perform this surgery, it won't be reversible. What is more, I won't give you any guarantees that it would succeed."

I knew that making the right decision won't be easy for me. And yet, the words that I heard right after that made even more hesitant.

"Also, take note of a certain risk it involves."

"What do you mean?" I asked.

"After such a surgery, there is a risk that the muscle responsible for keeping your face all together could get damaged and cause it to sag. There are also cases where there's a permanent metallic taste you would have to live until the end of your days. You are the one to decide. The surgery is not complicated and it doesn't take long."

In just one moment, my sister's good intentions went down the drain. I knew that nothing in life comes easy, which was even more true in my life. I saw in my head the woman I had recently met, deprived of her good looks by Lyme disease that caused her facial muscles to go completely weak, thus making the skin on her face sag inertly; I didn't want to experience something like that. I knew that I had to put that decision aside hoping that Rife's machine would do the job and my ears would regenerate on their own. However, I was glad that finally, there was someone who understood in detail what I was suffering from. He confirmed my diagnosis, which proved too difficult a task for most experts I had the pleasure of seeing. In all that stress, I forgot to mention my purulent cyst that started growing once again when I quitted antibiotics. However, it was addressed shortly after.

Despite the noticeable progress, my body and mind were still very tired. I was happy as a kid, though, as I knew that I was on the right way to recovery. This was evidenced also by a clearly visible decrease in flu-like inflammations that had been tormenting me notoriously, which evidently subsided with the beginning of the antibiotic treatment under Helen's supervision, and didn't come back. It all made us smile more often.

And yet, it was difficult for us to feel happy when we were seeing others in pain, sometimes unable to afford to even begin a therapy with Rife's machine or those who had to discontinue it for some time for the same reason. It weren't only our lives that were getting ruined by Lyme disease and the bacteria that go along with it. It's a completely different feeling when you read comments of people who suffer like you do, listen to stories about mothers who committed suicide and left two toddlers behind because they had no money to get treatment, or when you talk on the phone to those afflicted by *Borrelia,* and when you talk with them in person. The suffering written all over their faces the pain in which the eyes cannot weep anymore, and, most of all, the story that they tell you, are all so similar to your recent life experience that you both know a better listener couldn't be found anywhere else in the world. In a moment like that, you feel as if you were two best friends who have known each other backwards since childhood. Throughout my years of illness, I had no chance to exchange a word or two about my disease with anyone in a way that would make me feel completely understood, until I started meeting them during the therapy sessions using Rife's machine. The more I knew about Lyme disease and its coinfections, the more I had a feeling that it was a taboo, a topic that's not to be openly discussed or, God forbid, mentioned in the presence of any random doctor. I had the exact same feeling when someone mentioned religion or started talking about God; this subject was simply of no interest to me, and to many, it wasn't worth a discussion. Anna had similar thoughts to mine until the moment a girl infected with the same monster package who was sitting with us decided to share her extraordinary story with us, unaware that her words would have a dramatic impact on our lives, turning all our beliefs upside down.

After some time, Anna and I started considering our weekly trips to Czestochowa an entertainment of sort. We couldn't hop on a bike or go on a spontaneous sea-side excursion every weekend. We had to continue our therapy hoping that one day, Mayer's wife would tell us, "Dear ones, it's over." At the same time, we considered our sessions time well spent, which we didn't have much of in our lives back then. To us, having to sit down for an hour-long session with Mayer was like hitting downtown with a good buddy of ours. I think that it wasn't only me who longed for the company of others, but Anna did, too. Quite easily and quite soon, after many sessions, Mayer, Anna and I found some common ground and made friends. We found it just as easy to converse with Ela, a girl who was showing up for a treatment using Rife's machine together with her brother. On one occasion, we told them that we were spending quite a long time in-between sessions in Jasna Gora.

"Have you ever been to a healing mass?" she asked.

"No. What's that? Some special type of a church mass?" I asked.

"Yes. There are many Christian communes that hold prayer meetings, that is, a Holy Mass combined with the Eucharist. It differs from that we all know in that it is often varied with Prayers of Adoration, Release, Healing or the Calling of the Holy Spirit."

"What's so unusual about it that makes it different to what we know from church meetings on Sundays?" Anna asked.

"People are said to experience the presence of the living Jesus Christ, who heals them. Some fall asleep while standing up and collapse on the floor. Seriously! I've seen it with my own eyes!"

"They collapse on the floor, in a church?" I asked in disbelief.

That must be a hoax! I thought. *First of all, how can they experience the presence of Jesus if he's long gone?* I couldn't understand Ela.

"They do, they fall asleep and fall down on the floor like timber, and when they get up, there's not one bruise to be found on their bodies, and their illness or life problems are often resolved."

"Have you experienced that yourself, too?" Anna asked.

"I haven't fallen asleep, but I've experienced something else."

Highly intrigued by what Ela was saying, with due account of what I had lived through in Jasna Gora, we wanted her to spill the beans.

"Go on!" my fiancée asked.

"I saw people putting hand on themselves and praying for themselves, and then inexplicable things happened. I attended that mass by accident. I went there with my friends. At first, everything seemed inauthentic and staged to me, but after what I felt at a certain point I was sure that it was real and had nothing to do with any pre-planned turn of events."

"What happened?" I asked, the burning curiosity evident in my voice.

"In the course of the healing prayer, the priest who was offering the mass told us to close our eyes and say a prayer in the name of Jesus for the person in front of us. In that large gathering, there were many people in front of me. I don't know why but there was only one individual who caught my eye, though. I had no clue what problems that person was struggling with but I started praying for her. I asked Jesus to heal her from everything she was suffering from, saying, "If you are really here, help her.""

"And then what happened?" Anna asked, unable to wait patiently.

"All of a sudden, inside my head, I felt someone putting thoughts in that weren't mine, stating, 'Put your hand on her.' I got scared a little, but I felt I had to do that. So I placed my hands on the woman who started crying desperately, and then fell down on the floor and was just lying there still. It made me even more scared, but in just a moment, that fear was replaced by an odd sensation of calmness. I wasn't healed but it seems to me that by the means of my hand, that woman experienced that which everyone gathered there expected."

Anna and I were very touched by Ela's account. We had no idea what happened in our hearts that started beating stronger having heard that brief story, but we both had the same feeling. We knew that we definitely had to attend a healing mass, previously unaware it even existed. Soon after I realized that on numerous occasions I had been passing by posters with the likeness of Jesus displayed over church doors, saying, "I am waiting for you". Back then, I never cared for them, and these words written in bold seemed abstract. Mayer, who took part in that conversation, was also very excited because of what he heard a moment ago. Unlike us, he did know about the prayer meetings that draw thousands of people every month who come there to meet Jesus a stone's throw away from the place where we had our therapy sessions. As you can guess, just as in the case of the monastery in the village of Gidle, Anna and I didn't waste any time and decided to experience everything Ela told us about firsthand.

I'll never forget the day when for the first time in my life, we weren't on our way to a bio-energy therapist or a healer with great online reviews, but we were on our way to meet someone whose 'reviews' were higher than those of any competitive healing practitioners. We were on our way to meet the pioneer of healing. We were on our way to meet the living Jesus Christ. Regardless of what that really meant, it definitely made us very excited, intrigued, and at the same time, somewhat fearful of yet another disappointment. Up until that time, I didn't know much about Jesus. My strongest association was that of Baby Jesus lying in the stall, an image that was part of Christmas decorations at my church, the very same in the basement of which I used to play table tennis most passionately. And, above all, that of His passion and eventual crucifixion, which I saw on many occasions during Easter, for instance. It was at that time that I watched movies showing the biblical scenes of people being healed by His hands before He was crucified. Back then, I didn't realize what actually happened two thousand years ago. I didn't understand the message that movies about Jesus conveyed, a couple of which I watched in my life during holidays, while the Resurrection, which I had been celebrating every year, naturally, was insignificant to me. The things that mattered were the Christmas tree, presents, the Easter Bunny, and good food. However, in a short time, it was all about to take on a completely new meaning in my life (and not only mine, for that matter).

Since we had always assumed that God is everywhere, a theory that had been unsearchable to us, we went to the place mentioned by Mayer, though Ela experienced some extraordinary things elsewhere. We were totally unaware of what awaited us there and, having nothing but the address, we set off to the unknown.

And so, I took Anna and my mom, always in for a new experience. My mom had always been a religious person, but neither her nor my dad could attend the holy mass on every Sunday. Ever since I can remember, she'd always expressed much grief that for many years she and dad had been living in sin that made them unfit for participating in the Eucharist according to the religious law. My parents were one of those people who give priority to rules and never break them. I couldn't understand that since many times, I saw people receiving the host without going to confession beforehand and I am very open about the fact that I've done that, too, if I ever felt like going to church, that is. Their wedding outside of Church due to my dad's first marriage became to them sort of a brake that had been hindering their contact with Jesus for many years. The place where I took the two women who had been always accompanying me not only did change my life, but shortly after, also the life of my parents.

Yet again, it turned out that Mayer was telling the truth; the story about thousands of people flocking in to meet Jesus was not a theory. The Christian community that organized monthly meetings in a small church had grown so big that every month ten thousand believers came to see the love, power and mercy of Jesus Christ. In the spring and summer seasons, crowds that the temple was unable to hold inside would gather in a vast green meadow amidst grass and crops. As it was till wintertime, we happened to experience all the miracles mentioned by Ela in a spacious sports venue the size of which could ensure everyone got a warm seat. At the very beginning, trying to find a parking spot, we could already feel as if we had come there for a concert of some top-notch pop singer whose numerous fans were doing their best to get a slot between a hundred of parked cars. All of a sudden, at one point, a man in a hi-vis vest emerged from behind a long row of vehicles, trying to stop me with a gesture of his hands. I brought the car to a halt and rolled the window down.

"Brother! Go there, exactly that spot! That's where you can park!" he said to me. "Sister! You have a free spot, too, right next to it!" he addressed a woman searching for a parking spot who was right behind me.

We didn't even get to enter the building but we could feel the air of that place already, which only assured us that we had come to a very unusual location.

I didn't recall any stranger addressing me in such a kind, joyful manner, as if we were family. We couldn't wait to see the 'fireworks' we got there for. A moment later, we managed to take our seats. Anna and I experienced such massive crowds gathered in a single place only twice in our lifetime: first time at Bryan Adam's concert, and second time at Jon Bon Jovi's concert. Both these singers delivered a sensational show on stage, performing their most popular music hits. This time, we were about to see Jesus on the stage, whose marvelous performance and presence had been experienced by Ela.

The girl suffering from Lyme disease wasn't lying, either. The air of that place was nothing like the regular Sunday holy mass that I knew. The thousands of people in the grandstands who came there to meet the living Jesus Christ were just part of what immediately caught our eyes. The air of kindness that we were shown back in the parking lot was omnipresent. The joy and the smiles you could see on people's faces made us unsure whether everyone here was 'sane'. Priests who were preparing for the commencement of the mass took their positions by the altar with a huge icon depicting Jesus that was set up on the stage situated at the end of the court, where most likely just a week before young basketball players earned three points by shooting the ball through the hoop. It all was even more alluring owing to a music band with back singers praising Jesus to no end, with the entire hall raising their hands up to the rhythm towards Heavens, as if wanting to touch the feet of God above.

It all was affecting us in a way we had never knew before. We felt amazing, as if we had always belonged there. Although initially, each of us was somewhat holding back, unwilling to put their hands up, we soon gave in to the rhythm and started praising Lord Jesus in this way together with the crowd, as if we always did. I didn't understand what was happening to me; I needed no instructions, I just knew what I was supposed to do.

We were sitting there, praying harder than ever before. The voice of the father who was conducting the meeting was so warm that each of us was imagining the sound of Jesus Christ Himself speaking right to our ears.

"The mission of Jesus Christ is to let you live in abundance; to give you a new mind and a new heart. He wants you to be re-born as the true child of God, so that you can be a brother to others. He wants you to be in perfect health, both on the inside and on the outside. He wants you to have a sound relationship both with Him and others. Jesus was sent by His father to make you healthy. Yes, you!" he said during the release prayer.

Listening attentively to the words uttered by the presider, each person in the audience had a feeling that they were getting straight to them. Never before had I experienced such a great power of words at any mass. Had I received Holy Communion in that moment, I could've suspected that I got intoxicated with something together with thousands of people who took the host from the priests.

"'When you have lifted up the Son of Man, then you will know that I am he'," he added, quoting Jesus. "If you have any cross or a rosary with you, take it now into your right hand and lift it up! Renounce the evil that stands in your way to the real life. Show Jesus, that this act of recognizing the crucified Jesus as your Lord, you want to show Him that you need Him, that you want His love and that your believe in the power of His cross!" he added.

For most of my life, I had been wearing a small cross on my neck, a gift from my sister. Throughout that time, I had no clue what it was for and what power it had until that day, when I took it off my neck for a specific purpose for the first time ever. I raised it up and repeated all the words the presider was saying. I looked over at Anna, who was shivering from the cold while all the other people were taking their coats off because of the heat in the hall. The presider continued.

"Do not be afraid of prayer; do not be afraid of what is about to happen soon, for the Lord will walk among us; he will touch those tormented by all the evil. Much good will take place. It will be audible and visible. We will all experience the good that comes from a release. The evil will try to disturb it, but have no fear!"

I looked over at my mom, praying for our health among thousands with her eyes closed, tears falling down her cheeks.

I took another look at Anna, whose lower eyelids were like a tub full of water, struggling not to let it spill with the one last tear. Suddenly, a terrible shriek of a woman coming from the nearby section of the arena filled with about a hundred people made us all three stand up, our hair almost turned to gray. It was only a prelude of what unraveled at the sports hall, where on that specific day witnessed something we certainly were not expecting.

"Lord, free them from evil, from sin; make them free from all addictions, make evil spirits go away with your blood and wounds," the leader of the community said.

Then, horrific cries of despair and pain started coming from each section. If you could identify what suffering sounds like, I imagine it would sound just like that. Among the people wailing there were also some who were laughing at the top of their lungs as if they heard the funniest joke in their life just a moment ago.

"Come, Holy Spirit! The Lord releases you with His breath. Now, you all will rest in the Holy Spirit," the presider continued, exhaling the air out of his lungs towards the microphone and the audience.

After these words, we saw some unbelievable scenes. Many people, not only those who came to this meeting, but also those who were part of the community, were touched by something extraordinary. For the first time in my life experienced something so astonishingly mystical and mysterious. The people sitting in the sections of the arena simply started falling asleep, leaning on one another; some of them even fell unconsciously onto those sitting in the row in front of them, while those on the floor and right before the stage with the altar collapsed with a loud thud, just like

Ela described to us. I started looking for cameras, extras, actors; it was all there, it all could be staged, but our feelings and emotions could not be imitated.

"Say the names of those who suffer, those you're praying for. Give them to Lord Jesus. Introduce yourself to the person next to you. Ask them, 'Brother, sister, where are you from? What's bothering you?' Let them put their hands on you where your pain is, where your illness is!" the presider exclaimed.

Taking a quick look at the sections crowded with hundreds of people, I realized that most likely, the common denominator that brought us all to this place was pain and suffering.

What would happen if everyone here were nothing but strong, healthy and successful? I wondered. In just one moment I recalled where Jesus was in my life when everything else seemed beautiful and trouble-free. I didn't need to introduce myself to my mom or Anna, or tell them what was bothering me. They knew it perfectly. Then, each of us put their hands on one another. They were holding me by my head, my beck and my ears, which wouldn't leave me in peace.

"The Holy Spirit will now come and walk among you to make you free. Monika, Bartek, Krzysztof, rest in the Holy Spirit. The Lord sets you free, rejoice! Ewelina, the Lord sets you free with His gift of joy! The Lord touches Beata and Grzegorz, healing you and making you free from alcoholism, prostitution and cancer. Lord Jesus is now healing epilepsy, neurosis, depression; He's making your ulcers disappear, He's healing your liver, your eyes and ears, your disease-ridden joints and hips. Some of you will now feel warmth, cold and tingling. The Lord is healing you; believe and be healed! The Lord sets you free by tears; some of you are experiencing this for the first time!" he went on.

Out of the blue, in just one moment, I couldn't hold back the tears, too. With my mom and Anna, we were standing there, the three of us among thousands of people, who came there to beg Jesus for health and aid in their daily lives they were struggling with, just like we did. We were standing in a place free from differences; a place free from shame; each of us was just the same.

For the first time in my life I wasn't ashamed for being a grown man shedding tears of suffering in a public space. Emotions such as embarrassment, humiliation, disgrace simply didn't exist anymore. No one was paying any attention to us and we, too, weren't gazing at the people around us. We were all focused solely on one person, Jesus, whose extraordinary presence we could feel at the very first mass of this kind in our lives. Despite what I had experienced, there was a question arising in my head whether it all really came from God.

Lord Jesus, does all that I'm seeing here really come from you? I asked in my mind.

My doubts were swiftly dispelled by testimonies of people in the final phase of the meeting, who were sharing their private life, in many cases very intimate, too awkward to mention even to a close friend, with the ten thousand strangers gathered there. Standing by the microphone, one by one, they were thanking God for what He did in their lives. Some were grateful for being allowed to rest in the Holy Spirit, which made them quit alcohol addiction, while others showed their test results proving their brain tumor simply vanished. When I saw a young highschooler who was thanking the Mother of God with tears in his eyes for saving him from attempting suicide after his mom died, I knew that the hand of God must've been involved in it all.

Before we knew it, the charismatic prayer meeting came to an end. In each of us, the things we experienced on that day evoked a deep reflection on our lives and faith so far. On that day, however, something else that was extraordinary happened, which Ela forgot to mention. When we arrived at noon for the holy healing mass, we knew very little about such phenomena. When we were leaving the building, it was already after nightfall. Feeling no hunger, it seemed to all three of us that we had spent inside the building only an hour longer than usually at the regular Sunday mass at the church. When we checked what time it was, we couldn't believe our eyes, as it was one a.m.

Having returned home, each of us had difficulties to fall asleep; we were thinking about what we had experienced on the previous day and about how engaging that meeting was. I didn't know what to make of it all. One thing was certain, though. From then on, I couldn't stop thinking about Jesus and His healing. I believed in the magic of that place so much that from then onwards, I knew that my fight with *Borrelia* and the other monsters would be equal. My inner strength, my boundaryless will to resume training and Rife's machine gave me hope that I could get my former lifestyle back. However, the biggest ace card I could play from then on in the war against the enemy was my faith and the support of the Almighty.

To explain in scientific terms what really happened on that day and where did the time go, the passing of which we were completely oblivious of, I'd have to ask Albert Einstein himself and delve deep into his theory of relativity. He claimed that the reason why he was the one to come up with the theory of relativity was probably because unlike normal people, who believe they are done reflecting on time and space as they already did that in their childhood years, his intellectual development was slow enough to keep him busy with matters like that even when he turned into an adult man.

From the moment I appeared before the holy icon in Jasna Gora, I felt that I was very similar in that respect; I felt like a child whose intellectual development has just begun, with virtually no life experience. Following the healing mass we could participate in I realized that the image of God and His presence, formed in my mind back at the youngest age, came down like a house of cards in just one moment to be then rebuilt in a completely different form.

Just like Einstein, Rife did much good for humanity, and Anna and I could experience that firsthand. Sadly, the time at our sessions dragged on and wouldn't flow as fast as when we were on the healing mass. Nonetheless, despite of our weekend trips to meet Mayer, we didn't regret it, as subsequent sessions brought nothing but positive news.

"I don't detect any *Yersinia* or *Riketsia* anymore. The only thing that's left is to fight *Borrelia* and *Bartonella*," Mayer's wife said during one of our follow-ups.

Moments like that were hard to put in words; the awareness and joy that finally, our treatment yielded positive results was simply indescribable.

Although the list of our experiences with the force that was hard for us to comprehend was getting longer, back then, I didn't attribute these good results with God's intervention in any way.

One thing was certain: all three of us were inexplicably drawn to participate in another prayer meeting. We started looking for God wherever we could, going from one Christian community to another, having outstanding experiences and listening closely to accounts of people touched by God, which was charging our batteries of hope and faith each and every time. At one of such masses, we encountered a young Christian, charismatic Marcin Zielinski, who showed me how wrong and lost I was to believe the stereotype that God should be sought only at a regular Sunday mass offered by an elderly priest. The first time I saw that young man preaching God's word in church before hundreds of people, who was younger than me and studied at the Academy of Physical Education, I realized that age was completely meaningless and that my previous view on faith, which I associated mostly with old folks such as my grandma, may she rest in peace, was turned upside down. The way that young man was talking about Jesus and the miracles He performed with His hands made me want to become part of it.

"True healing is for those who want to renounce everything to seek Jesus, following His voice without fear. The Holy Scripture says that who seeks God with all his heart will find Him. Jesus is not in hiding; He wants you to find Him," he said.

"I felt like I've never heard of it before. I want it, too!" I said.

"'As Christians, we must be people whose spiritual eye see deeper, below what's visible physically. God wants to communicate with us and give us a prophetic insight into the reality we live in.'[28] You only have to tell Jesus, 'Lord, use me! Do not pass me by!" Marcin Zelinski said.

---

[28] M. Zielinski, *Rozpal wiare*, Lodz 2017, p. 21.

Despite the good news we were getting from Mayer's wife over time and the receding herxes noticeable in the course of the week after every session, I was still in pain and I didn't feel healthy. I was looking for God as if He was a painkiller; I wanted Jesus and the Holy Spirit that were mentioned to come to me like a delivery driver that leaves my beloved pizza at my doorstep whenever I have a craving for it. Self-centered, I hoped that I'd get physically healed. From one meeting to the next, I imagined the Jesus I knew from paintings on all the walls at my late grandma's apartment, dressed up like Dr. Armani, with a stethoscope on His neck. I hoped that He would show them all how it's done and in a snap of the fingers, He'd simply take all my ailments away. I wanted Him to take away all my other symptoms, just like He did with all the other people sharing stories of their healing, waiting for one of the priests to say the words, "Michal, Lord Jesus is now healing you from Lyme disease!" I didn't give much thought to whether the fact that other symptoms had subsided was because of Him. Back then, I didn't understand yet that my presence there and then was not accidental, and that Jesus would not heal me by following the plan I devised. Shortly after, I realized that it wasn't me who had the plan. "'For my thoughts are not your thoughts, neither are your ways my ways,' declares the Lord. 'As the heavens are higher than the earth, so are my ways higher than your ways and my thoughts than your thoughts.'" (Isaiah 55:8-9), I heard during a mass.

We didn't give up and continued our new journey without stopping at only several healing masses. Despite the odd cold that touched my Anna and the strong desire to cry out all the tears that all three of us experienced, we still wanted something more; something that we call the proof of Jesus's presence. We were dreaming of the gift of rest in the Holy Spirit that people among us were graced with. We went for another trip in search of Jesus, an event organized – yet again – at a sports venue, and my aunt, my mom's friend, tagged along, eager to experience what we told her about. Again, each of us had a feeling that time passed instantaneously and when there came the moment to leave the building, my aunt cast a glance at a small line of people waiting to meet the community leader.

"Why do you want to leave so soon? Let's line up with them. The priest will say an extra prayer for each of us," she said.

None of us came up with that during our previous trips. Therefore, we approached the presider who was putting his stole on every individual, placing his hand and praying to Jesus.

Sadly, though each of us wanted to feel anything physical, nothing like that happened. Somewhat disappointed, I was heading to the door to leave the building. All of a sudden, in the vestibule leading to the exit I saw another priest and over ten people lined up in front of him, collapsing onto the floor like dominoes in the same moment when the clergyman grabbed each of them by the head. Though it seemed to me that some of them were lying down only to feel what it could be like if the Holy Spirit really put them to rest, I knew that some of them weren't faking it.

"Girls, let's go to him! He's decking them all down like a champion!" I said with a smile.

So, we join the line where every other person had already been put to rest, and the closer to the priest we got, the more Anna and I were stressed up. We grabbed each other's hand and stood together before the priest who reminded me a little of actor John Leguizamo.

"God bless you, Father! My fiancée and I are suffering from Lyme disease. Please say a prayer for us," I requested.

"That's interesting! It's a small world, isn't it?" Father John said.

"I don't get it," I replied.

"I have Lyme disease, too. I've been treating myself with antibiotics, among others, for a couple of years now, but with poor results, and I can't get rid of it. It sucks! Of course I'll do that, lean forward, you two! I am blessing both of you!" he started a brief prayer.

It was still too early for me to understand that on that day, it wasn't me who was supposed to be healed. It was a time when I still wouldn't comprehend the words of Marcin Zielinski; back at that moment, God used me to find among several thousand people that one person who was suffering from Lyme disease, too, and I had more than just one solution for that.

Shocked by what Father John revealed to us so unexpectedly, we thanked him for the prayer and we headed back towards the exit. Then, at one point, something stopped me.

Rife's machine! I thought. I approached the clergyman again and shared my story with him, telling him about the results I got using that device. The priest thanked me most earnestly for sharing that knowledge and gave me his phone number. Although back at that moment, I didn't see anything extraordinary in that situation and considered it happened by chance, to my mom, it was an unusual encounter. I had a feeling that just like Einstein, she believed that "Coincidence is God's way of remaining anonymous." However, shortly after, I verified that the Almighty acted incognito indeed, or at least that's what I strongly believed in.

Though many could regard that ordinary meeting with Father John as a coincidence, to me, it was just another reason to wonder. Despite the skeptical element that was rooted deep inside of me, some part of me that I'd always called my intuition (the very same that didn't fail me when I was ardently seeking a solution to my problems) was telling me that there was more to come.

"Michal, when are we going for another meeting?" my mom asked me; I'd never seen her so fascinated.

I'm not using the word 'fascinated' for no reason. From then on, it was something my mom and I had in common. Anna, who felt cold on many occasions and wanted to cry at nearly every meeting we attended, didn't say much. Unlike her, I wanted to experience more and more, as if I was hypnotized. The time I would previously dedicate to watching Hollywood movie productions or the boxing matches I adored so much was now replaced by viewing recorded prayer meetings available online. Despite good results and herxing, which I was still experiencing, *Borrelia* and *Bartonella* were still doing their job. Though some days were giving me a particularly hard time, my companions and I would go meet Jesus, nonetheless. But sometimes I just couldn't go, unfortunately. On such days, I'd just put on a mass that was being broadcasted live on the Internet. I realized why they had all the cameras put up there.

"I believe the Lord is now healing those who are watching this meeting online."

"Yes! He's healing you, Przemek, from your hernia!" the clergyman said.

The accounts the healed were sharing during the meetings we had attended so far started appearing also in the comments of the viewers.

Incredible, I thought. I wanted to have the same experience so bad; I wanted to share my testimony so bad; and yet, sadly, I didn't feel anything aside from the suffering that was still annoying me caused by the ideal destructive duo of *Borrelia* and *Bartonella,* still present and wreaking havoc inside of me. I had no way to win with time, which was running forward ceaselessly with a wide smirk, not taking even just a moment to look back at me when passing me by year by year, always disease-ridden. I hardly even noticed when it was June knocking on my door, intimidating me with grass and cereal pollen allergy that was murdering me. Though I was taking medications intended to stop these allergens, in critical situations I had to stick tissues formed into tampons up my nose, and after spending even several minutes in nature, my eyes and nose were turning into Niagara Falls. The thing I experienced on yet another charismatic meeting that involved prayers for healing made my need for a relationship with God even greater.

On that day in June, the weather across Poland was beautiful and sunny, promising a perfect day. It was time we could praise the Lord outdoors; the space among fields and trees was filled by an extraordinary numerous crowd. Several months earlier, there was not a single chair in the sports hall stands that wasn't taken. Gathered in front of a small church, we couldn't wait to celebrate Jesus, particularly the healing prayer and the release prayer, during which unearthly scenes were taking place. Delighted by the location and the ambiance in which we could pray to God, we were nothing less but hypnotized. My mom and Anna were worried if I'd endure the event. They were concerned because of my allergy, which on that day was put to a hard test. The green lavish canopies brought back to life from dormancy, the flowering acres of cereals and square miles of green grass were only waiting for me to appear among these several thousand people to strangle me and force me to have an endless sneezing fit until eventually I'd retreat hastily. As usual, the three of us drifted away in the prayer, addressing their intentions to Jesus so fervently that in a blink of an eye, we had to get up of our foldable chairs, as the clergyman gave us all a sign that it was time to say the healing prayer.

At one point, Anna and I realized that my mom wasn't with us anymore, and that her spot was taken by some elderly lady.

"Ask the person next to you what's their name, ask what's bothering them, put your hand on them and pray in the name of Jesus. God wants you to collaborate with Him on Earth. He wants His creation to take place "as in Heaven, so on Earth." "They will place their hands on sick people, and they will get well,"[29] the community leader said.

We were looking for my mom but we couldn't spot her anywhere. Therefore, Ana and I introduced ourselves to the unknown lady and asked her to take our hands. Excited, the woman told us her name.

"Is it your first time here, too? Have you experienced anything unordinary yet? They say extraordinary things happen here! I'm very curious. I'm not much of a believer," she went on with no intention to stop talking.

Not wanting to let this most important moment that we came here for pass us by, I interrupted her.

"Give me your hand, and take my fiancée's hand with your other one. Let's pray. It's that time now."

"God, why is your hand so cold? And you, yours is completely opposite, so warm."

---

[29] Mark 16:15-18.

I smiled at the chatty lady and cracked a joke.

"That's perfect, ma'am, now we're like a battery, positive and negative; maybe it'll turn up the voltage that's about to go through us!"

I didn't even accentuate the final syllable as I intended, when the woman's body pulled Anna down on the grass with all its weight. Since I was stronger, I managed to dig my feet in the ground; still holding the inert lady's hand in mine, I let her lie down slowly on the grass, so that she could rest in the Holy Ghost peacefully.

This time, Anna and I didn't get touched by anything unusual, such as tears, sadness or incredible joy, that could be expected; something that could be described as a subjective, inner experience of God. We were both shocked by what the lady experienced, which we definitely contributed to. It was only then that I believed that there was a reason why of the several thousands of people, it was her who appeared by our side exactly when my mom was not there anymore. It was an incredible feeling.

Looking for my mom, we eventually spotted her. I couldn't believe what I saw, which on that day made me even more certain that God exists. For the first time in my life, I saw my mom kneeling before a priest, confessing all the accumulated sins that throughout these years she was unable to let out, though she wanted it very much at every Sunday mass.

"You can't even imagine how much I needed it! I felt that I had to do that today! I really don't know why! I just had to! I wanted the Eucharist today so much," my mom said on our way back, tears in her eyes.

On our way back home from yet another mass that involved a healing prayer, we were so caught up in the events of that day we totally forgot about something we were all very concerned about when we were heading to the mass.

"Michal!" Anna shouted, as she recalled what it was.

"I know," I replied.

Unable to explain why sitting throughout the entire day among cereals and grass in flower I didn't shed even one tear and I didn't sneeze even once, I was driving home, contemplating.

All these extraordinary situations evoked something unusual inside of us; something that I started referring to as a 'fascination' with God. Though initially, we were attending a healing mass only once a month, after some time, we started going there more often. As my mom would say, "I miss the mass." Despite still not feeling well, I was watching people falling asleep in the Holy Spirit and listening to accounts of people who overcame various diseases. I didn't lose my faith in that one day, I'd get touched by the grace of God, too. I was still waiting for the two words I was yearning to hear so bad to be mentioned among other conditions by the clergymen who were experiencing the Word of Knowledge[30] – Lyme disease.

It is impossible to explain what was going on with me. I could feel that there was some kind of transformation happening within me. Aside from the healing masses that I participated in and the live broadcasts on the Internet, I started listening to testimonies of people who were sharing their stories online. There was a growing desire within me to be in contact with Jesus more often. A rosary, which had been completely unfamiliar to me for most of my life, and which I saw for the last time in the cab of the taxi driver a couple of years ago during our minor fender bender, was now in my backpack, always with me during my sessions using Rife's machine. I'd never imagine that the very same boy for whom training his chest was the most important thing in the world just a few years ago would ever pray the Novena to Our Lady of Pompeii[31], which takes fifty-four days, or that instead of blasting Bryan Adams in his car he'd be humming songs that praise God.

To this day, among my friends, I'm sometimes met with skepticism of those who don't believe in the source of my issues for some reason and who never believed that Rife's machine worked,

---

[30] The Word of Knowledge – the information from the Holy Spirit, a revelation of what the Holy Spirit is doing at a given moment – M. Zielinski, *Rozpal wiare*.

[31] Novena to Our Lady of Pompeii – a form of a rosary prayed to Mary, Our Lady of Pompeii written in 1884.

on top of that, not to mention divine intervention or divine action that were manifested at 'mysterious' meetings. I will never forget words of one of my 'friends', who on one day decided to visit me with Tomek, whom he was seeing more often than me although Tomek was living broad. Seeing me with a catheter in my arm, hooked up on an IV drip administered by Helen, he said, "Get your shit together, man! You're not sick!"

In situation like that, what was left of my mental health was calling to the universe for strength and the power of love for my neighbor, for although it seemed to me that unlike others, I had a bit more of it, it turned out that I was wrong. I couldn't forgive my buddies that they were absent in the moments I needed them the most. Many times, during my meetings with Jesus I heard that giving yourself up to the Holy Spirit is something more than just praying a novena on a rosary or putting a sticker with the ichthys[32] on your car, but I struggled to do so. However, there came a moment when words uttered at one mass started working in the background like an antivirus software on a PC; or maybe it was my awareness becoming mature enough to allow me to notice the more significant matters in life?

"Hate and resentment indicate that the Holy Spirit is absent in your life. You have to forgive everyone who wronged you, just like Jesus did. Give yourself up to the Holy Ghost and let Him act in your life; seek to benefit your neighbor rather than yourself, renounce sin, egoism, forgive like Jesus did on the cross. Only then you will be healed!"

And that's exactly what happened. I can't recall the specific moment when my emotions linked to my resentment towards my buddies subsided. One thing is certain: the meetings at which I experienced the love of many people or even nice moments spent in Mayer's company showed me that the world doesn't end on a few acquaintances and that there are numerous people who need to be in contact with their neighbor, who can become my

---

[32] In Old Greek, it means a 'fish' (□χθύς, ΙΧΘΥΣ). It is the sign of the first Christians and a symbol of Jesus Christ.

friends. I also came to understand how wrong I was about myself. Although I was resentful towards my friends, I realized that I was far from being able to call myself their friend, too. When Tomek got injured at work and ended up in hospital for three months with his leg crushed as a result, I wasn't there for him. When another guy from our pack was struggling with mental issues, we weren't there for him. When yet another of us was asking for support and for his time and mind to be filled with anything else after his long-term relationship fell apart, we weren't there for him, likewise.

My massive resentment towards my buddies simply disappeared, though this (and not only this) happened owing to God, predominantly. There was some force that was repeatedly trying to take away the moment of my life I found myself in and what I started believing in. There were days I felt awful, wrestling with my thoughts and my egoism, crying to God, *Where are you? Why are you healing them all, but give no damn about me?* I kept asking, astonished, listening to the accounts of people who were thanking God for relieving them from knee aches or elbow aches that seemed nothing compared to what I was suffering from. What is more, sometimes, I had a feeling that Tomek (and not only him) thought I lost my mind.

I started sharing my story and telling what I saw Jesus do with my own eyes. Oftentimes, some of my listeners were my buddies that I wasn't resentful towards anymore, whom I had a chance of meeting occasionally.

Those who were going to church every Sunday from the time they were kids, unlike me, calling me a 'godless man' who'd only stick around behind the walls of the temple, were the most surprised, and their faces were saying one thing: You're talking nonsense! Things like that don't happen.

In moments like these, I had no clue what to say. I felt like a kid mocked by his peers for telling stories about monsters under his bed that didn't exist; what's worse, the foundations of my faith that I had been putting in place were getting demolished. It was just like Marcin Zielinski says in his book, "When you'll start walking on the path of faith, people can be surprised. Don't get offended by that, don't be afraid they will reject you. You have faith, a deep belief inside of you, and on these grounds, you go forward. God respects and rewards that. Faith allows you access to things that are concealed. Faith is a vehicle for revelation that you can catch in your hand. Don't let it be torn out of your hand regardless of what stands in your way."[33] Whatever the listeners I confided in were thinking, I knew what I felt, I knew what I experienced and what I was allowed to see. Although on the eyes of my peers you could see traces of sarcasm, it didn't stop me from walking forwards in the path in Jesus's footsteps, whom I was still looking for and whom I wanted to experience firsthand so bad. The thing that we experienced at the next meeting broke down all remaining elements of disbelief that were still dwelling within me, which still had the power to persuade me that everything I had lived through was a hoax and a manipulation of my feelings that generated the desired result like a placebo would.

The prayer meetings we were attending more and more often weren't taking place only at sports venues or in a field of grass. There were also ordinary masses held in the very same churches that parishioners were attending every Sunday, which every once in a while ended with an additional prayer of healing and adoration. I had a feeling that cases of healing of relief were most common at the meetings with the biggest audiences, where several members of the community and the priest had to intervene and take away individuals who were shaking violently, screaming, as they couldn't calm down. This time, I learned that I was wrong.

They must be doing that for the public, I thought on occasions when I wanted to be touched and saved from my issues so bad but nothing spectacular was happening to me.

For some reason, Anna and I didn't make it in time for the meeting. Having reached a massive, gloomy cathedral whose two giant towers were scratching the sky that was getting darker and darker, we saw a gathering seemed to have no end. On that evening,

---

[33] M. Zielinski, *Rozpal wiare*, p. 76.

my mom was not with us and I ended up regretting it a lot. Also, we had virtually no access to any free spot inside the temple, and so we had to participate in the mass outside the cathedral.

It was only us, the dark night that in a blink of an eye replaced what was a gray evening just a moment ago, and a young woman who just like us most likely was late for the first half of the meeting. It wasn't very pleasant to stand behind the doors, listening closely to the voices of clergymen and what was happening inside. Though it could seem that the power of the Holy Spirit touches only those who gathered inside the church like the limited range of Rife's machine whose frequencies were affecting only those who were at a specific distance, we couldn't have been more wrong. We didn't even notice when the woman who was standing right next to us was lying flat on the concrete floor. The rain that started falling a moment before she collapsed made the sound of her hitting the wet floor muted so that we barely noticed it. Watching her, many would think that something might've happened to her, but we knew that what just happened must've been positive. Standing on the doorstep of huge, closed church doors, feeding the blame of my faith so that it burned even stronger, I was looking to the sides, wondering, *What if something happened to her? Where are those crowds of people for whom you collapsed for to do your little performance? What's the point in lying down in the rain just for the two of us to watch?* I didn't have the answer to these questions; however, standing in the darkness in which no one else would notice that woman resting, I knew that it wasn't for show. As it is often the case, many people leave a holy mass before it's over for different reasons without waiting for it to end, and so it was in this case. Yearning for the touch of God, impatient, we stepped forward toward the altar and the clergymen who were praying for the sick. Perhaps it was not by accident that at that time, there was already some space in-between the people gathered in the church and we could find a spot for us.

"The Holy Spirit is now touching you by means of the breath!" the presider said, holding his mouth close to the microphone and blowing some air onto it.

I will never forget the moment when on that day, on every other bench, I could hear the sound and see bodies collapsing to the floor, predominantly bodies of elderly people. Special effects had always been an element of cinematography that I found most alluring, aside from a good story and a dramatic plot twist that was giving me goosebumps. What happened on that day in that church not only made my hair stand on end, but also changed my life forever.

"The Holy Spirit is moving among you!' the clergyman added, continuing to blow air.

All of a sudden, at that moment, Anna and I felt a breeze that tingled our noses and lifted my bangs for a second.

What the hell? I thought, aware that I was standing away from the priest, who didn't even do his best to make his lungs exhale the air as strong as they could.

Looking around for an air conditioner, some half-opened stained glass windows or a draft caused by open church doors, confused, I was wondering where did that gentle, cool breeze come from. It was just as if the Holy Ghost was really passing between the benches at that moment, stopping by those who were about to be graced with a rest. Excited and somewhat flabbergasted, I was standing there listening to the mass, oblivious to the fact that in just a moment, I was about to experience something that would make me a completely different man when I will be leaving this church.

At each of these meetings, it was hard not to notice people suffering for various reasons. Some of them were standing with crutches, some were sitting in wheelchairs, and many others were visibly ill.

Most likely, every participant was struggling with some issue. Perhaps many were suffering from Lyme disease that, as in our case and the case of Father John, usually wouldn't let anyone know we could be suffering, carrying a highly destructive occupant around. On that evening, there was one attendee who stood out from among us all in an exceptional way, and for some reason, Anna and I could see him closely.

Surrounded by many different people, we were sitting behind four completely unremarkable individuals. Though I never wondered who came to Jesus with what kind of a problem and whether they have any at all, I wasn't even trying to assess these four people. You could even assume that the elderly man and his wife took to Jesus their very young, pregnant daughter and her partner to ask for a healthy delivery. Meanwhile, it was the opposite; from one minute to the next, I realized that something was wrong. The young girl was holding her boyfriend's hand all the time, who started acting weirder and weirder as the mass went on. She was letting his hand go from time to time to caress his neck and right shoulder, whispering into his ear, "Hold on, love! Just a little more. Everything will be fine." Initially, you could think that the young man was suffering from some disease and that it was some pain that was bothering him incessantly was making him sigh and flex his neck all the time, which reminded me of one of my symptoms of Lyme disease. The thing that was bothering him was not Lyme disease, though, or any other health condition I had ever read of, for that matter.

"I can't do this anymore!" the young man turned towards the pregnant woman, holding in his hand a First Communion prayer book.

Anna and I looked at each other somewhat baffled.

"I really can't take it anymore!" the young man continued explaining himself to his companions, trembling and sweating like a marathon runner.

I had no idea what I was witnessing. Never before had I seen a young, well-built man sweating so fast while standing still. I trained many years and I knew that was impossible. His gray jacket was turning darker and darked in front of my eyes due to unbelievable amounts of sweat. It was just as if obscure rainclouds gathered above him only, leaving him soaked to the bone.

"It's almost done, hold on, please!" the girl wailed terribly, fearful, her fear infecting all other attendees near her.

At one point, the boy's companions realized that they couldn't wait any longer and started walking towards the clergyman to ask for help.

In that moment, Anna and I were still unaware what we were about to participate in, and what up until that point, I had seen only in movies. Never before had I seen a priest not hesitating even for a moment, like a true doctor, and immediately attending to the young boy who was suffering for some reason unknown to us. We soon came to understand what was happening.

"Damned spirit, in the name of Jesus Christ, I command you to leave his body!" the clergyman said.

Anna and I weren't the only ones who were terrified by what we were seeing. All the people who gathered in that church on that evening, looking for God and the answer to many questions just like I was, were profoundly moved by this scene.

What's actually going on here? I kept asking myself. The more fervently the priest was praying over the young man, the more the latter screamed and moaned, until eventually he started vomiting with nothing at all.

"Let it out! Leave this body! In the name of Jesus Christ, I command you!" the clergyman continued to shout, holding the man who was leaning to his knees.

The sound of vomiting coupled with the boy's agonizing cries and sighing echoing in the church, and his companions' despair gave us goosebumps.

It's all extraordinary, it's really happening! I thought, still trying to spot cameras and a director.

At one point, it wasn't only the boy who was all wet, but the clergyman, too. Minute by minute, vast amounts of sweat appeared on the priest's forehead to be then rubbed off by a deacon.

After a struggle that lasted for over ten minutes or maybe several tens of minutes, eventually, there was some positive result. The young man eventually started vomiting when he was still in the same pose, his head supported by his knees.

"God! That's impossible! What a relief! Much better! Thank you! Thank you, honestly!" he said.

Unquestionably, that evening changed me, but it also awakened in me some fear of the world we live in; though it is shown to us often by means of movies or other sources we don't believe, it cannot always be experienced in our daily life. Therefore, I started confessing my sins most ardently. My confession was like a weekly shower I took whenever I felt like I needed to. I was doing that not only because of my fear of evil, the battling of which I witnessed at the last mass or during other relief masses. My goal was to come into contact with Jesus, whom I couldn't experience firsthand, most likely because of sins I still had on me. Like one of the clergymen said, admitting your sins can be the key to healing. And so I was driving every week to go to church, entering the confessional like a shower cabin to wash away all my dirt, oblivious to what confession really was. Maybe I didn't always need to confess, but merely to talk to those who were closest to God. To those who knew how to contact Him. "What am I doing wrong?" I kept asking, wanting to finally get touched and healed, wanting Anna and my mom to not have to cry anymore, and my dad to finally feel calm. Sadly, I didn't get Jesus's phone number; I did, however, hear a very important line, "Being a Christian doesn't only mean being a good man; it also means making others happy." Back then, I realized that my pain was inevitable, and my misfortune is just a matter of how I approach the situation at hand.

Then, I thought, *I will mourn my condition and I will become a victim of my own fate for the rest of my life; or, I will accept it and resist it even stronger than before, helping other in the meantime until I will be saved. If I can't be happy, I will make sure that others are happy because of me!* I said to myself. It was just like in the case of the elderly man who helped me on the road a few years ago without much concern for his own loss or benefit despite all the evil he had met on his way. I started following his footsteps. Wherever someone needed help, I was doing my best to help. I came up with an idea of writing a several-pages-long manual on how to diagnose Lyme disease and its coinfections, as well as treatment methods that might prove helpful.

I did it with those people in mind who encountered that problem just like me, looking for the answer for six years. It wasn't easy. Writing down even one page of a well-though-out content proved highly strenuous for me, both physically and mentally. What is more, while hanging out on various online forums, I started sharing my experience. One day, my eye was caught by a comment that I found exceptionally touching. "Please, help! My eight-year-old daughter is losing her vision and the use of her legs. No one knows what's going on with her. I don't know what to do. Please, help!"

I didn't know why but I could vividly feel inside of me the suffering of that woman, whose daughter had some mysterious disease. Some part of me felt that I knew what the cause of her problems was, and urged me to talk to her. Giving it little thought, I grabbed my phone and dialed the number I got from the desperate woman. Overwhelmed by emotions, hearing a voice of a complete stranger in her phone, the woman paid no attention to who she was talking with, grateful for anything fate would give her on that day. She shared her horrible story with me. The woman's young child was passed from one doctor to another like I was with the standard diagnosis I knew all too well, which didn't surprise me. The only thing I couldn't comprehend was how could anyone presuppose that the only issue that eight-year-old was struggling with was a mental issue. What her mother must've felt when she heard her kid saying, "Mom, I can't see you, mommy dear, it hurts so much." What experts offered the child was psychoanalysis; meanwhile, *Borrelia* and Co. were having a ball inside that small, young body, which was revealed shortly after – something the woman couldn't stop thanking me for.

It was very easy for me to forgive my buddies; however, I still struggled to cope with my negative emotions towards doctors and their attitude towards the patient. Stories like that one, where even the little ones were affected, were making me even more contemptuous and repulsed by that specific group of people, which I then would go confess in church. Primarily, I would get overwhelmed by a feeling of compassion for the sick who, like me, probably had to handle not only their suffering but also the world that for some reason closed the door before each and every one of them when they were calling for help, labelling them 'crazy'.

There's a common phrase in my country that refers to many Catholics. It took on a completely new meaning for me. Previously, I'd often say, "I believe, but I do not practice my religion" whenever someone asked me if I believed in God.

Now, however, I was not only a believer but I also started practicing what I experienced at the meetings that involved healing prayers. I'd never been indifferent to the suffering and illness of other people, but also, I'd never given much thought to how to help them. Now, however, something inside me changed. All the suffering I saw on the streets, all the illness, poverty or simply sadness on the face of another human being would immediately put me into a state of a brief prayer for that person or make me ask for a proper medical doctor to be put on his or her path.

"Lord, whatever that person is struggling with, help them, please," I'd pray.

Only a couple of year earlier, I didn't understand the phenomenon of Golgotha, I didn't realize what really happened two thousand years ago, what took place back then. To this day, I wonder why my grandma, may she rest in peace, cried while looking at crucified Jesus, shedding the biggest tears I've ever seen in my life.

Did she misinterpret the work of God? Or maybe knew more than we do, and this is how she was thanking for everything God did for her? I wonder to this day.

As Marcin Zielinski informs us in his book, "We do not appreciate the power of the cross; we do not appreciate the goodness that Father showed us by His Son's death. Hanging on the cross, Jesus said these promises over your life and mine. He said to you and to me, 'Everything was now finished. Trust Me. Everything you would like to pay for has already been paid for.' To get a better understanding of this, you can imagine a scene at a store. You're dreaming of the best plasma TV. You chose a cutting-edge model, the biggest, the most expensive. You head towards the checkout and want to pay for it, and the clerk says, 'No need, it's already been paid for.' And you're hell-bent on convincing her that you have to pay. Likewise, in our Christian life, we say after a confession, "God didn't forgive me. I can't feel it,' or, 'I guess God can't heal me completely.' Our doubts then undermine the mission of the cross, the power of the blood that was spilled for us. This shows we haven't understood the completeness God gave us by dying on the cross."[34]

---

[34] Ibidem, p. 29.

Marcin was right; despite all the confessions, despite all the extraordinary situations that I was lucky enough to experience at the meetings that involved healing prayers, despite all those numerous accounts and, most of all, despite what I was feeling within, I still couldn't comprehend the completeness bestowed on us by God.

Please, heal my Anna instead of me. If you're planning to heal me at today's mass, don't do it; heal that person with cancer! I requested during yet another healing mass that took place at a sports hall near my house, in the very same hall where my journey into the world of weightlifting started back in the past.

I still was not aware yet that I was just a character in a game, a script that God prepared for us all, written down ages ago. I was still unaware that it wasn't the first day Jesus started influencing my life. Back then, I didn't even realize that my egoistic drive to recover or, more specifically, the sudden absence of it, was caused by Him, for, as I heard at one of the healing masses, "The Holy Ghost is a remedy that you need to complete your mission; a mission of recreating the image of Christ in your life. When Jesus died on the cross and then rose from the dead, he sent the Holy Spirit onto each of us so that we would preach the Gospel wherever we go.

Lord Jesus lets you know that you have to muster the strength and lift your cross. He won't leave you alone in that difficult experience; He'd always carry the heaviest part for you, He'd always support you and make you keep it together. This way, Jesus wants you to grow in love and strength, getting closer to perfection, 'for my power is made perfect in weakness'!"

Everything changed within me when I heard one of the clergymen saying these words, which were yet again addressed by Zielinski, who claimed, "Our bodies have become living temples of the Divine Spirit and it is there that His presence dwells. This truth hides an extraordinary message. If only you realize that God has made you His dwelling, and you start caring for the close relationship with Him, everyone who meets will have the opportunity to experience His power and closeness that can radically transform them. Each and every one of us is the priest in his own temple. It is you who decide whether the fire that is burning within you will be only a faint-glowing ember or a flame of a torch that will ignite others. Father seeks worshippers, and if He seeks them, it means there are few of them out there. He seeks those who will understand that wherever they go, they carry His valuable presence with them, and others need it badly."[35]

From then on, my audience was not just Tomek and my buddies, who considered me somewhat of a madman, or at least that's how I felt about it. I had a conviction that I had to share my testimony of faith with others, because maybe this was the only way I could come to understand the completeness that Zielinski wrote about. From then on, I wasn't only asking God to heal the sick I was letting cross the street while I was driving my car, but I started sharing my experiences with others. My audience included my neighbors, relatives, but most of all, those who were attending therapy sessions with the use of Rife's machine, since among them there were those who needed God's presence the most, or at least that's what it seemed to me.

My stories about people wailing or collapsing onto the church floor weren't always making a big impression on everyone, but I'd try talk these individuals into attending a mass, regardless. However, there was something else, something remarkable, something that made every listener drift away in their thoughts for a moment, just like I did when I heard of it for the first time. Surfing the web, I stumbled upon a video recording of a talk delivered by Pastor Louie Giglio on Jesus and the symbolism of the cross, in which he shares a story of his extraordinary, 'coincidental' encounter with a complete stranger before an event on his tour that he was about to preach the word of God at. This reminded me of my situation with Father John, the difference being that their encounter was even more incredible.

As I have already mentioned, a certain man approached Louie completely 'on accident'. He introduced himself and asked him where he was going on from there. Louie replied he was on his way

---

[35] Ibidem, pp. 98-99.

back home and that on that Sunday, he was about to preach the word of God, tell others about His creation and, most of all, the human body. The man said, "That's really amazing! I'm a molecular biologist at the university down the road. Give me your talk!" Louie was flabbergasted; not quite yet ready to deliver his monologue yet, he was concerned of making any slip-ups in front of the professional who was dealing with biology on a daily basis. Regardless of it all, he decided to give the inquisitive lecturer a sneak peek to his talk; listening to the abridged version of the speech, the latter failed to find it as powerful and moving as it could be perceived by the audience at the catechism class on Sunday.

"What's your big left hook? You gotta have a left hook, a big finish, right?" the biologist asked.

"I don't have a left hook yet," Louie replied.

"Oh, Louie! Oh, man! Your left hook is laminin!"

Louie didn't get it, though. "Louie, it's a cell adhesion molecule. Protein molecule. Do you know about proteins?" the charismatic biologist asked.

"No," Louie replied.

"Louie! Cells organize into certain molecular structures and that determines what protein they are. There are between ten and sixty thousand proteins in the human body; we don't even know how many proteins are in the human body, but one of them is a cell adhesion molecule . It's organized into this certain structure and that tells the cell what its job is in the body. And this one is a cell adhesion molecule!"

"Alright!" Louie said, not understanding the biologist fully yet.

"No, Louie! It's like the rebar of the human body, the steel they put in the concrete when they lay the foundations of things – it's that stuff. It's holding your membranes together. It's the glue of the human body, Louie! It's laminin! You've got to tell them about laminin!"

Louie was still far from getting what the excited biologist was talking to him about.

"I promise you, I'm going home and tell them about laminin," he said with a hint of irony, "And I'm sure when I do, revival is going to sweep across the church and probably around the world when I tell them."

"No, no, no! You've got to see laminin!"

"Okay. Let's see it."

"No, no, no. You need to go look it up online. You need to go google laminin ."

"I don't even know how to spell laminin," Louie replied.

The biologist wrote down the correct spelling on his card for him; when Louie got home and typed the name on his keyboard to enter it in the search engine, he was struck dumb.

"Woooow! That's laminin?" he asked himself in disbelief.

He couldn't believe what he was seeing. He couldn't hold his emotions in. His excitement was sky high and it was only then that he realized what the biologist meant.

"I love laminin! I'm so fired up!"

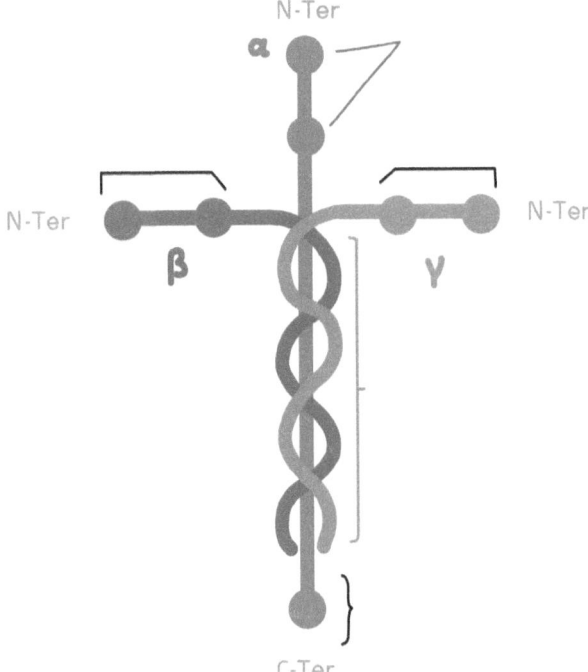

The structure of laminin. https://en.wikipedia.org/wiki/Laminin

Just like Louie, I couldn't stop myself from eulogizing over that moment; I just couldn't believe my eyes that the protein that keeps all our organs together is shaped like a Latin cross. Meanwhile, he kept on talking.

"And immediately, I'm thinking about the words of Paul in Colossians 1. You know, this beautiful passage where Paul's talking about the supremacy of Christ and the sufficiency of Christ. He says, 'For by Him,' talking about Jesus Christ, 'all things have been created. Things in heaven and things on earth; all things were created by Jesus and for Jesus.' But then, the next verse goes on to say this – it's crazy, 'and he, Jesus, is before all things, and in Him,' that is, in Jesus Christ, 'all things hold together.' That's right! It's right there!" he pointed at the Holy Scripture he's holding in his hand. "I'm like, of course they do! Of course they do. Everything holds together in Jesus Christ."

Then, Louie asked a question that was perfectly accurate for the situation I was in at that time.

"So you're at the toughest place in your life. How can you know that God is going to hold you together and bring you through? You know because there is a cross standing over history (...). (...) But the cross is also proof that God always has a purpose in the circumstances and that His purpose and His plan will prevail and will triumph through any circumstances in this world,[36]" Louie said.

I was so absorbed by Louie's speech that I didn't have to come to understand anymore that God dwelled within me, that I was part of the greatest plan in the world's history. Some of my symptoms that I was still suffering from seemed to have become a little blurry. It was as if part of my awareness was focused on something completely different. It was exactly like he said – it was amazing. At that point, I meaning behind Marcin Zielinski's words became clearer to me; the authority of the believer, the power bestowed on us as Jesus's heirs. As His children and, at the same time, His heirs, we have the authority to speak on His

---

[36] https://www.youtube.com/@LouieGiglioOfficial – "How Great Is Our Good"

behalf, to drive away diseases, for instance, like He did himself. Back then, I came to understand where did all those cases of healing come from. As Roger Carswell writes in his book, God's greatness is manifested in the entire world, and just like a designer makes his mark on his work, so does God. Every creation has its creator, be it the smallest molecule of the human body or the tallest mountain.[37] I believe that God left His copyright mark in each of us, and that mark is laminin.

There were days when I thought all those cases of healed people that I witnessed at prayer meetings were not a work of God but merely a placebo or some hoax. I realized that even if during these masses people did experience feelings that could be referred to as a placebo, which was effective, it started inside of us. In movies that I've been always watching most passionately it was only superheroes or simply gods who had divine powers. Now I knew that each of us could be a superhero together with laminin, with Jesus. Although to the mother of the bacteria-ridden eight-year-old girl I was a hero already, I received the same label shortly after from Father John's colleague, who was ordered by the priest to call me to talk about Rife's machine and its capabilities. For nearly two hours, that man was discussing that with me, pondering on his future and his desire to open up a business based on non-conventional methods for helping others. I couldn't discourage him from doing that, especially that in the very same time, we heard Mayer's wife saying the words we had been waiting for for ages.

"Dear ones, I do not detect any bacteria in you two. It's over!"

I cannot put in words what hearing this diagnosis was like to us. I cannot recall the euphoria that filled the office back in that moment.

After the relatively long trips to Czestochowa that we had been on, in contrast to other sick carriers of bacteria and with due consideration of our Lyme disease experience as a whole, all we could fell was joy. Our happiness didn't last too long, though.

---

[37] R. Carswell, *Pytanie o wiare*, p. 5.

CHAPTER VI

Unlike Anna, who was feeling better, I was still wrestling with my problems.

Though most of my symptoms ceased and I don't even recall the moment when the painful prickly sensations inside my head and groin simply disappeared, I didn't feel any better, still experiencing weird symptoms when focusing on creative or mental tasks, for instance. My ears continued to bother me big time. I was also unable to make any physical effort due to the persisting unease in my neck and all the sensations that it involved. With all this taken into consideration, I couldn't believe Mayer's wife was right. My intuition, which never failed me, was telling me that likewise, something wasn't right here. Therefore, I decided that we'd get additionally diagnosed at other facilities offering bio-resonance diagnosis. Since I was aware that there could be more methods such as that offered by Natalie, I knew that it wouldn't be an easy task.

After all, we could've go back to the place recommended by the carpenter's 'on-eyes' daughter where we received a very detailed diagnoses; however, in my view, such an opinion wouldn't be reliable. I needed a specific test administered by someone who had never seen us before; someone who didn't know our story; someone who would confirm my suspicions that we hadn't been fully cleansed of all the bacteria that were ruining us; that Mayer's wife was simply wrong. We received some help from Father

John's colleague who recommended a certain place that we headed to right away. As it turned out, the woman who was offering bio-resonance diagnosis was using the exact same device that was used to test us in the venue recommended by the young woman who almost lost one eye due to *Borrelia*. Although I've always considered lying repulsive and I knew that withholding truth would take a toll on me, in this case, Anna and I had to lie again.

"We've come here for a bio-resonance test. We've heard that this device allows you to tell us if my fiancée and I are carrying anything that could be the reason behind the allergy we both have," I lied, intertwining truth with untruth.

"Of course, that's right. That exceptional device allows me to do that," she replied. "Please, take a seat. Who's first to go?"

I didn't hesitate and I sat in the chair. I put my hands on my knees, pretending I had no idea what to do next.

With her short haircut that made her remind me of actress Julianne Moore, the woman commended the diagnostic process and started administering acupressure by gently prickling one spot.

For over forty minutes, she was carrying out the procedure very diligently and meticulously; throughout my diagnosis and, later, during her own, my Anna was asking her questions that we already had the answers to to make herself more plausible during our minor provocation. Then, there came a moment of truth we were waiting for most impatiently.

"Have you been taking any antibiotics lately?"

"No, why?" I lied, yet again.

"Both of you are carrying a fungus called *Candida,* which can be dangerous to your bodies if it grows in excess. However, I'm most concerned about the fact that you carry bacteria *Borrelia* and *Bartonella*, which can make your lives very unpleasant," Julianne said.

Hearing the woman's diagnosis, as usual, Anna and I gave each other a look, this time smiling confidently. If there was still any skepticism for this type of diagnostics left within us, at that very moment, they all simply disappeared.

"It's not that bad, though. It could've been worse. It's a rare thing for *Borrelia* and *Bartonella* to coexist without their other regular companions," she added.

Julianne not only did confirm Helen's words, but also to some extent the diagnosis issued by Mayer's wife whose device wasn't most likely as sensitive as this one. There was nothing else Anna and I could do but to admit what really brought us to Julianne and continue our therapy with Rife's machine while getting diagnosed from time to time in some new place.

"Meeting Jesus gives us a new identity. What you did in the past becomes meaningless; the weight of your baggage of experiences and grief that you were carrying around becomes unimportant; that meeting makes you a new creation."[38] Marcin and the clergymen I had the pleasure of hearing inform that if you only allow Jesus to act in your life, miracles and inexplicable things will start taking place. I believe this is what happened in my life. I guess that He was acting even when I wasn't asking anything of Him, when I couldn't have cared less about Him. I believe that it wasn't just a coincidence that my intuition, which had always guided me like a navigation system, made me oppose the theory that Mayer's wife put forward. Perhaps it was also a product of my subconsciousness; either way, there's no doubt that it was one of the works of God that He shares with us in ways that are not always obvious, albeit always serve a specific purpose.

When I heard Marcin Zielinski's story for the first time at a prayer meeting, which he also described in his book, I thought, "What a load of bull." Shortly after, I went through a very similar one myself.

One summer, being a very devout man who believed that God wants to act and use us every day, Marcin was desperately seeking a means to get used by Jesus in any way possible during his stay by the sea. In his service to God, he experienced healing, conversion, and miracles of all kind many times, but on that particular day, he didn't.

---

[38] M. Zielinski, *Rozpal wiare*, p. 30.

Somewhat frustrated, Marcin argued with God to make Him put on his path someone he could help. On the last day of his stay in the seaside town, Marcin felt an immense desire to pray; he knew and he could sense that the Holy Spirit was up to something. He knew in his heart that he had to be vigilant about what was going on around him. Then, something happened; as he put it, "Thousands of people were passing me by left and right. Suddenly, my gaze fell on a man who didn't stand out from the others by no means. I knew that I was expected to approach him, but I had no idea at all what I was expected to tell him. I felt weird, because at that moment he was talking to someone, so I told God that if that man was there on my way back, I'd approach him. I secretly hoped that I wouldn't encounter him the second time I got there, but he was still there, talking to someone. I discussed this with God again, telling Him it wasn't that inappropriate for me to interrupt someone's conversation. At that very moment, my sister came to me and said I should go back to the store, because we didn't have much time and we had to leave soon. Disappointed with myself and my lack of response to God's incentive, I went to do some shopping. I started apologizing to God for not doing anything about that. What I saw a moment later was inexplicable to me. To this day, I have no clue how could it happen – the man whom I failed to approach earlier was the first person standing before me in line to get checked out. I was so grateful to God. I thought: Lord Jesus, let him only wait in front of the store, so that I don't have to run after him. That's the man of faith I was... He went outside the store and was standing there; he didn't go away. I didn't know what exactly I should say to him or how to strike the conversation. My only feeling was telling me that this man had some issues with narcotic drugs and alcohol. I told him, 'Listen, maybe it sounds stupid, but I have to tell you that Lord Jesus loves you very much, he died for you on the cross, he spilled his blood to make you free from alcohol and drugs.' He smiled and said, 'You know, that's not stupid at all, because three years ago, I met Jesus, and he made me free from drugs and alcohol. Thank you for telling me that. It's profoundly reassuring.' I was overwhelmed with happiness. I asked if I could pray for him. I put my hands on him and proclaimed God's victory over him, so that it would never be stolen from him, and so that he would never think that he did it all on his own merits. Of all the people in that crowd, God chose one person to give him his love and reassure him how much he loved him. It was an extraordinary encounter for that man, and for me, too."[39]

When I was standing with my eyes wide open, listening to Marcin telling this story at a holy mass in my city, I wasn't ready yet to believe it. I considered a 'yarn' like that like a good script for a comedy. But today, I had my new identity, owing to which I know that my encounter with Father John or any other was not a mere coincidence. The one I experienced shortly after closed the door to all disbelief behind me, turning me into a brand new 'creature', as one more time, I became a tool in the hands of God; a tool that played a role in one of the key foundations of our faith, my faith – the first successful evangelization.

I would always ask myself, *Why me? I've never stolen anything, I've never did anything my peers were coercing me to do if I considered that to be wrong. I didn't break women's hearts, I didn't hurt animals, I conducted myself well. I've always stayed clean, I've never been a bad son, a bad partner or a bad friend. Since childhood, I've been able to tell good from evil, also on the big screen, so why do I have to be sick?* I pondered. Though I was closer than ever to reaching the understanding that made me capable of feeling happy again, I was still wrestling with the egoistic nature of the disease, desperately attempting not to bring my issues back to the epicenter of my attention. Everything changed, though, once I saw on the Internet a testimony of faith of a priest who was offering a Healing Mass. He provided an extraordinary account of experiencing Jesus's presence at the age of twenty on his path to a life in a seminary. Planning to offer and trust his entire life to God, he missed His presence, and so he got overwhelmed by massive fear and uncertainty. This concern about the

---

[39] Ibidem, pp. 59-60.

lack of evidence, that fear of the void that he felt every day led the young priest in the making to suicidal ideation. Wishing fervently that he could offer himself to the Holy Spirit, he asked time and time again how to live with Him; sadly, he didn't get the expected response until the moment when he put his hands on a book by Jose H. Prado Flores originally titled *Jesucristo Sanador de mi persona*. The priest told me about the zealous commitment he read that book with and how reading it, he immediately felt a noticeable change. He shared the information about the unusual prayer that book contains that allows you to experience Jesus Himself, as he felt His presence in the most extraordinary way while saying that particular prayer.

"While I was praying, I had my eyes covered with my hands and a moment later, I couldn't take them off. I could feel they weren't mine; I could feel they belonged to Jesus. The vast warmth and love I experienced at that moment defied description. I felt like a little child surrounded by paternal love. I started crying, I howled for joy, for infinite happiness. I couldn't take His hands off, I didn't want to; I was afraid that the feeling would disappear, that I wouldn't see Him again. The joy and the mercy Lord immersed me in were indescribable. My problems were gone, and each time after that wonderful moment when I entered the chapel of the seminary I could feel Jesus's presence in the Eucharist stronger than ever before."

> "Do not fear your weaknesses. Everything within you is mine and I use everything according to my plan, for you insist on offering yourself to me and desire to carry out My plan."[40]

I need to get that book! That was the first thought that came to my mind. I didn't have to put as much effort into finding it as I did on identifying the cause of my issues. All it took was entering the title in the search engine and click enter. A few more steps

---

[40] A. Lenczewska, *Slowo Pouczenia*, Poznan 2021, pp. 439-440.

later, I was already counting the days to the moment a courier would show up at my door.

I will never forget the day when I got the package with the book I yearned to be my remedy, which was about to connect me with God Himself, with Jesus, whom I was meeting for one purpose only; so that I would be healed and receive a relief from all my problems. It was one of those days when I was rubbing my watery eyes just to ensure that the man who was handing me a package wouldn't notice I had been crying. If he would, I always had a reply, "That allergy is killing me!"

On that day, my desire to break free from my world was through the roof. Though the ailments that were causing me derealization largely ceased already, on the day that I hung my astronaut's helmet on a hanger, I was still experiencing the ramifications of all I had been through, primarily the highly subjective sensation that was annoying me when I was looking at my hands. Back in that moment, my emotions were giving me a really hard time, making me blame all the evil of this world on one person who eventually gave me a reply.

I opened my package, grabbed a very thin, small book in my hand and, giving it little thought, I started looking for the prayer the clergyman mention. I didn't care for the content of the book; I wasn't interested in what was it about. I wanted to feel the exactly same thing that man was talking about as soon as possible; I wanted to feel Jesus's presence. I was turning the pages hastily, as if in a frenzy, to find it as soon as possible. Finally, I saw the longest text of a prayer I had ever prayed. The empty house and the vast silence disturbed by nothing except for my tinnitus was adding to the ambiance of that moment.

That's it! That's the moment I've been waiting for! I thought.

Like never before, I focused all my attention, I muted everything else that was boiling within me, as if I knew that it was my last opportunity, the one chance in my lifetime that I couldn't blow. I wasn't hoping for connecting with God in the same way the clergyman did. I imagined anything would happen, even just a rest in the Holy Spirit that people mentioned repeatedly while sharing their accounts of falling asleep while reading the Scripture, for instance. I started reading.

With every word of the prayer, I tuned myself to it as if it were my words that I had written down beforehand. The more spellbound by the read I was, the more emotional I got and the only one thing that was distracting me were my tears, as I didn't want them to fall on the dry pages of the book. Then, the moment arrived, the very same that the priest who had shared his account of faith and meeting with God mentioned; the moment when you had to put your hands on your eyes; the very same moment when he felt Jesus's touch. I couldn't do it, since the prayer went on, and I needed to continue reading it with my eyes open.

So I prayed on, covering one eye and squinting the other a bit, so that the task was done properly at least to some extent. Once I finished reading, I closed my eyes and, just like the clergyman, I placed both my hands on my face to cover it, waiting for anything to happen.

Never before had I wanted the Almighty to interact with me more, regardless of what form it would take. Sadly, in the course of the first seconds, nothing happened. I could feel all the doubt that was dormant within me like an old volcano, waiting for the right moment to explode with massive amounts of anger, grief and rage, trying to come out. I managed to hold back the words that were already on the tip off my tongue. However, I didn't manage to hold back tears, which I continued to shed throughout the day, additionally intensified because of my deep disappointment.

"What am I doing wrong? What have I done wrong? Why can't you see me? If all that is true, give me a sign!" I wailed like a baby.

When all my hopes packed their bags and headed to the exit, my eyes had no more tears to shed and I put Flores's book away; in the moment when I got up and made a step forward to fill my mind with something else, a thing I will remember to the end of my days happened. My phone started vibrating, letting me know that someone texted me. I grabbed it and looked at it to see who that was. I saw an unread direct message sent by some complete stranger on one of the social media websites. Somewhat confused, I read it and I didn't really know what it was all about. "Read about Kambo," the unknown man wrote.

Ka-what? Who are you, anyway? I thought, tossing my cell phone aside.

Slouching around the empty house, I had no idea what to do with myself and my thoughts were centered on what had just happened. As usual, I went online; this time, I entered into the search engine the word 'Kambo' I never heard of before. I opened the first website that came up among many others dedicated to this subject. What I saw made me a bit concerned, and then overwhelmed by a feeling of tranquility, as I started reflecting on not only what was before my eyes, but also the fact that eventually, my prayers were answered and I received the sign that I had been asking for. "Kambo – the remedy for all maladies," said the headline on the website I visited. These several words already sparked my interest, though I recalled the headline in the newspaper that was promoting the Philippine healer as the last resort. This time, I knew that it wasn't just a coincidence, especially after what was written below the headline. Despite all the information contain there that now everyone would be fond of, the only thing I was interested in was the list of diseases that you could treat using Kambo. Of all the conditions mentioned on a very long page that I was scrolling down using a computer mouse there was only one that was highlighted in bold – Lyme disease.

When at the end of the day I told my loved ones what happened, they were all stunned. We didn't know what to do. Not because we didn't believe in the thing that happened or whether it was really an act of God or not, but because Kambo, also known as the Amazon frog poison drug, proved to be a treatment that wasn't entirely safe. To make the attempt at regaining full health, restoring the body-mind balance, purging toxins from the body, and strengthening the immune system in general, I had to make one of the most difficult decisions in my life. It involved taking one of the most powerful antibiotics that are present in nature, that is, the poison of the Amazonian tree frog.

I didn't know what to do. On the one hand, I really wanted to fully recover, and the strong anti-inflammatory and antibacterial properties of Kambo could help me achieve that. On the other hand, I was very afraid of the unknown, and of coming in contact with a substance as strong as Kambo was, since it contained over two hundred chemical compounds, some of them highly toxic. Though Julianne included some herbs into our therapy with Rife's machine, and we also started taking highly antibacterial Manuka honey from New Zealand, which also gave me additional herxes, I felt that I didn't get the information about Kambo for no reason.

What to do? Give me a sign! I begged God.

"I'll go with you! I will always go where you go! I will hold your hand when I'll be taking Kambo, too, if you want," Anna said.

"What? You'll go with me?" I asked, not wanting to take Anna into a territory that was yet unknown to us.

"I will. We're in this together, and we will overcome it together!" she said.

I didn't know who the man who DM-ed me on the social media website was. I could only guess he was one of those people I had been turning to for help for years, asking them to give me an answer to my problems. Also, I didn't feel like striking a conversation with that man to ask him why he decided to contact me at that specific moment. Though you could reflect for ages whether it was a mere coincidence or not, shortly after, I realized that Anna's decision and everything that I had gone through up until that point was not a coincidence, but part of God's plan.

Lord, if that's your will, I will go there, I thought.

We barely even noticed when it was almost the end of the year 2016. The unpredictable weather that November brings is one big mystery. To me, that month became synonymous with significant moments of my life, and what we were about to do was undoubtedly an important part of our story. On our way to the so-called Kambo ceremony, we all had the very same feeling of uncertainty.

I wouldn't be myself if I didn't check what I was probably about to face this time beforehand. With due account of all the information, especially scenes from recorded Kambo ceremonies,

I wondered many times on our way if we shouldn't go back. Despite believing that I didn't get DM-ed merely by chance, I had never been so stressed up in my entire life. However, once I got there, the stress started going away.

Our destination was not accidental, either. These people were virtually the only Kambo practitioners I stumbled upon online; what bought me was predominantly their website, on which among various diseases, the only one in bold was Lyme disease. For some reason, I could feel that I had to choose that specific place. Back then, I didn't know yet why but everything got clear just a moment later.

We arrived at an ordinary detached house with a utility building in the back, where a young married couple was performing Kambo ceremonies.

Anna and I were invited in, and so we entered, leaving our parents behind, who were about to come fetch us in a couple of hours. At the doorstep, we were greeted by a young married couple with genuine smiles on their faces and their charismatic helper who reminded me of king Ragnar Lothbrok from the TV series *Vikings*. He stood out not only from the spouses but also all the other people who gathered there on that afternoon. The whole group of over ten attendees who were awaiting the ceremony was invited into the biggest room where mattresses and empty buckets were provided beforehand. We were shown to our respective seats and asked to sit down comfortably, though it wasn't easy. Being the only person 'qualified' to apply the poison of the Amazon tree frog and the only Kambo shaman present at the ceremony, the young man introduced us into the process we were about to subject ourselves to. He mentioned that traditionally, the prerequisite for commencing the ritual is that each participant shares with everyone why they decided to come there and what they expect from the 'holy' frog. As he claimed, the ceremony was not only about injecting the poison that was intended to make us discharge all the toxins from our bodies, but it was also about raising the awareness of coming into contact with the Spirit of the Frog and directing to it all the intentions and requests that dwell deep in our hearts.

He asked the first person to share her brief story, stressing that she didn't have to do that in front of everyone. To my surprise, no one had any problem to do so. Starting from the first person asked all the way to my Anna, who was sitting to my right, they all confessed their secrets and expectations.

"I am an alcoholic and I came here on my daughter's request. I'd like to get healed," an elderly man said.

"I've been doing this for a couple of times now and I'm feeling better and better," the next person said.

"I came here driven by curiosity," a young girl said.

"I am suffering from Lyme disease and I'm giving everything there is a try," another female said.

"I have Lyme disease, too, and I came here with my fiancé," Anna said.

When it was my turn to share my story with the people who gathered there, I felt that I had to tell them all the truth. I didn't know why, but I just felt I had to do that. Despite still feeling somewhat resistant, and not brave enough to rise to the challenge and share if nothing than just my account of faith I experienced at healing masses, I mustered the courage.

"Like my fiancée, I am suffering from Lyme disease, but there is yet another reason why we came here to see you," I said.

Telling them a much abridged version of my story took ten minutes of the ceremony time; when I finished, the room was filled with an odd silence and an air of contemplation. Having listened to the rest of the participants, the ritual began.

The shaman and his wife divided us into groups. One group was tasked with drinking more than half a gallon of water in twenty minutes so that they had something to vomit with into the buckets sitting by the mattresses, as it was the only way the body could discharge all the toxins that were leaving the body after the poison was administered. Meanwhile, participants from the other group were burned with a hot wooden stick by the shaman, leaving a mark of several red dots of burned skin on men's arms and women's calves, which was then removed to administer the frog poison; this was the only way Kambo could enter the bloodstream to then spread throughout the body. When Anna was having her small wounds burned on her skin, me and the other members of my group had to drink the most water I had ever drunk in such a short time. Ragnar had several tasks to fulfill in that time. Aside from letting incense spread across the room to add to the ambiance of the ritual, he was refilling one-quart plastic cups for everyone with any water that had been already drunk. When he realized mine was about to get empty, he approached me and kneeled in front of me to refill it.

"It's amazing, you know," he said to me.

"What's amazing?" I asked, surprised.

"That we've met."

"I don't understand."

"Man, I'm telling you, for the last couple of years, I struggled to find my place in this world. I joined a seminary with a plan to offer all my heart to the God you speak of, whom I've grown to love dearly. And yet, at the same time, there was that woman who turned my world upside down. I fell head over heels in love."

I continued to drink my water while he went on, still refilling my cup.

"I had to make up my mind: to serve God whom I loved or to give my heart to the woman who became all my world. You know what I did?" he asked.

"You chose her?" I replied with my mouth full of water, already sick of having to drink it all.

"I did. I left God and went followed her. And you know what she did to me?"

"No idea."

"She cheated on me with another man and that hurt me so bad that I buried myself alive. Back then, I hated the entire world and turned my back on the Lord even more. For a couple of years, searching for my place on Earth, I was trying to get my shit together spiritually. I was wandering from one religion to another. You know... Harry Krishna, Buddhism, now even Kambo. I intended to become a shaman, but when I heard your story and you told us everything about Jesus and how you got here... It... It all made me want to go back. I need to go back. You have to tell me what's that book called," he wrapped it up and stepped away on the shaman's mark that it was time.

What Anna and I experienced a moment later at the Kambo ceremony was indescribable; undoubtedly, both for me and for her, it was the hardest thing we had ever gone through. However, the young man whose looks reminded me of the Viking heathen with his perfect characterization and his words allowed me to make it through that painful initiation. In one moment, I realized that God used me just like charismatic Marcin Zielinski described it.

"Now, I will ask the Spirit of the Frog to hear our requests and act. You, dear ones, can do the same, and those who believe in other deities of this world should not hesitate and ask them to be present, as well," the master of the ceremony said while commencing the prayer.

Making the incense smoke even harder, Ragnar and the shaman's wife started playing Peruvian music on wooden instruments. At that point, I realized why the entire Kambo process and its setting are called a 'ceremony'. Then, there came the time we all had been waiting for. Singing some Indian melodies, the master of the ceremony started applying the frog poison prepared beforehand onto our tiny wounds.

It took only a couple of seconds to make the thick secretion reach the bloodstream. Since in men, the wounds were located closer to the heart, the reaction in males was much quicker than in women.

The thing that each of us felt was the worst feeling of my life.

I could feel my entire body going numb and a wave of extremely high pressure hitting my head. In one moment, I got awfully hot. I felt as if all the veins in my head started swelling as if filled with vast amounts of blood in just one moment that was pressing on the walls to no end. My heart was pounding at the speed I'd already known from my anxiety seizures; this time, however, it was trying to surpass its limits. I felt that my head was very close to exploding. It was just like that moment when you're inflating a basketball and can already tell that there's too much air in it.

It seemed to me that either someone or something was trying to rip my extremities off my body, particularly my arms and hands. It was as if some force was twisting them like a wet towel until every thread in it was dry again, until finally, I felt they were completely gone; exactly like you feel when you've been laying entire night in the same position with your hand underneath, and wake up feeling like it's not there anymore.

The fear that overwhelmed me at that moment was beyond words. Still, I knew and felt that it all served a specific purpose and was not happening for no reason.

My blurred vision didn't allow me to tell anything more than the color of clothes of the master of the ceremony walking past us; then, I started feeling that all those sensations intensified even more, making me gradually lose my vision.

I'm probably dying, I thought.

Sharing virtually the same sensations, Anna and I were praying in our thoughts to Jesus until in just one second, an immense relief came upon us, which could mean only one thing. I came back to life on the spot, hoping that it was the end; sadly, though, the most strenuous and time-consuming part of the Kambo process was just about to begin.

When it seemed to me that it was all good, my stomach proved me wrong, starting to cleanse and expel all the filth that Kambo encountered on its way. For the next thirty, maybe forty minutes I was spewing out green-and-yellow vomit while Ragnar was handing me gallons of water, forcing me to drink it all.

"You're almost done, pal! You're doing great, you can do this!" he said.

With no more strength inside of me, looking at the bucket that was almost full, I peeked at Anna and the other participants who were already done, lying down to have some brief rest. I knew that something was wrong with me. Unlike the others, I could keep vomiting like that to no end until I would feel that I couldn't do that anymore. It wasn't only the willingness to keep on vomiting that made me stand out from everyone else gathered there. I was the only one who expelled something reminiscent of yellowish-green scrambled eggs floating on the surface in my bucket, while my body was so weak that I could barely get into my car. At that moment, I realized why prior to the ceremony, Anna and I had to sign a document that confirmed our awareness of the risk Kambo could involve, that is, a risk of losing one's life or health. Though we had some concerns as regards that event, the young shaman reassured us, claiming that he had performed two thousand 'rainforest vaccinations' and that nothing bad ever happened. Sadly, as it is often the case in life, there's a first time for everything.

Having returned home, we were exhausted on the next day. Though many people after the ceremony immediately feel tremendous progress and an unparalleled zest for life, in our case, as usual, it was all backwards. It wasn't anything serious though compared to what happened at Ragnar's event with a young married couple who were about to go through their Kambo initiation on the next day.

"Michal, come, see what's on the news!" Anna shouted, terrified.

We were standing gazing at the TV screen, paralyzed, unable to believe our own eyes and ears. It turned out that on the following day, after our Kambo ceremony, a tragedy happened in the same place.

A young woman blacked out and died after being taken to hospital. It was the first case like that.

When I learned about it, I had no clue at that moment what to make of it all. It was publicly stated that the young shaman would have serious problems.

Deep inside, I was convinced that my presence there just before this tragedy unraveled was part of God's plan not only with regards to Ragnar. The moment when I saw the young married couple contemplating and smiling, which let me know that they, too, must have heard my words, I felt that they'd face these upcoming problems more easily.

The last six years of my life were a very tough time for me, but they also taught me a lot. I began the year 2017 as a completely different person than I was before, not only mentally, but also spiritually. After all Anna and I had gone through, I burned all the bridges of hate and resentment towards the people who hurt me.

By 'the people' I mean the doctors participating in the system of treating the sick that was incomprehensible to me, who were unable to help me. The thing that I experienced when talking to Ragnar assured me in my approach to life and that I was going in the right direction. I stopped living only for myself and started living for others.

"Whoever wants to be my disciple must deny themselves and take up their cross and follow me. For whoever wants to save their life will lose it, but whoever loses their life for me will find it. What good will it be for someone to gain the whole world, yet forfeit their soul? Or what can anyone give in exchange for their soul?" (Matthew 16:24-26)

In his book, Jose H. Prado Flores says that there is much more to giving yourself to the Holy Spirit than just praying a novena.[41]

To reach peace, happiness and health, one has to follow His rules. These include, among others, seeking to benefit your neighbor rather than yourself; most of all, it's forgiving others like Jesus did on the cross. My forgiveness and, primarily, my strong position in my new life arrived on the day when I realized we all make mistakes and we're all just humans.

From time to time, Anna and I would have a blood test done along with a check-up of the liver and other organs, which is recommended especially after undergoing a long-term antibiotic therapy like the one we both subjected ourselves to.

After six years, we visited my uncle's friend, the cardiologist, who was the first person who recommended me to see a psychiatrist and who gave me his colleague's phone number. As it turned out, in the recent years, his wife fell prey to Lyme disease, while he fell victim to the criticism of his fellow psychiatrists who claimed his wife should undergo psychiatric treatment. When my uncle asked me for help and some advice for his friend, I knew that the latter had no courage to ask me for it directly. As an understanding person, I didn't hesitate to do so.

---

[41] Thomas Forrest CSsR and Jose H. Prado Flores, *Jezus Chrystus Uzdrowiciel Mojej Osoby*, Lodz 2015, p. 120.

At that point, I realized that if that man was capable of going back in time and giving me a different advice, he would've certainly done that; I also came to understand that he would give up everything to save his wife now.

I would give up everything to make my fiancée healthy, too, without staying focused only on my condition. I wanted Anna to recover so bad; then, Julianne read to us the results of the most recent bio-resonance test.

"I cannot detect any *Bartonella* in you anymore, sir, but *Borrelia* can still be observed, unfortunately." Then, she proceeded to diagnose Anna. "You, on the other hand, are free from bacteria now; my device shows none of the two bacteria. Congratulations, I'm very glad for you, miss."

Although *Borrelia* was still with me, I was more than happy that we managed to eliminate pathogens from the body of my Anna. However, she wasn't as ecstatic as I was, as she hoped for things to turn out the opposite way. Despite the fact that no one could guarantee that these devices are completely reliable, just like serology, I believed that Anna was cured. I didn't know whether that was due to Kambo, our long-term therapy with Rife's machine or the other supplements and herbs.

Nonetheless, I was convinced that Jesus played a part in it, too. Perhaps I wasn't destined to fully comprehend His sacrifice that happened two thousand years prior, and for this reason, I wasn't fully healed.

Or maybe I was? I pondered.

With my new identity, I took on a new belief that in our story, it wasn't me who was supposed to be physically cured. I believe that God used me, once again, and put Anna on my path so that with our love for each other and our strength, we both could overcome the bacteria that were putting her life at risk. Why else would I miss a bus on the day I met her for the second time, 'accidentally'?

What happened 'by chance' in the life of the person who held number fifteen, who for some reason had to leave the line and thus let Anna take his or her place? Why did the fate make it so that Tomek's bad luck made my life gain meaning? I believe that

He chose me so that I could help not only her, but also others who needed it. Many times, He'd put signs on my way that I was unable to decipher, like back when He was leading us to the cross on the mountain summit. I know a couple of cases of people encountering some signs on their path time and time again, some recurring numbers that wouldn't leave them be. Some consider them to be attempts made by angles who wish to communicate with us. It's remarkable what the number fifteen hides. *Angles want you to make necessary changes in your life and they will support you throughout the upcoming transformation process. Very soon, they will prove highly beneficial not only for you, but also for others. Gradually, you'll leave old, bad limitations behind to make room for the new to enter your life.* Although many may consider numerology and all other sources of mysticism a kind of hypocrisy when it comes to Christianity, I think that as long as you believe that what you're experiencing here and now is God's plan, nothing bad would happen. Subjecting myself to healers, I never wondered if they could make things worse for me. I was glad that in this world, there are people who give me any hope for a better tomorrow; a hope that was so hard for me to find among doctors practicing conventional medicine. Did any of them do anything wrong, something that could and can still have impact on my life further down the line? I don't know that. One thing is certain, though: that was the plan.

    As Muhammad Ali once said, "God gave me this illness to remind me that I'm not Number One; He is." I didn't get my illness from God. There are too many mosquitos out there in the world for me to blame Him for that. I do know, however, that I needed it to trigger some transformations within me. I realized what was really important in life, who was a true friend of mine and who I could always count on. Wasting my time at the gym back in the past, I didn't pay attention to the things that are really significant in life. Throughout that time, I thought I was ill due to Lyme disease. However, I came to understand that that I was always ill, all that time, because there was no Jesus in my heart. That was my most severe condition.

When I was ill, I used to wonder how many years I had lost due to Lyme disease. Today, I wonder how many years I could've gained had I had Him in my head all this time. Perhaps I lost a lot, but I know that today, I gained much more. *Borrelia* and Co. took a lot from me, but at the same time, they guided me to where I am today. I realized that faith does not always come with physical healing, and that there is something much bigger behind our suffering and the cross we bear than just subjective, most often unpleasant sensations. Power is honed in moments of weakness, and the part of Jesus we carry inside (most of all, that tiny building block of His suffering inside each one of us) allows us to be part of the greatest victory of all time, to add our own experiences and our own personal cross to that beautiful story.

I realized that despite our closed eyes, Jesus had been with us all this time, everywhere. Though I felt really bad, my suffering was not in vain, and Jesus was with me throughout that time in the form of my loved ones. In those moments when I could count on my dad, for instance, who was giving me a lift here and there regardless of his own ailments; in those times when my mom was massaging my head despite the pain in her wrists, gritting her teeth to bring me some relief, if nothing else than for just a second. With Anna by my side, who was dedicating her life and investing her time into the progressively collapsing foundation that I was, regardless of it all, I still wanted something more; I wanted to be touched like many were during healing masses or simply fall asleep with the Holy Spirit guarding me. I didn't realize, though, that back then, I already had more than others.

We waded through the year 2017 until the very end with much hope that I, too, would finally get some positive news from Julianne. I deeply believed that I would, since my neck pain subsided, at last. It didn't happen overnight; it was a strenuous process during which I resorted to various methods. I do know, however, that what contributed the most to this success was Rife's machine. Month by month, I was testing my own abilities, making more and more intense physical effort, and the horrific sensations I had been having for several years simply eased up. The day on which I was capable of doing pushups again effortlessly, hoping that I'd be able to enjoy sports again, was one of the best days of my life. Tomek was right saying that I'd get back to training again; he believed that more than I did. It was only on that day that I felt I was recovering, which others starting sensing much sooner than I did. As you can imagine, nothing could beat my purulent cyst until the thing that had to happen happened, and it eventually broke open.

Although it could be unimaginable to many that I had been carrying it inside my throat for so long, what was unimaginable to me was that none of the doctors I had met on my path wouldn't do anything about it until I had to ask God for help again.

Give me another sign, just one, that one last time, I thought.

Sitting in front of a computer monitor at work, I wondered which hospital I should go to. I was concerned, though, that I'd be assigned, yet again, to a medical doctor who'd conclude it wasn't as bad as I thought. And then, something extraordinary happened; something I knew all too well already.

Out of the blue, after my brief prayer, an e-mail arrived at my inbox, reminding me of the laryngological appointment I ended up not showing to several years ago. Back then, I went to meet with the laryngologist and ended up in the middle of nowhere, and the doctor himself called me to apologize.

That's impossible, I thought, a smile appearing on my face, since I knew what I had to do.

We called right away to ask if there was any vacancy by any chance, as I was struggling with a terrible issue. It turned out that the laryngologist could see us on the next day. Therefore, we set off to the location which was several hundred miles away from my home. As soon as that man saw what I was suffering from, he became very blatant.

"I'm so sorry for my colleagues!" he said overtly. Then, he asked me to sit on his other chair which back then didn't give away that anything unordinary was about to take place.

I took a seat then, and a moment later, the doctor, who looked much like a young version of Ed Harris wearing black plastic glasses, retrieved from a nearby drawer the biggest forceps I've ever seen in my life.

"If I don't remove it in this moment, you can get some bigger problems. It's a miracle that puss didn't cause you more hurt. You're an adult, you decide."

"But here, now? I thought maybe you'll refer me for some surgery to a hospital," I was terrified.

"Young man, my colleagues should've removed the thing inside your mouth long ago. We can eliminate your problem here and now. It will hurt only for a while and you'll go home."

I put my trust not only in him, but also in God and His plan. I opened up my mouth and the laryngologist ripped the vesicle that had been growing in my mouth for several years out in a few motions, without anesthesia, and cleaned it all up. It was so painful and exciting that on my way back, I fainted twice due to extreme emotions.

Throughout all these years, suffering had become a kind of inherent part of my life.

In the worst moments of going through Lyme disease, when I was lying down, crying for the universe to help me, when my 'self' disappeared completely, I felt suspended between one world and another. It was just as if despite the terrible state I found myself in I could feel the presence of some great power. It was not the same thing like seeing light in a tunnel or the other side on your deathbed; it was as if I suddenly became my own soul watching my suffering body from the inside, unable to get out, but feeling that moment would come. Perhaps only people who are highly sensitive to stimuli get impressions like these?

Nonetheless, I learned to stop listening only to my ailments and ceased to pay attention to the constant wailing of my body. Instead, I started listening to Jesus with faith, doing what He told me to do. I hoped that one day, I'd fully recover and Christ Himself would be living inside of me.

I took another attempt at telling the world about God who did so much good in my life when after a couple of years, I was back at the office of the neurosurgeon who was the first one to not claim I required psychiatric treatment and one of the few who didn't make that recommendation. Since the situation still was not what it should have been, I hoped that perhaps after all this time, something changed in conventional medicine.

To my surprise, I heard words that could serve as a reason for reigniting massive hatred within me.

"There's no such thing as Lyme disease. I don't believe it exists," the neurosurgeon said, now a couple of years older, yet still reminiscent of Al Pacino.

"Do you believe in anything? I bet you don't believe in God, either," I asked him.

"I don't. Because when I'm doing my best and the human in my hands dies regardless, there's no God in that," he said.

I recalled him telling me at our first session about the lifeboat that appeared out of nowhere to save him and his friends from a sinking yacht.

"Do you think that was a coincidence?" I asked.

"Of course I do."

"I have a different view on that. I believe God saved you so that you can save others. Save those destined to live. You're not the one who decides who should live and who should not. You're only a tool in God's hands; a tool that God needs."

Though I ran out of arguments, I hoped that I managed to convince him, even a little bit.

I did not convince Anna, though, to forego seeing an expert in infectious diseases. Although she was right that we both should try make any entries in the history of our disease recorded in a book of infectious diseases every patient has kept for him, I knew that no one would help her.

I was certain that the words directed to Anna after she begged for any Lyme disease test would fall, just as certain I am that it will rain in November.

"You have no Lyme disease and you never did," the female infectiologist said, handing Anna back her Western blot results.

I received the diagnosis the doctor issued for my Anna composedly despite the fact she was very wrong. A colleague of Father

John uplifted me, calling me after a long break to thank me for our precious lengthy conversation that made him decide to venture into self-employment based on unconventional methods.

"Thanks to you, I've managed to help a few people already. Thank you!" he said, setting my heart on fire.

I consider this book my votive offering, my testimony of how I experienced the work of Jesus Christ in my life. A testimony that I should have proclaimed long ago in front of several thousand people, for instance on the day when I didn't sneeze even once among millions of blades of grass. It is said that those who didn't live fully didn't experience anything at all. I think the opposite is true. I think that those who didn't experience Jesus in their lifetime didn't experience anything at all.

I didn't have it all, I didn't travel the world, but that one sign, that one answer was enough to compensate for everything that many consider to important, everything that in truth, is completely meaningless. Today, being thirty-three years old (coincidence?), I want to share my story.

Just like the main protagonist in a movie production (though I wasn't one here, that's for sure) changes because of his experiences, I changed, too. Throughout my life, I've been trying to live by the principles of a righteous Christian that my parents instilled in me in my childhood years. And yet, it didn't protect me from a failure that transformed me and changed itself into a victory. If not for the suffering, if not for Lyme disease, I wouldn't have met Jesus, I wouldn't have experienced His presence. People are oblivious to how massive a toll this disease takes. Seeing young, well-looking individuals, they can't believe they could be suffering from something. Leaning against the walls at my home due to inexplicable weakness on many occasions, my shoulder leaving a mark that was saying, "help me", I regretted that I didn't have some cancer, because then I would at least know what the cause of my anguish was. That devastating disease was taking everything away from me; *Borrelia* and Co. were depriving me of the most beautiful years of my youth, making me aware of the world around me too soon. I definitely matured too soon, sometimes feeling older than my parents. Sending me off to an expert in human mind, completely unnecessarily at that, most doctors must have assumed that our happiness is determined by how we see the world and with what eyes we look at it, thinking that all my problems would disappear once someone taught me that. There's some truth to that, undoubtedly. However, on that day I realized that being a good, sensitive person is not enough to live a fully healthy, happy life. It's not enough to pick snails that go on the sidewalk after the rain or walk around them. God wants something more from us.

If I could turn back the hands of time and have two paths to choose from, the one filled with suffering with my experience of encountering Jesus at its end, and another one in excellent health and subjective happiness but without the opportunity to experience God, I'd have taken the first one. Even if you haven't experienced Him here and now when you needed Him the most, do not give up; pray, and your time will come, for what you will experience is worth every price and all your suffering, too, even if it lasts forever.

When it comes to medicine, it was hard to come up with the answer as to what disease I had; when it comes to religion, I found it hard to come up with the answer as to how God works.

"I'm arguing with God, Father," I told a priest in a confessional.

"You can't be arguing with God, son; God doesn't reply."

"What are you talking about, Father? He did, twice already!" I said.

"Seek and you will find" and "You will do miracles. Not like those I have done, but greater," are my two favorite quotes from the Holy Scripture. Today, owing to the Internet and books, we can go further than Jesus did, who was limited to his region only for some reason (and, after all, "everything happens for a reason"). This allows the memory of Him and the faith in Him to be present in every place in the world, whereas we are able to strengthen them to continue his work. You may ask me, "Why do you cite the words of people who follow other religions?" The answer is simple: it doesn't matter. Jesus loves us all regardless of our denomination or beliefs; we are all equal, every one of us has laminin inside, and He died for us all regardless of who we are and what we represent.

To this day, I've never heard the words, "Michal, God is healing you from Lyme disease" at any holy mass.

Nonetheless, writing this book, I do believe that I was touched by other words, spoken by another priest at a mass, "Lord gives you the gift of persuading people to pray; go and preach the Gospel."

If anyone told me at any time before that I'd be telling people at my own bachelor party about Jesus and what He did in my life, I'd say, "you need serious help!"

Yes! It's exactly what you're thinking. Anna finally had her dream wedding ceremony. It wasn't the only wedding that happened owing to God. My mom and dad, who were estranged from God throughout these years, remarried in the Catholic Church. It's astounding how much God did for us all. After establishing my 'new' relationship with God, I was provided with many blessings. To this day, my mom cannot imagine her day without a rosary; perhaps one day, I'll receive that grace, too.

You must wonder why it's only now that I professed my faith in writing. First of all, because it is only now that I can do that without a burdensome mental and physical effort, which was persistent for quite a while, making my brain subjectively torpid. I also hope that if you're going through what I have gone through or if you're suffering from any other disease, you'll find in my story that tiny element that will help you endure it all better and (who knows?) maybe even overcome it. And maybe you'll find an answer to questions that have been tormenting you, perhaps the very same questions I was asking myself. However, the answer to this question is completely different. Immediately after our wedding that we had been dreaming of for years, some of my previous symptoms were eliminated; I acquired another ailment, though, which caused me much discomfort in daily life – I started experiencing the so-called floaters. My eyes turned into a glass Christmas snow globe, the one with Santa inside, filling with floaters like a Christmas snow globe fills with fake snowflakes floating around after it's shaken.

God, why? It was supposed to be better now.

You have to write a book! That was the first thing that came to my mind.

But how am I supposed to do that? I've never been a straight-A student, I've never read books, I just watched movies, mainly!

Sit down and start writing. That was the next thing that came to my mind.

If you suspect you might have Lyme disease, remember that none of the methods you've read in this book is not the one proper solution to your problems. I wasn't lucky enough to meet on my way the right person who would've directed my life on a different path so that today, I would've been a perfectly healthy man. It might not happen to you. I have one piece of advice for you, and, unfortunately, it's not exactly my own words: "Never consent to being less than healthy in the way you understand it."[42]

***

In 2020, we all experienced yet another pandemic, though more transparent and, seemingly, more terrifying than the one caused by the bacteria called spirochetes. Sadly, Anna and I didn't get to steer clear of COVID-19. Having been isolated for six months, the vast majority of that time spent on lying in bed, I was taken to an ER where I got admitted to hospital because of suspected stroke. For some unknown reasons, I got an aphasic seizure of the mouth. Losing my memory as if I were a PC hard dive that wiped itself clean, I couldn't recall my dad's name, and when I was saying goodbye to my family, frightened, I was unable to tell them how much I loved, as all that came out of my mouth was a slurred speech with syllables all jumbled up.

---

[42] S.H. Buhner, *Leczenie boreliozy*, Olsztyn 2015, p. 15.

What's astonishing about it is, the only thing I was capable of spitting out without getting my tongue all twisted was the prayer Our Father. I had a feeling that *Borrelia*, which I haven't defeated until this day, and which can still make me withdraw from life from time to time, like a perfect host, it welcomed a traveler who got in, thirsty after a long journey – COVID.

Already in the ER, for a few hours I was unable to utter anything. Doctors contacted my wife, who told them briefly what had happened, mentioning the highly significant, destructive time bomb called *Borrelia* that was still ticking inside me. One of the medics leaned over me.

"I've no idea who told you all that nonsense about Lyme disease and bio-resonance. If not for COVID-19, I would've concluded you were severely mentally ill and required psychiatric treatment. You're a convalescent patient, you have the antibodies, you should be donating your plasma instead of lying here. We'll take you to the ward to get some additional testing done, but only because of the virus."

Unable to say anything, trembling because of the cold, I didn't know what to make of it until the next day, when I was capable of speaking again and my mom texted me. "Rest well, son, lie down and have some sleep." "I can't, mom. I'm telling a boy with glioblastoma about Jesus!" I texted her back.

"It will be beautiful in your life, regardless of it all. Just make sure the shoes you put on are comfortable, because you have a long way to go - your entire life."

John Paul II

ACKNOWLEDGEMENTS

Although it could seem that writing a debut book is the most difficult task to carry out, there's nothing further from the truth. This part is much more difficult. At the very beginning, I must thank my beloved Wife, who regardless of everything took up the risk and invested her love in me, and never stopped believing in a better tomorrow, following me in my footsteps.

Also, I'd like to thank my Family and my true Friends who have been always supporting us and sharing their positive energy with us. In particular, I'd like thank my Parents, who proved to be my best Friends, and whom I've never referred to using this title. I'd like to thank them for everything. I'd like to thank everyone without whom this book would've never happened. I'd like to thank everyone who over these years had their share, even if just a minor one, in keeping my hope alive; all the enthusiasts of non-conventional medicine who contributed to our recovery and better wellbeing, and those who still give hope for a better tomorrow to everyone struggling with health issues. Despite appearances, I am grateful and thankful to the medical doctors who, though they did not try, they did their duty very well. If not for them, most likely, I'd have never found God in my life.

Most of all, I would like to thank God for my Cross, for if not for Him, I wouldn't have experienced it all and I would've probably be still looking forward to connecting with Wi-Fi networks more often than with Him.

Contents

CHAPTER I	7
CHAPTER II	117
CHAPTER III	193
CHAPTER IV	255
CHAPTER V	319
CHAPTER VI	375
ACKNOWLEDGEMENTS	405

www.ingramcontent.com/pod-product-compliance
Lightning Source LLC
Chambersburg PA
CBHW031604210526
45464CB00004B/1427